SPECT

TECHNOLOGY, PROCEDURES AND APPLICATIONS

BIOMEDICAL DEVICES AND THEIR APPLICATIONS

Additional books in this series can be found on Nova's website
under the Series tab.

Additional e-books in this series can be found on Nova's website
under the e-book tab.

MEDICAL PROCEDURES, TESTING AND TECHNOLOGY

Additional books in this series can be found on Nova's website
under the Series tab.

Additional e-books in this series can be found on Nova's website
under the e-book tab.

SPECT

TECHNOLOGY, PROCEDURES AND APPLICATIONS

HOJJAT AHMADZADEHFAR
AND
ELHAM HABIBI
EDITORS

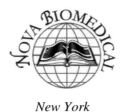

New York

NOTICE TO THE READER

The Publisher has taken reasonable care in the preparation of this book, but makes no expressed or implied warranty of any kind and assumes no responsibility for any errors or omissions. No liability is assumed for incidental or consequential damages in connection with or arising out of information contained in this book. The Publisher shall not be liable for any special, consequential, or exemplary damages resulting, in whole or in part, from the readers' use of, or reliance upon, this material. Any parts of this book based on government reports are so indicated and copyright is claimed for those parts to the extent applicable to compilations of such works.

Independent verification should be sought for any data, advice or recommendations contained in this book. In addition, no responsibility is assumed by the publisher for any injury and/or damage to persons or property arising from any methods, products, instructions, ideas or otherwise contained in this publication.

This publication is designed to provide accurate and authoritative information with regard to the subject matter covered herein. It is sold with the clear understanding that the Publisher is not engaged in rendering legal or any other professional services. If legal or any other expert assistance is required, the services of a competent person should be sought. FROM A DECLARATION OF PARTICIPANTS JOINTLY ADOPTED BY A COMMITTEE OF THE AMERICAN BAR ASSOCIATION AND A COMMITTEE OF PUBLISHERS.

Additional color graphics may be available in the e-book version of this book.

Library of Congress Cataloging-in-Publication Data

ISBN: 978-1-62808-344-6

Library of Congress Control Number: 2013942947

Published by Nova Science Publishers, Inc. † New York

BIOMEDICAL DEVICES AND THEIR APPLICATIONS

Additional books in this series can be found on Nova's website
under the Series tab.

Additional e-books in this series can be found on Nova's website
under the e-book tab.

MEDICAL PROCEDURES, TESTING AND TECHNOLOGY

Additional books in this series can be found on Nova's website
under the Series tab.

Additional e-books in this series can be found on Nova's website
under the e-book tab.

SPECT

TECHNOLOGY, PROCEDURES AND APPLICATIONS

To our lovely children Niyousha and Ariya

Contents

Preface   ix

Chapter I   Physics, Instrumentation   1
                   Karl Reichmann

Chapter II   The Impact of SPECT on Medical Internal Dosimetry   37
                   Michael G. Stabin

Chapter III   SPECT in Primary Hyperparathyroidism   45
                   Paloma García-Talavera San Miguel

Chapter IV   SPECT in Malignant Bone Diseases   75
                   Ali Gholamrezanezhad, Edward Pinkus and Rathan Subramaniam

Chapter V   Ventilation/Perfusion Tomography in Diagnosis of Pulmonary
                   Embolism and Other Pulmonary Diseases: Methodology
                   and Clinical Implementation   91
                   Marika Bajc

Chapter VI   Imaging of Neuroendocrine Tumors with SPECT   109
                   Thorsten D. Poeppel, Ina Binse, Andreas Bockisch,
                   James Nagarajah and Christina Antke

Chapter VII   Tumor Imaging with $^{123/131}$I-MIBG SPECT   133
                   Verena Hartung, Marcus Ruhlmann, Andreas Bockisch
                   and James Nagarajah

Chapter VIII   Cardiac SPECT   147
                   Tomoaki Nakata and Akiyoshi Hashimoto

Chapter IX   The Story of Myocardial Infarction - Before, When it Strikes,
                   and Afterwards: A Tale in Images   159
                   Elly L. van der Veen, Hans J. de Haas, Artiom D. Petrov,
                   Chris P. M. Reutelingsperger, Jos G. W. Kosterink, Clark J. Zeebregts,
                   René A. Tio, Riemer H. J. A. Slart and Hendrikus H. Boersma

Chapter X   Cardiac ^{123}I-MIBG SPECT   189
                   Ji Chen and Weihua Zhou

Chapter XI   SPECT in Parkinson's Disease   **201**
                  Hong Zhang, Mei Tian and Ling Wang

Chapter XII   SPECT in Epilepsy   **221**
                  Hojjat Ahmadzadehfar and Michael P. Malter

Chapter XIII   SPECT in the Evaluation of Brain Tumors   **235**
                  Yasushi Shibata

Index   **249**

Preface

Single Photon Emission Computed Tomography (SPECT) cameras have revolutionarily changed the nuclear imaging techniques and given us new diagnostic possibilities. They provide images that reveal subtle information about physiological and pathological processes. For some indications like cardiac and brain imaging, as well as tumor imaging, the importance of SPECT compared to planar imaging is beyond words.

This book covers a broad spectrum of clinical applications of SPECT in the diagnosis of benign and malignant diseases. The opening chapters discuss the technology and physics of SPECT and its use in dosimetry. Applications covered include, among others, imaging of the bone and lungs, imaging of neuroendocrine tumors, cardiac imaging and brain SPECT for different indications like brain tumors and epilepsy. In each chapter, different radiopharmaceuticals for SPECT imaging were discussed and the scan procedures described. Readers will find this book to be a useful source for often performed SPECT imaging in the clinical routine.

We wish to sincerely thank each and every author for generously contributing to this book.

H. Ahmadzadehfar, M.D.
Associate Professor

E. Habibi, M.D.

In: SPECT
Editors: Hojjat Ahmadzadehfar and Elham Habibi

ISBN: 978-1-62808-344-6
© 2013 Nova Science Publishers, Inc.

Chapter I

Physics, Instrumentation

*Karl Reichmann**

University Hospital Bonn, Department of Nuclear Medicine, Bonn, Germany

Introduction

SPECT means: Single Photon Emission Computed Tomography [1]. In this introduction to SPECT we will follow the above words:

Single Photon means that we are dealing with radioactivity that emits a single photon per decay. The alternative to this is the annihilation radiation in PET, where two photons are emitted in virtually opposite directions. What is the consequence of this single photon case for imaging? The answers will be given in this chapter of this book.

Emission means that the source of radiation is within the body of the patient. It is emitted to the outside so that it can be detected there by a gamma camera. As α and β radiation have very limited ranges in tissue (microns or millimeters, respectively), they are not suitable for imaging of organs not being at the surface. Thus, for imaging in SPECT the only alternative is γ radiation with a range in tissue of several centimeters. Emission also means that the radiation has to be incorporated into the patient. Thus the radioactivity may be used in conjunction with tracers. What is the consequence of this fact compared to transmitted radiation? In this case, the answer has to involve physiology, but this is beyond the scope of this article.

Computed Tomography is, in a sense, the opposite of planar imaging [2]. If acquired with a gamma camera the resulting planar images - the scintigrams - display the distribution of counted photons translated into grayscales or colors. The scintigrams are projections from 3D space into the 2D image plane. In other words, photons emitted from the source are counted. This is not the case with (transaxial) computed tomography. The resulting tomograms exist only after execution of a mathematical reconstruction algorithm in a computer. The acquired planar images are used as the input data. The values we obtain from these reconstructions are

---

* Email: karl.reichmann@ukb.uni-bonn.de.

actually "funny numbers" that don't, by themselves, have any meaning. They only make sense in relation to each other. To obtain equivalent count values that can be used, for example, in uptake calculations, they first need to be normalized.

SINGLE PHOTON IMAGING - THE NEED FOR COLLIMATORS

The intention of imaging in nuclear medicine is to acquire information about the distribution and quantity of the incorporated radioactivity. This means we need to know the paths of the incoming γ. To determine the path for each γ, which is a straight line in three dimensional space, we need the coordinates of two points, P1(x1, y1, z1) and P2(x2, y2, z2), as shown in Figure 1.1.

In the case of PET, we profit from the fact that the two gammas of the annihilation radiation are emitted from the patient in virtually opposite directions. Thus we can determine the resulting path by detecting γ_1 at detector 1 and γ_2 at detector 2, respectively (Figure 1.2).

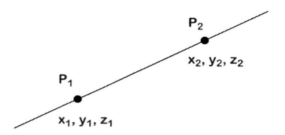

Figure 1.1. To define the path of a straight line in space, we need the coordinates x_i, y_i, z_i of two points.

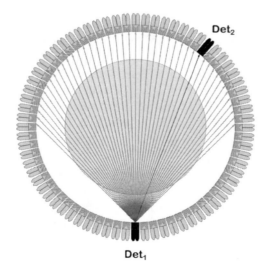

Figure 1.2. In PET the path of the annihilation radiation is defined by two detectors Det_1 and Det_2 that are electronically connected in coincidence.

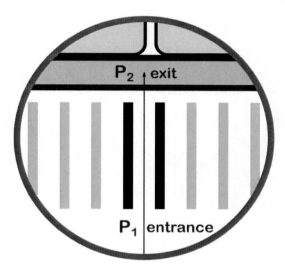

Figure 1.3. With a long bore collimator the path of the gamma is defined by the entrance (P$_1$) and the exit (P$_2$) of the hole.

Unfortunately, we are not that lucky in the case of single photon emitters like [99m]Tc - because we have just one γ that has to be detected by a single detector (Det. 1). If we were to put a second detector (Det. 2) in the path of the gamma, we would inevitably have compton scattering. But this means we would "destroy" our straight path from the source to the detector.

Therefore we need to introduce a collimator (Figure 1.3) [1] where, with a longbore collimator, the entrance into the collimator hole is the first point, P$_1$, and the exit is P$_2$ (cave: with a pinhole collimator it's somewhat different).

To "destroy" the straightness of the path does not necessarily mean that we have a problem. For example, optical lenses do just that - and they are good! In nuclear medicine a similar approach has been explored several times by different groups [3, 4]. These groups indeed put a detector ahead of the (uncollimated) gamma camera. Like a lens, it diffracted the gamma that was eventually detected in the gamma camera. This camera was called a "Compton Camera". It unfortunately had several fundamental problems. Therefore it existed only in prototypes and we've seen only imaging of point sources. As this camera could have been the difference between a pinhole camera and a camera with an optical lens, we wanted to mention it, but we are not going to delve into this topic.

Components of a Gamma Camera

The characteristics of SPECT depend on the nature of the underlying planar images acquired by a gamma camera [5-7]. The main features we are interested in are the energy and spatial resolution of the gamma camera and its sensitivity. We therefore would like to give a basic overview of the gamma camera and its components since they are the subject of these attributes and the quality of SPECT.

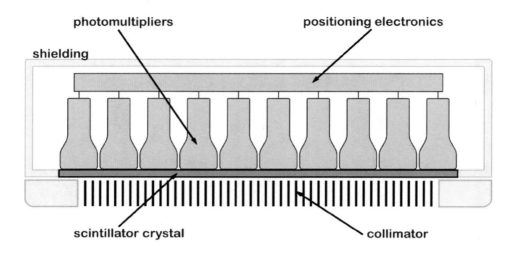

Figure 1.4. Components of a gamma camera.

For convenience we would like to break down the gamma camera into its functional components:

The *camera system* (Figure 1.4) is a combination of the following two functional units:

The *camera head with computer* is the unit that detects and localizes the incoming gammas. It is, in a way, the body of a digital photographic camera, including film and development. The camera head itself is divided into the following components:

The *scintillator crystal* converts the incoming gamma radiation into visible light. To increase the probability of the photo effect its material needs to have a high number of protons, therefore NaI(Tl) is by far the most often used scintillator material for gamma cameras not used for PET. Tl is blundered into a very small amount (10^{-3}) of the scintillator NaI. It shifts the wavelength of the scintillator light of pure NaI to a higher value (meaning to lower energy), so that it can leave the crystal. Pure NaI would be opaque to its own scintillation light, but when doped with Tl the crystal is clear for the shifted wavelength. The outcoming light is visible (blue, 420 nm) but, with only about 4000–5000 photons per event, very faint (that's about 1/2000 of a firefly!). To be able to process it electronically, it has to be converted to electrons and electric current and afterwards amplified by photomultipliers.

The *photomultipliers* convert the visible light into electrons to obtain a reasonable electrical output. A fraction of the photons generated in the scintillation process emit (about 400) photoelectrons out of the photocathode of a photomultiplier. These are multiplied by the high voltage in a cascade of dynodes by a factor of about 10^6 to 10^7.

The *positioning electronics* calculate the coordinates of the distributed scintillator light. The computer stores and processes the data coming from the camera itself.

The *collimator* is, so to speak, the lens of the camera. It produces an image of the three dimensional activity distribution by projection into the two dimensional plane of the scintillator crystal.

The *gantry* is the flexible mounting of the gamma camera. It gives the camera the ability to rotate around the patient to perform SPECT data acquisition.

Resolution and Sampling Theorem

As the spatial resolution of a SPECT system is one major issue, we will discuss this topic now.

Definition of (Spatial) Resolution

There are different ways to define the resolution of a system. The one that is less intuitive for "non-engineers" is the modulation transfer function (MTF), which is - just to say it - the Fourier transform of the point spread function (PSF). As this approach leads us into signal processing and the associated mathematics, we will follow a more intuitive approach here.

Spatial resolution may be defined as the ability to identify two points or line sources that are very close to each other. The easiest and most commonly used method is to image bar phantoms with different spatial frequencies (Figure 1.5a). The problem with this approach is that we don't really measure resolution but only report which of the bar segments can still be resolved. Due to the frequency nature of this definition of resolution, its unit is [1/cm], very often written as [cm^{-1}]. In this case higher values mean better resolution: the more bars you see, the better. To assign a number to the resolution there is another, also quite convenient method. Resolution just means that an ideal point source (δ (delta) function) turns out to be a distribution in the real image: the broader the distribution, the worse the resolution. Therefore we only need to figure out how broad the distribution is and we have the resolution (Figure 1.5b). As there is not "one" broadness to this function, we just define the FWHM (Full Width at Half Maximum) as the broadness of the point spread function. The FWHM is a distance, therefore it's unit is [cm]. In this case higher values mean poorer resolution.

Using the point spread function for the determination of resolution, often an additional parameter is given: the FWTM (Full With at Tenth Maximum). This parameter is often given to characterize the amount of scattering in a system.

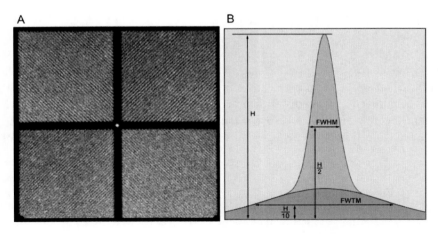

Figure 1.5. A: Measurement of resolution with bar phantoms. B: Point spread function (PSF) of a point source with scattering. The "full width at half maximum" (FWHM) is a measure of the resolution, the "Full Width at Tenth Maximum" (FWTM) for the scattering. In this example the amount of scattering is overemphasized compared to usual circumstances.

Imaging Matrix - Sampling (Shannon) Theorem

To make the images acquired by the camera durable we need a recording medium. In an earlier era recording was totally analogue in its operation. Today in nuclear medicine - like in many other faculties - the whole imaging technique is digital. There is one major error in digital imaging that may be a cause of medical malpractice: under sampling.

But let us start at the beginning: what is sampling? Sampling is, generally speaking, a topic of signal processing and may be, from the point of view of non-engineers, highly academic, or let's say "completely incomprehensible". Therefore let us start with a realistic example. We have a bar phantom as shown in Figure 1.6a. It is divided into 4 segments, each with a different structural width and is used for quality control (which we will talk about later). For this example we will take segment C, which has a structural width (lead + plastic) of 6.36 mm. This pattern has to be reproduced by the digital matrix in the computer. Let us assume the matrix is able to cover the whole field of view (FOV) of the camera, which has a width of 500 mm. If in the acquisition parameters we select a matrix of 128 x 128 pixels, then each pixel has a width of 500/128=3.9 mm. This pixel size is obviously unable to reproduce the black - white pattern of a 6.36 mm structure. The question now is, how small the pixel size has to be to adequately image our 6.36 mm structure. The answer from the point of view of Claude Shannon would be [8]:

-    Sampling theorem by Shannon: the pixel size needs to be smaller than half the width of our structure

As our structure has a size of 6.36 mm, our pixel size thus has to be less than 3.18 mm; with an actual size of 3.9 mm it is too large and therefore unable to resolve the 6.36 mm structure.

Harry Nyquist viewed the same concept from the point of view of frequency. Therefore the expression "Nyquist frequency" is often used but, without illustrating this here, it's the same idea.

Take care: the word smaller in the Shannon theorem means smaller! It does not include terms like equal or "about".

As we have already seen above, the resolution of a system may be defined in different ways. For convenience we choose the bar phantom and the FWHM of a point source. We explained the Shannon theorem by means of a bar pattern because we feel this might be the most intuitive approach. Instead of "structural size" we could also have talked about FWHM. The Shannon theorem, in other words, means if you have an FWHM of your planar or tomographic imaging system, then your acquisition matrix needs to have a pixel size of

width of pixel [mm] < 1/2 FWHM

If the FWHM of your SPECT is 10 mm, then your pixel size needs to be less than 5 mm! In Figure 1.6c, especially in segments B and C, it can be seen what the technical term "aliasing artifact" means. The structures of segments B and C in Figure 1.6a are well reproduced and we can see an undisturbed image of their frequency pattern. As the imaging matrix in Figure 1.6c is too coarse to adequately reproduce B and C, we obtain an incorrect frequency that in reality does not exist. It is only an imaging artifact due to undersampling. We could also say: due to this undersampling we give the right frequency another name, an alias.

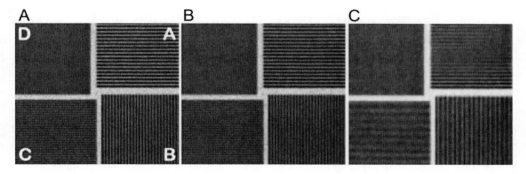

Figure 1.6. Acquisition of a bar phantom always under the same conditions. The only difference was the acquisition matrix: A) 512x512, B) 256x256, C) 128x128. Please note: the phantom has never been rotated!.

Camera Head – Intrinsic Resolution

The basic part of the camera head is the scintillator crystal. After interacting with compton or (preferably) photo effect, gammas are converted into visible light, the scintillation light. As the intensity of the light pulse is very faint, it has to be amplified, and in order to know the position of the interaction, it has to be localized [9].

Both amplification and light gathering for localization are performed by photo multipliers (PMs). These multipliers have a diameter of several centimeters. Therefore, to determine the exact position of the scintillation process it is not enough to know which of the photo multipliers has been activated. As the scintillation light in the crystal is emitted from the point of interaction isotropically in all directions, the surrounding PMs will, in dependence of the distance from the scintillation center, also be illuminated. We thus get an activation pattern over several PMs that corresponds to the distribution of the light. The position of this distribution is represented by its center of gravity and has to be determined by the adjacent electronic microprocessors.

The problem in exactly determining this location is that this light distribution is not smooth but disturbed by the limited Poisson statistics of the photons (meaning, the light distribution itself is noisy). Additionally, the initial number of electrons generated by the light at the photocathode is limited. For gamma energies common in nuclear medicine this may represent only a few hundred electrons - and they follow Poisson statistics. As an example, we might have in the mean 400 electrons at the photo cathode. Their statistical fluctuation would be about ± 5%. We again have a statistical error that prevents exact localization of the point of interaction. Another additional fact limits the accuracy of spatial resolution: the thickness of the crystal. The best values for intrinsic resolution are obtained for cameras that are mainly optimized for use with ^{99m}Tc. Usually crystals for these cameras have a thickness of only 3/8" (about 9.5 mm). In this case nearly 90% of the incoming gammas are detected in the photo peak. It would not make much sense to increase the crystal thickness to gain a few percent more.

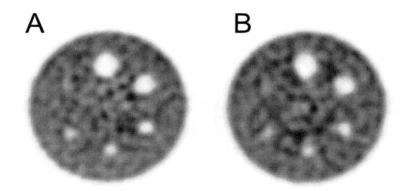

Figure 1.7. SPECT tomograms obtained with a 3/8" (A) and a 5/8" (B) crystal.

But with ^{131}I or even ^{18}F detection would be only about 22% and 12%, respectively. For these energies thicker crystals would be useful to increase sensitivity. Therefore, if a camera is designed for additional use of ^{131}I or even as a PET system, the crystals have a thickness of 5/8" (15.9 mm) or even 1" (25.4 mm). For the 1" - crystal the fraction of the gammas detected in the photo peak would rise for ^{131}I and ^{18}F to 54% and 36%, respectively. But in these cases the engineers have to work hard to obtain a good compromise between absorption of high energy photons and resolution.

Thus the true position of the scintillation process may not be determined closer than several millimeters. This resolution is called the "intrinsic resolution" R_i. Sometimes it is also called the "inherent resolution".

The value for the intrinsic resolution is unique for a camera head. Depending on the purpose the camera is designed for, it may vary from 3.4 mm to 4.5 mm. The comparison in Figure 1.7 shows different tomographic results obtained with a 3/8" (A) and 5/8" (B) crystal. In both cases everything was identical but the thickness of the crystal.

The rotational radius was 14 cm, which is the radius that can be adjusted for tomography of the brain.

Pinhole Collimator

As we have already seen, the gamma camera has to use collimators for imaging. The possible materials for collimators are lead, gold and wolfram. Lead is used almost exclusively, because it's the cheapest and the one that is best to be treated.

The easiest and probably the oldest method to generate images is the pinhole camera [9]. The underlying geometry is the central projection. As seen in Figure 1.8, the size of the imaged object depends on its distance from the collimator. Furthermore, the overlapping of structure depends on the lateral position.

The interpretation of these images is thus somewhat complicated. For these reasons, imaging with a pinhole has been established in nuclear medicine only for very special clinical investigations. In the early years this type of collimator was also used for longitudinal SPECT (see under that section).

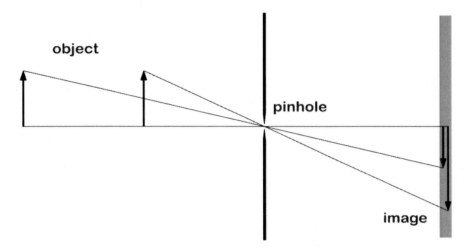

Figure 1.8. Geometry of imaging with a pinhole camera. The imaging scale depends on the distance of the object from the pinhole. This makes the interpretation in diagnostics complicated.

Long Bore Collimator – Geometric Resolution

The origin of the name "Long Bore Collimator" (Figure 1.3), sometimes also called a "Multihole Collimator" is obvious: long, thin lead blades, called septa, define the geometry of the holes and thus the imaging characteristics of the collimator. The resolution and sensitivity of a SPECT – system, for example, are given by the different geometries (here the lengths) of the holes [1]. Short holes define broad cones and thus higher sensitivity and vice versa. The more the cones of adjacent holes overlap, the poorer is the resolution.

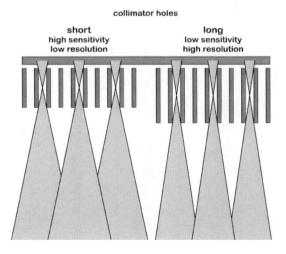

Figure 1.9. The geometry of the collimator holes defines the imaging characteristics: short holes have a broad cone and thus high sensitivity and low resolution. For long holes it's the other way round.

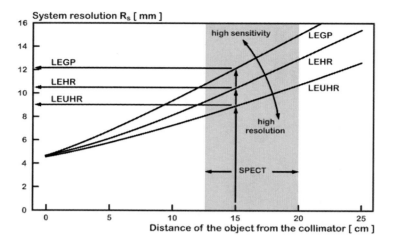

Figure 1.10. A collimator has either high sensitivity but low resolution and vice versa. Therefore the characteristics of a collimator are always a compromise between resolution and sensitivity. In SPECT an MEGP collimator has about 3 mm less of resolution compared to the LEHR collimator.

The overlapping of the cones in Figure 1.9 shows that in the case of broad cones, overlapping occurs more close to the collimator rather than with narrow cones. As the resolution of the collimator depends on this geometry, it is called the geometric resolution R_g.

From what we have said and from the geometry shown in Figure 1.9, it is obvious that either you get a high sensitivity but then the resolution is poor or the other way round. It is not possible to simultaneously make both parameters better: collimators are always a compromise between resolution and sensitivity (Figure 1.10).

LEHR - MEGP - HEGP Collimators

The cones shown in Figure 1.9 assume there is no septal penetration. Even if we would accept "nearly no" septal penetration, this could make the septa unreasonable thick.

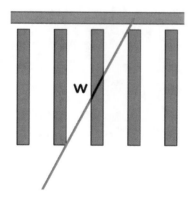

Figure 1.11. The septal penetration is defined by the path „w". This is the shortest possible path of a gamma through lead, when only one septum is penetrated.

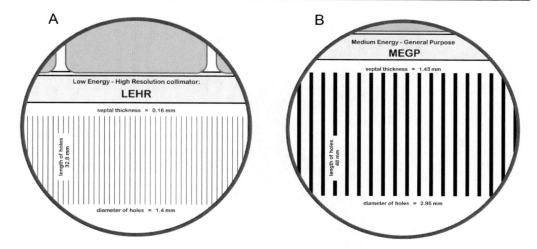

Figure 1.12. Collimators LEHR for low (up to 200 keV, A) and MEGP for medium (up to 300 keV, B) gamma energies.

The calculations for designs of low energy collimators therefore usually accept that about 2.5% of the gammas having the path shown in Figure 1.11 may penetrate the septum.

But nuclides used in nuclear medicine may have very different gamma energies. The most commonly used isotope, ^{99m}Tc, has a low energy of 140.5 keV. The half value layer in lead in this case is about 0.3 mm. Accepting the above penetration of up to 2.5%, septa, LEHR (low energy-high resolution) collimators, often also called "Tc-collimators", have a thickness of less than 0.2 mm, sometimes even 0.14 mm.

If we take ^{111}In instead, whose gammas used for imaging have energies of 171 and 245 keV, then the septa have to be thicker. In Figure 1.12, sections of a LEHR and a MEGP (medium energy – general purpose) collimator are shown for comparison, respectively.

The spatial resolutions of these different collimators will be discussed later.

Very High Energy Gammas

Sometimes nuclides [10] used for imaging have gamma energies well suited for imaging with a LEHR collimator and with a good abundance. But very high energy components with much greater septal penetration make a large difference for imaging, even if their abundance is very low. In planar images you will have a quite well resolved image with a lot of apparent scattering, but much of it is septal penetration. A well-known example is ^{123}I, which has a gamma energy of 159 keV (abundance 83%); but it also has a lot of higher energies, above all the energy of 529 keV with an abundance of only 1.4%. But when imaging using a LEHR collimator with 0.2 mm septal thickness, the broadening of the cone (Figure 1.13) virtually increases the abundance by about a factor of 20. Thus, depending on the activity distribution of the source, SPECT may be obsolete with ^{123}I and a LEHR collimator.

Another example is [186]Re. Its peak used for imaging has an energy of 137 keV (just like [99m]Tc!) with an abundance of 9.42%. But unfortunately there are two other energy peaks at 630 and 767 keV, respectively.

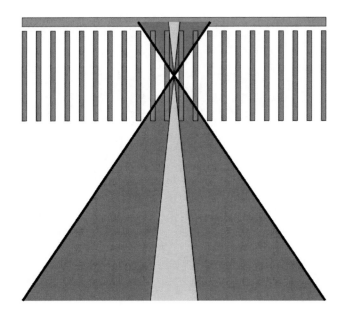

Figure 1.13. Septa define the cone for imaging low energies (light gray). Due to septal penetration the cone of high energy components may be very broad and thus the sensitivity for these components very high (dark gray).

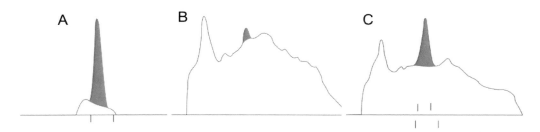

Figure 1.14. Spectra of ^{186}Re obtained with different collimators. a) no collimator, b) LEHR collimator, c) MEGP collimator. The dark area represents the photo peak of 137 keV.

Their combined abundance, compared to the 137 keV transition, is only about 0.66%. This sounds negligible, but spectra obtained under different conditions may be seen in Figure 1.14.

In Figure 1.14a we see the spectrum we obtain without a collimator. There is no geometric effect that modifies the acceptance of the camera due to energy dependent sepal penetration. The only difference between low and high energies is that the acceptance of high energies in the crystal is less than for low energies. Based on this spectrum we wouldn't suspect a problem for SPECT due to high energy photons.

But Figure 1.14b shows the spectrum acquired with a LEHR collimator. The dark area represents the photopeak, the rest is scattering and septal penetration, which winds up being background. So in this case the signal is about only 10% of the background! Taking into account that the phantom used didn't have significant scattering or absorption, the situation would be worse in the clinical situation.

To diminish this *insanely* high background, we repeated the acquisition with a MEGP collimator, which improves the situation a lot (Figure 1.14c). The signal is now 50% of the background. For clinical SPECT applications with ^{186}Re, the collimator of choice would thus be the MEGP collimator. As we didn't have a HEGP (high energy – general purpose) collimator, we could not make that comparison. On the other hand, the resolution would again worsen by about 1.5 mm. Therefore appropriate tests would have to be performed to determine which of the collimators would be better for SPECT: MEGP or HEGP.

We have already mentioned ^{123}I, ^{177}Lu has a similar problem. As the problem depends on the distribution of the activity - small sources have fewer problems with high energy components than large ones - in cases like these, preliminary studies have to be done to decide which collimator should be chosen.

System Resolution (R_s)

The resolution defined by the properties of the camera head is called the "intrinsic resolution" R_i. For each combination of nuclide and brand it has a unique value and lies in the range between 3.0 and 4.5 mm.

The resolution defined by the collimator depends (mainly) on its geometry and is called the "geometric resolution" R_g. As can be seen in Figure 1.15, it depends on the distance of the organ from the collimator.

Generally speaking, a limited spatial resolution is the measurement error of an imaging unit - our gamma camera. The resolution of the whole system is called the "system resolution" R_s and is a combination of the resolutions R_i and R_g. As each is independent of the other, the resulting resolution R_s (Figure 1.15) has to be calculated following the rules of error propagation

$$R_s = \sqrt{(R_i^2 + R_g^2)}$$

The example shows the values of the PRISM 2000 (Picker) camera with a mounted LEHR - collimator. The abscissa represents the distance of the activity from the collimator, the ordinate is the resolution (FWHM) in mm. The system resolution R_s in dependency from the distance is shown by the slightly bended upper curve, the contribution of R_g by the straight line and the contribution of R_i by the gap between the lines for R_g and R_s. As R_g increases linearly with distance and R_i remains constant, the influence of R_i becomes less the greater the values of R_g are. This means the gap between R_g and R_s gets smaller with increasing distance. Directly at the collimator we get a resolution of about 5 mm. But this may be realistic for "hands on the collimator", at most. At a distance of 15 cm we get a resolution of about 10 mm. Typical distances in SPECT may range from about 13 to 20 cm. Even for SPECT of the brain the rotational radius cannot be adjusted to much better than 14 cm. For these distances the resolution range from about 9 to 12 mm.

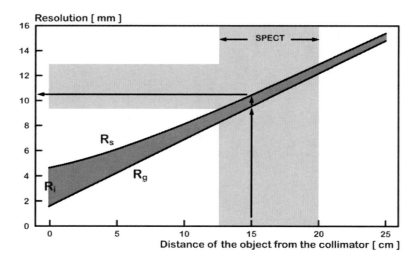

Figure 1.15. The spatial resolution of a gamma camera system (R_s) is a composition of the intrinsic resolution (R_i) of the camera head and the geometric resolution (R_g) of the collimator. As a consequence of the distance dependent geometric resolution the system resolution varies for SPECT distances from about 9 to 13 mm.

Depending on which collimator is used, the resolution may differ from these values. Especially for low energies, often different collimators with different resolution - sensitivity - characteristics are offered. In our example (Figure 1.10), the resolutions at 15 cm from the collimator vary from 9 mm (LEUHR) to 12 mm (LEGP). If, especially due to very high energy components, medium (MEGP = medium energy – general purpose) or even high (HEGP = high energy – general purpose) energy collimators have to be used, the resolution of SPECT worsens to values up to 13 mm or even 15 mm.

Recovery Coefficient

Talking about resolution doesn't only mean talking about the detectability of structures, but also about visual and quantitational assessment [11]. To understand this topic, let's first of all look at an example that has nothing to do with nuclear medicine.

For a test of analogue photographic materials the resolution chart "USAF 1951" [12] was photographed and scanned under different conditions (Figure 1.16).

The well resolved "4" on the chart is shown in Figure 1.16a, a badly resolved "4" in Figure 1.16b. In both cases it is the same "4" that has been reproduced; the only difference was resolution. So, why this difference!?

In Figure 1.17a we see the resolution of a system: the intensity profile through a true point source is the vertical line, often called the δ (delta) - function. The profile of its improperly resolved image is the overlaid Gauss - function. Limited resolution means that we have an increasing slope on the left side and a decreasing slope on the right. Usually this is called the point spread function (PSF). Let's look at Figure 17b. The profile of a large, homogeneous object is represented by the large rectangle.

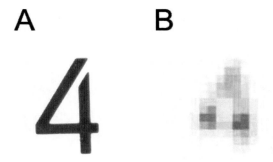

Figure 1.16. Demonstration of size dependent intensities: in (a) the scanned object was large and could be well resolved, in (b) the same object was small (at the limit of scanner resolution). The result was the intensity pattern seen here.

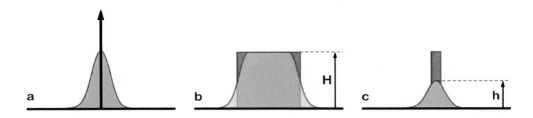

Figure 1.17. Illustration of the recovery coefficient. In a) we see the point spread function (PSF) of an ideal small activity (δ-function, delta-function). In b) the profile of a large distribution is shown. The object is large enough that the profile can reach the plateau H. But in c) the object is too small, so the profile achieves only the height h. The ratio h/H is called the recovery coefficient.

The profile of the image shows an increasing slope at the left edge and a decreasing slope at the right - just like with the δ - function. But we should take notice of the extended plateau with height H. Now let's look at Figure 1.17c. Here we have an object that's smaller than in Figure 1.17b. Again the profile of the image has increasing and decreasing slopes on the left and right sides, respectively. But the size of the object is too small for the slopes to be able to reach the plateau H. The profile of a small object will be limited to the height h. The recovery coefficient RC is defined by:

RC = h / H

and always has a value of less than or equal to 1. The smaller the object, the smaller the RC. The problem in medical imaging is that the physician or investigator may be led to believe the activity density in a small organ, and sometimes he doesn't know how small it is, may be less than that in a large one. For very small organs, especially for spheres less than about half of the resolution, its apparent size remains constant. In this case there is essentially no correlation between its size in the image and its true size. A very small hot spot with very high activity may appear as "just a small spot with mean uptake". In the case of a tumor this might be a fatal misinterpretation. If the real activity of that very small tumor only had a mean value, it probably wouldn't be detected.

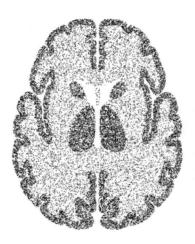 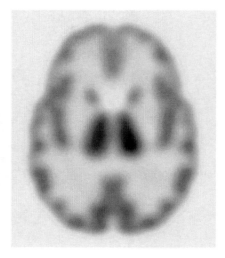

Figure 1.18. Recovery coefficient: In this simulation (left) grey matter, nucleus caudatus and thalamus have four times the activity of the white matter. In the right image the resolution of about 10 mm was simulated by gaussian filtering. It is clearly to be seen, that the resulting grey levels depend on the structure size and distribution..

Remember that the system resolution of a SPECT - system varies from about 10 to 15 mm. "Small" or "large" is always in relation to this resolution. As a formula of thumb it may be stated that organs need to be about 2 to 3 times the size of the resolution to obtain a recovery coefficient of more than 90 %. For line sources it is more like 2, for spheres more like 3. If we assume a resolution in our system of, for example, 13 mm, then this means that a spherical metastasis needs to have a size of more than about 40 mm to see its "true" activity!

In Figure 1.18 a simulation of brain SPECT is shown. If we normalize the activity of the white matter to the value of "1", then all other structures, grey matter, nucleus caudatus and thalamus have an activity of "4" (Figure 1.18 left). It is easy to see that the resulting activity intensities shown in (Figure 1.18 right) are very dependent on a structure's size and folding. Only a minor part of this effect is due to statistics.

Statistics and Sensitivity

As we know, radioactive decay follows Poisson statistics. We also know that statistics plays a major role in SPECT. In the following two sections we will show the reasons for that.

Overall Sensitivity of SPECT

Before we approach SPECT, let's first look at CT: only the investigated volume is irradiated by X-rays and only for the duration of the data acquisition. Furthermore, the absorption of the X-rays in the tissue is not a "loss of X-rays" but the information we need to in order to obtain Hounsfield numbers. As dosimetry of the patient is the limiting factor for the allowed amount of X-rays, this is all good news.

In SPECT, on the other hand, we have, compared to CT, bad news. Only a minor part of the injected activity is really used for imaging of the target organ. Let us try to give an answer to the question, how much of the injected activity is really used for imaging. As an example we will use investigation of regional cerebral blood flow in the brain (rCBF) with ^{99m}Tc-HMPAO or ^{99m}Tc-ECD. The injected activity is about 740 MBq, and the physical half-life of ^{99m}Tc is 6 hours. From this we make the following rough estimation:

- *Injected nuclei:* The integral (or area) under the decay curve from t=0 to infinity gives us the number of injected nuclei. Ignoring renal (or other) elimination this is the number of decays that irradiate the patient. The result of this is *2.5 10^{13}* nuclei.
- *Uptake:* In the case of rCBF, the uptake of activity into the brain is only about *5 %.*
- During the *duration of acquisition* of 30 minutes only about **4%** of the activity decays. The residual 96 % are not used for SPECT.
- *Absorption* of activity in tissue: after transition of the gamma rays through about 5 cm of tissue we lose about 50% of activity. If we assume the head to have a radius of about 10 cm, then only *about 25 %* of the radiation comes out of the head of the patient.
- *Collimation:* The standard LEHR - collimator has a sensitivity of about 10^{-4}. This means that from a point source in front of a camera only about 10^{-4} of photons are used for imaging. The rest is lost.

Taking these four factors of activity loss into consideration, only 5 x 10^{-8} of the injected activity is used for (brain) SPECT of the rCBF. This means, that from the injected 2.5 x 10^{13} nuclei, only 1.25 x10^{6} are used for brain imaging. If we assume a resolution in SPECT of 10 mm and that the human brain has a size of about 1600 ml, then in 1 ml of the brain we have on average fewer than 900 decays during SPECT data acquisition. If we assume this number to be Poisson distributed, then the statistical error in the decays per ml would be about 3%. Just because of physics and statistics there is unfortunately no way to be better than this. But, are we as good as this?

Statistics in SPECT, Budinger formula

Unfortunately we are not! To imagine why not, let us go back to data acquisition with a gamma camera. What we get there are projections of three-dimensional organs into two-dimensional (planar) images. Doing this we lose the depth information for each volume in the patient. Not only that, all the counts of the organs at different depths are superimposed onto one single element in the planar image: what we acquire are integrals of counts (see Radon transform)!

The tomographic reconstruction restores this loss of three-dimensional information. But, however this restoration of information is done, we have to pay for that gain of information - and the currency for that is statistics.

In 1978 Th. F. Budinger et. al. [13] gave a formula for the root mean square error (rms) in emission tomography:

$$\text{rms \%} = \frac{120 * (\text{number of resolution cells})^{3/4}}{(\text{total number of events in a resolution cell})^{1/2}}$$

Sure, and we already knew that, the fewer "total number of events" we have, the worse our statistics is. But the formula also tells us that the statistics depends on the "number of resolution cells" - and that's in the numerator. This means the more resolution elements our reconstruction volume has, the worse are its statistics.

Let us take SPECT of the brain as an example. Let's assume the brain to be 1600 ml, our resolution is 1 cm and the slice thickness is about 2 cm. This gives us about 8 slices. Then the volume of the largest slice is 335 ml, which means we have 335 resolution elements in this slice. The number of counts per resolution element is about 1000 if 740 MBq ^{99m}Tc-HMPAO was applied. From the presented charts in this paper [13] we would get an rms error of about 20%, but from the Poisson statistics of 1000 events we would expect an error of only 3% instead. The same activity in a volume with only 200 resolution elements would give us an rms error of only about 10%.

On the other hand, this means that small volumes, children, are easier to be reconstructed than large ones, adults. This may either result in in better images or the ability to administer less radioactivity (children).This also means that the virtual or effective sensitivity of the system is increased.

By the way: not talking about SPECT but about Time of Flight (TOF) in PET we have the same fact: Using time of flight information in PET, the uncertainty of depth is reduced to 5–10 cm. By doing this, we essentially reduce the size of large organs to the smaller "TOF – volume" and thus get better statistics in the reconstructed tomograms. Once again this results in better images or in less activity needed to be administered.

The SPECT Method

At the beginnings of SPECT with a gamma camera we identified two different kinds of tomography: limited angle- and transaxial- tomography. Today's SPECT [14] is nearly exclusively transaxial with a rotating gamma camera. To understand the need for transaxial, we would like to briefly introduce limited angle tomograpy.

Limited Angle Vs. Transaxial SPECT

In the early years of SPECT, when most cameras did not have rotating gantries, this kind of imaging was used for limited angle tomography (Figure 1.19). If there is an organ that is small compared to the field of view (FOV) of the camera (for example the myocardium), then it is possible to use the multiple pinhole technique. Compared to transaxial tomography, multiple pinhole tomography belongs to longitudinal tomography.

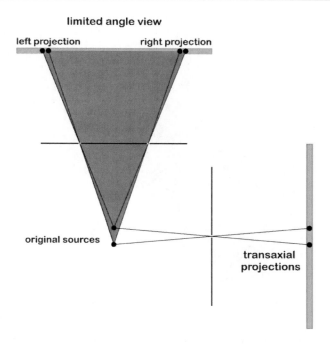

Figure 1.19. Limited angle tomography: in the left and right projections of the limited angle view the images of the original sources can only fairly or not be resolved. In the transaxial projection instead, the resolution of the point sources is clear.

As projections 1 and 2 "look at the two spots" from two different directions, it is possible to separate them – but not really good. The reason for this restriction is the fact that the angle between projection 1 and 2 is limited by the FOV of the camera. The lateral resolution of the resulting tomograms was fine, just like the resolution of the camera itself. The main limitation was the resolution in the longitudinal direction. To get a clear separation of the two spots we would have to look from another direction, as indicated by the "transaxial projections". In order to do this, we would need to rotate the camera by 90 degrees - but our camera was fixed.

As more and more cameras had rotating gantries, longitudinal, limited angle tomography became obsolete and was replaced by the transaxial SPECT with a rotating gamma camera. The collimator of choice for this kind of tomography was the long bore collimator.

SPECT Acquisition for Transaxial Tomography

In planar scintigrams we lose one space coordinate because we don't look at the object from different views. As we just saw, the first step toward getting different views was limited angle tomography. As this didn't give enough depth resolution, the rotating gamma camera was introduced to be able to acquire data from all views around the patient (Figure 1.20). The incremental steps are 3°, which gives 120 projections when acquisition is performed over 360°. From the mathematical point of view the angular range of 180° would be sufficient if the opposite views would be identical. But due to absorption and resolution this is not the case. Therefore SPECT acquisition is nearly exclusively performed over a 360° range.

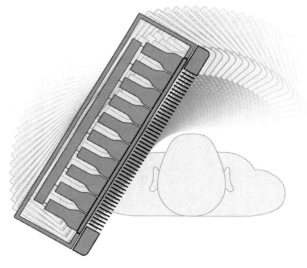

Figure 1.20. Gamma camera rotating around the brain of the patient in incremental steps of 3°. The result are projections from 120 different views in a rotation of 360°.

In SPECT with double or triple head cameras there would be no need to rotate each head by 360°, but sometimes even this is done. The reason is that each head has slightly different characteristics: sensitivity, homogeneity, linearity and so on. Therefore, to obtain a consistent dataset for tomographic reconstruction, the 360° data from the three heads are averaged to a virtual single head camera.

SPECT Reconstruction

In the introduction to this article we have already seen that scintigrams acquired with a gamma camera are 2D projections of an activity distribution in 3D space. The consequence of this is that all the activities lying along a single line are summed up to give the value we get in the projection: our projections are integrals of activity. But we don't want line integrals; we want to have the local activities. In other words, we want to get our lost dimension back! Is this possible?

The answer was given in 1917 by Johann Radon in his purely mathematical publication "On the determination of functions from their integral values along certain manifolds". The "functions" are the activity distributions that we only know from their "integral values", the projections. The "certain manifolds" [15] are actually the solution to the problem: we have to acquire the projections from different views. The idea of tomographic reconstruction will be presented here for SPECT, but actually the first clinical implementation was realized in CT by G. H. Hounsfield in 1973.

There are two approaches to reconstructing the activity distribution from its projections: the filtered back projection [16] and the algebraic (iterative) [17] solution.

Filtered Back Projection

Please note that the expression "filtered back projection" is a composite of two words. Let us start with the second term, back projection. In Figure 1.21 we show graphically what a back projection is. Let us assume we have an activity distribution as shown in Figure 1.21(left). Then one of our projections is the one seen in Figure 1.21(middle). As we lose depth when we acquire information with the gamma camera, this is all the information we have of our original activity distribution; it is what we usually call the planar image. The back projection shown in Figure 1.21(right) is the first step to determining where our activities were. What we have demonstrated here with graphite pencil on a sheet of paper is just what happens digitally in the computer. But unfortunately this step is as unsatisfactory as it looks: from this single projection we don't get any other information than this! The result obtained by superimposing back projections from different projections will be very confusing and doesn't really show us the positions of our initial activities. Therefore let us restrict ourselves to only one point source and make the following statement: if we know the result of filtered back projection for one point source, then we also know the result for a distribution. Mathematicians say the underlying algorithms are "linear". In Figure 1.22 we see the back projection of 12 projections. It can clearly be seen that the densities of the back projections are superimposed so that the hottest spot is where our activity source has been. In Figure 1.23 we simulate the back projection of the two point sources in 1-23a. In this simulation the point sources have a diameter of 5mm each and a distance from center to center of 10mm. If we have, like in SPECT, a resolution of 10mm, then the result, however it is obtained, should look like in 1-23b, where they can just be resolved visually. The back projection in 1-23c simulates angular increments of the gamma camera of 3° and the resolution of 10mm. This demonstration tells us that pure back projection is not enough to reconstruct a distribution of activities.

But even if it doesn't look that way, the information on the initial activity distribution is still in there – surely not better than the resolution of the camera. What we need to do now is to filter out that information. Unfortunately, this is not as intuitively demonstrated as back projection. So let's try it the other way around. If we have, like in Figure 1.17a, an ideal point source, the δ (delta) function, then imaging with any device will always be imperfect and the result is a distribution, our point-spread-function (PSF). Now, generally speaking, if we have the PSF of an imaging system, then we only need to know that there exists a mathematics that can simulate the limited resolution of that system. That's actually what happened from Figure 1.23a to 1.23b. The underlying mathematics is called "faltung" or "convolution" and the point-spread-function is the "kernel" of that convolution. The question now is, can we get our object back by something like a "deconvolution" of our image? Yes, we can! The only thing we need to know is the PSF of the system.

Thus the situation after pure back projection is that we want to get back our initial activity distribution. What is the PSF/kernel we need to know for our deconvolution? Let us go back to Figure 1.22 and 1.23c. The density distribution we get from that back projection has a $1/r$ – characteristic: twice the distance = half the density. In signal processing this knowledge ends up in a function for correction called "ramp" (also well known as the "ramp filter").

Now let's see if we have everything we need for SPECT acquisition and reconstruction. In Figure 1.24a we see three simultaneous projections of HMPAO-SPECT acquisition done with the CERASPECT (Figure 1.25). Pure back projection of these data is seen in Figure 1.24b.

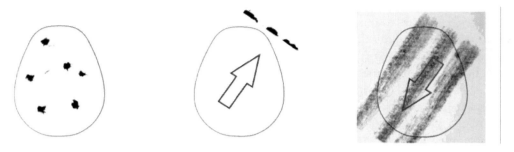

Figure 1.21. Demonstration of pure backprojection: left) small heaps of graphite (of a pencil) represents the spotted distribution of activity, center) by projecting the graphite the way seen, we obtain the "summed activity" of one projection, right) by backprojecting the graphite we get the streaks from figure 1-22.

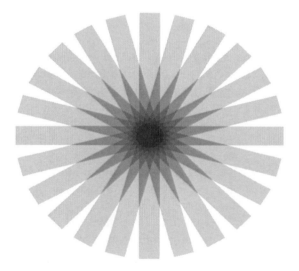

Figure 1.22. Superposition of 12 backprojections. The original spot is clearly emphasized in the center by the backprojections, but it is also distributed (stripes) over the whole matrix.

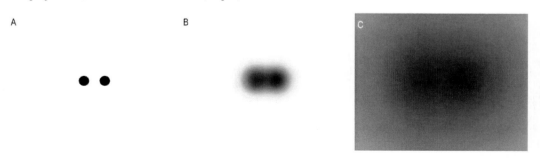

Figure 1.23. a) the original idealized object. The distance of the points is 10 mm. b) Image as expected after clinical tomographic reconstruction. c) Result after pure backprojection.

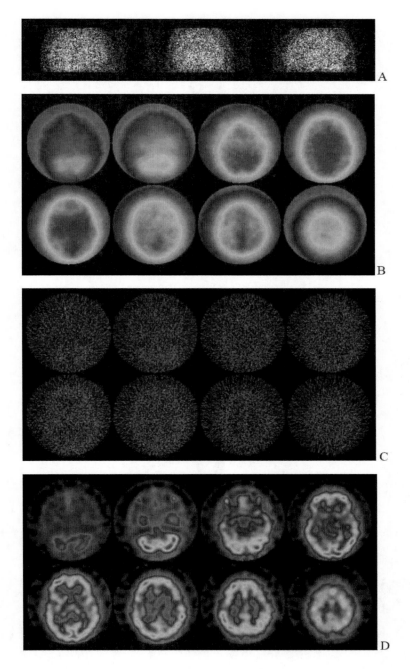

Figure 1.24. Steps of tomographic reconstruction: a) projections after acquisition with the CERASPECT, b) pure backprojection, c) correction with RAMP, d) clinical filtering with Butterworth filter.

As seen before, back projection only gives us very blurred results. But we have mentioned that we can obtain details of the activity distribution by deconvolution of the back projections with our "ramp filter".

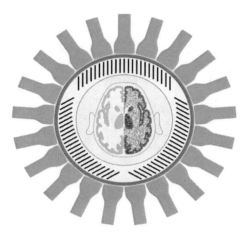

Figure 1.25. Cross section of the CERASPECT. The only moving part of the camera is the parallel hole collimator.

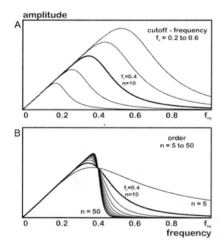

Figure 1.26. Butterworth filter often used in SPECT. f_{ny} is the Nyquist frequency, the highest possible frequency for a given imaging matrix. f_c = cutoff frequency; it defines the onset of the roll off. n = order; it defines the steepness of the roll off.

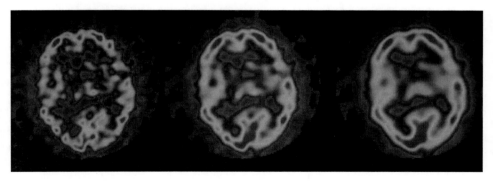

Figure 1.27. Butterworth filter with left) high, middle) medium and right) low cutoff frequency.

The result is shown in Figure 1.24c. But we don't like that either! What happened? To understand what's going on let's go back to the acquired projections in Figure 1.24a. We can see that they are quite noisy due to their Poisson statistics. And we already saw (see: Statistics in SPECT, Budinger Formula) that we additionally have to pay for recovering the lost 3rd dimension with poor statistics.

To understand the next step in tomographic reconstruction, in a more intuitive rather than mathematical way, let's see it this way (see also: "Space- and Frequency- Domain, Filters"): If Figure 1.24c would be an acoustic signal, you would say that what you hear is a faint signal overlaid by an overwhelming amount of noise. And in that noise there are a lot of very high frequencies. In the acoustic case the solution would be to diminish the high frequencies with the treble control, which is also called a filter. And in this case our filter was used to extract the signal out of the noise by suppressing high frequencies.

One very popular filter in SPECT is the Butterworth filter, because of its flexibility. This flexibility comes from its two parameters, the cutoff frequency and the order (Figure 1.26). The cutoff frequency, often named f_c, defines the onset of suppression of the high frequencies. The order, often named n, defines the steepness of the decline. With these parameters set to values appropriate for clinical use we obtain the final tomogram seen in Figure 1.24d. The effect of different cutoff frequencies can be seen in Figure 1.27. A high cutoff frequency gives us higher resolution tomograms but with a lot of noise. With a low cutoff frequency it's the other way round. Again, similar to the sensitivity-resolution compromise, here we have its counterpart, the noise–resolution compromise.

Iterative (Algebraic) Reconstruction

Instead of reconstructing the true activity distribution from the (just shown) filtered back projection, it's also possible to go the algebraic way. Let's again try to follow the intuitive way.

Let us assume we have our activity distribution in a slice divided into a matrix of voxels. Then for our projections we sum up all the activities lying along a single line of projection as:

$$P_{(with\ some\ indices)} = p_1 + p_2 + p_3 + ... + p_n$$

$P_{(with\ some\ indices)}$ is our measurement, the projection, and p_1, p_2 etc. are the activities of the voxels. If we want to know p_3, then we have to solve the equation:

$$p_3 = P_{(with\ some\ indices)} - p_1 - p_2 - ... - p_n$$

But unfortunately the only known value is our measurement $P_{(with\ some\ indices)}$. This means our equation cannot be solved without knowing all the other Ps. From the mathematics we were taught in school we know that we have, in this case, one equation with n unknown parameters. But we also know that we could determine the value for p_3 if we had n instead of only one (independent) equation. For a whole line this would be e.g. 128 equations! This might be fine for one line, but take into account that we have a lot of lines (128) for only one projection and additionally we have a lot of projections (128) – and all this for only one slice!

As we can see, this kind of calculation ends up with more than a million equations. The procedure to solve this problem is the iterative reconstruction method. What is done here is essentially similar to curve fitting, but in this case our function is not a curve like, for example, the function of biexponential decay [15, 18]. What is done therefore is the estimation of a model that only looks similar to the real activity distribution. The model and the real distribution are compared with each other. After this comparison the model is corrected in an iterative step and again it's compared – and so on. After a number of iterations the iteration by iteration improved model (best) fits the real activity distribution, so the reconstruction is done. The number of iterations needed for reconstruction is not unique for all algorithms and distributions. It therefore has to be defined in the reconstruction protocol.

Iterative reconstruction is, due to its many iterative steps, very time consuming. But with the processing power of today computers, this method has often been favored in recent years.

Attenuation Correction

Similar to radioactive decay, attenuation follows the exponential law:

$$A = A_0\, e^{\,(-\mu x)}$$

where μ is the absorption constant. For 150 keV in water it has a value of 0.149 1/cm. From this we calculate that, after passage through 4.5 cm of water or tissue, we have only 50% of the initial activity, after 9 cm only 25% and so on. This means that in the case of quantification, but also in visual assessment, the central organs of the brain are underestimated by about a factor of 4. If we assume the brain to be homogeneous (from a tissue density point of view), then it is quite easy to correct for that absorption [19]. The outline of the skull has to be defined by a given threshold (about 45%) or an ellipse. If scatter correction has been applied during tomographic reconstruction, an absorption coefficient of 0.149 1/cm is taken; without scatter correction, a coefficient of 0.12 1/cm is usually taken.

For the brain we just assumed homogeneous density of the tissue. If, as in the lungs, the tissue density is not as homogeneous as in the brain, then the result of attenuation correction by defined outlines is disturbed by unpredictable errors. In these cases tomograms of the local densities have to be created by transmission scans – and that's CTs! This may be done by external radioactive transmission sources (^{153}Ga) [20]. But we always have to keep in mind that the generated density maps have a lot of noise that is transferred to the corrected tomograms.

In the case of a SPECT-CT scanner [21], the CT modality is not only adopted for generating density maps, but also for diagnostics and overlaying. Therefore noise is less dominant in these cases; thus their Hounsfield numbers are the method of choice for attenuation correction of the emission scans.

Acquisition Parameters for SPECT

The acquisition parameters for SPECT with low energies (^{99m}Tc) when acquisition is performed with a low energy collimator and a camera with a large FOV are:

- Acquisition matrix: 128 x 128. In the case of a FOV of 500 mm, the pixel size is then 3.9 mm. From Shannon we obtained the formula that this gives us a resolution not better than 8 mm. For the already discussed resolution of 9–12 mm with the LEUHR – collimator (Figure 1.10) this would just fit. But anyway, for small organs like the brain, it would be better to make an acquisition in zoom mode (zoom = 1.6 or 2.0). This would give us the reserve not to suppress any existing resolution of the camera. And additionally, in the unzoomed images there are a lot of zeroes we don't need!
- Number of acquisition steps: 120 or 128. Usually, if the acquisition matrix has a size of 128 pixels, then the number of acquisition steps has to be similar. With 120 steps, which is widely used, we have an angular increment of adjacent projections of 3°.
- With modern cameras the usual rotation mode is "step and shoot".

For medium energies or, much more often, low energies but with very high energy components (e.g. ^{177}Lu) the MEGP collimator is used. In Figure 1.28 we can see that the resolution at a distance of 15 cm is about 13 mm. If, in this case, we could take a 64 x 64 matrix, our resolution would not be better than 16 mm – not enough to resolve structures of 13 mm. Therefore, even if the resolution of the MEGP collimator is worse than the resolution of the LEUHR, for the MEGP collimator we also need to adopt a matrix of 128 x 128 pixels.

The acquisition time needed to get good results depends on the organs, their sizes, the activity distribution etc.; this is the reason why it's not possible to make general suggestions here.

As a rule of thumb for filtered backprojection with the Butterworth filter, we can suggest the order of the filter be around 10. The fine tuning of the cutoff frequency has to be performed individually for each system and acquisition protocol, as this depends on the size of the voxels in the reconstruction matrix, the amount of activity and its distribution and so forth.

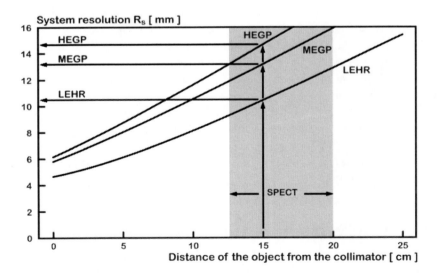

Figure 1.28. In SPECT an MEGP collimator has about 3 mm less of resolution compared to the LEHR collimator.

Space- and Frequency-Domain, Filters

Thus far we have neither mentioned frequencies nor used the expression "Fourier transform". This area of work is pure mathematics and signal processing – and not very intuitive for clinicians. We would prefer not having to talk about this, but unfortunately clinical routine is often confronted with "cutoff frequencies", "orders", Nyquist and so on (Figure 1.29).

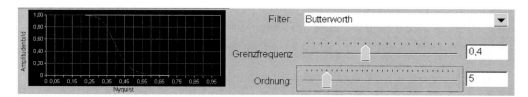

Figure 1.29. Parameters of signal processing used in clinical routine. Left: window function. Right: Grenzfrequenz = cutoff frequency f_c; Ordnung = order n; Filter = Butterworth filter.

Therefore let's put it this way:

1) There exists a space domain with the dimensions meter [m]. It's the space we live in and are familiar with.
2) There exists a frequency domain with the inverse dimensions [1/m]. Engineers and physisists, who talk about signals, noise and filters, usually work in this domain. Some kind of mathematics (convolution) is better performed in the frequency domain than in the space domain.
3) The Fourier transform (and its inverse) transforms any object from the space- into the frequency-domain (and vice versa). The fast Fourier tranform (FFT) makes it easy to switch from the space- to the frequency-domain and vice versa. This also is one of the reasons why a lot of work is performed in the frequency domain.
4) Large objects in the space domain are represented by low frequencies (long wavelengths) in the frequency domain.
5) Small objects in the space domain are represented by high frequencies (short wavelengths) in the frequency domain.
6) Raising high frequencies enhances spatial resolution, but you pay for this with noise.
7) Suppressing high frequencies diminishes spatial resolution, but you get smooth images.
8) The Nyquist frequency is the highest frequency an imaging matrix can represent (see Shannon theorem).

Quality Control and Quality Assurance in SPECT

To obtain reliable and artifact free results in clinical SPECT, the protocols of quality control (QC) are defined by law. In Germany the "Richtlinie Strahlenschutz in der Medizin" essentially tells us that for SPECT we have to use the DIN 6855-2 for QC.

The content of this standard is the QC for gamma cameras used for planar imaging, and for rotating gamma cameras for SPECT. Not only that, but for SPECT we need to control additional parameters (for example, the center of rotation (COR)); also, the necessity for high quality in cameras used for SPECT is much higher than with cameras used only for planar imaging. In the following we will discuss the most important parameters that have to be tested.

energy window	daily
background	daily
inhomogeneity	weekly
sensitivity	monthly
center of rotation	monthly
spatial resolution and linearity	every six months
imaging scale	every six months
tomographic inhomogeneity	every six months

Energy Window

The incoming gamma rays interact with the crystal either through the Compton effect or through the photoelectric process. In the Compton effect the gamma loses part of its energy and is scattered. The amount of energy lost depends on the scattering angle and varies from interaction to interaction. After the photo effect the whole energy of the gamma is lost and with it the gamma itself.

As "scattering" means to transfer information to other, wrong places, only the photo effect is interesting for imaging.

For these reasons, to obtain better images, processes that underwent Compton effect have to be eliminated. To do this, the transferred energy of the process is measured in a multichannel analyzer and a discriminator has to decide if the gamma has to be discarded or not.

This would be very easy if scattering only happened in the crystal and if the energy resolution of the camera would be infinite. In that case we would have a clear gap between the photo peak and the highest possible energy after the Compton effect, the Compton edge (Figure 1.30 solid line). But unfortunately that's not the way it is. First of all, our scintillation detector NaI(Tl) has a limited energy resolution of about 10% of the gamma energy. The gamma energy $E\gamma$ and the Compton edge, both well-defined from the physics point of view, are merged due to the limited resolution (Figure 1.30 dashed line). We additionally have scattering in the patient (not shown here) which itself smears the photo peak to lower energies towards the Compton edge.

The broadening of the photo peak due to limited energy resolution means, for ^{99m}Tc, that the photo peak reaches from about 126 (-10%) to 154 (+10%) kev. To eliminate counts that underwent Compton interaction from those of the photo peak continuum, we have to define an electronic discriminator that discards events outside of the photo peak. This is usually called the "energy window".

The problem with an incorrectly adjusted energy window is that it generates inhomogeneity. To eliminate this error, the energy window has to be adjusted daily for each nuclide used on that day.

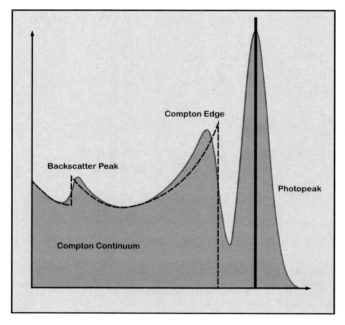

Figure 1.30. The effect of limited energy resolution of NaI(Tl) scintillators. Dashed and straight line (in the photo peak) would be the energy spectrum with unlimited energy resolution. The solid, curved line is the result of about 10% of energy resolution.

Inhomogeneity – Uniformity

Two definitions are usually used to define the inhomogeneity of a gamma camera: the integral and the differential inhomogeneity (in the NEMA *standard* called "uniformity"). Both of them are defined for the UFOV (Useful Field Of View) and for the CFOV (Central Field Of View). The UFOV represents the whole field of view of a camera. As the problems associated within homogeneity are greatest at the boundaries, and not always representative of the whole field of view, homogeneity values are also defined for the central part of the field of view, the CFOV. It is defined as being only 75% (linearly) of the UFOV. "Linearly" means that both the x- and y-dimensions are 75% of the extension of the UFOV (and not the area, which is about 0.6 of the UFOV).

The *integral inhomogeneity* is a measure of the largest deviation in pixel counts within the integral FOV tested. If the maximal counts of a pixel are MAX and the minimal are MIN, then the integral inhomogeneity is calculated by the formula:

int. inh. = (MAX - MIN) / (MAX + MIN)

and has nothing to do with the mathematical integral ($F = \int f(x)\, dx$). This value is totally insensitive to the distance and direction between the MIN and MAX pixels. Before calculation of the integral inhomogeneity the data have to be smoothed with an appropriate 9-point filter.

The *differential inhomogeneity* takes into account that due to the PM - structure there might be a visible inhomogeneity where we can "see" the PMs. In this case intensity gradients may clearly be recognized. To calculate the differential inhomogeneity, the same formula as for the integral inhomogeneity is used. But the pixels chosen for calculation should have a distance of about 30 mm, which is 5 pixels of 5–7 mm each in a 64x64 matrix and a FOV of 400 mm. As gradients have an orientation, the differential inhomogeneity is defined for both the x- and y- directions.

System Uniformity

Talking about SPECT with a rotating gamma camera, we have to take into account that these systems are much more sensitive to errors than cameras used for planar imaging only. Thus, in SPECT we need a higher quality standard. But the setups for QC of the gamma camera are very often defined for planar imaging only. The main difference is that quality control with a point source is suitable only for assessment of the intrinsic uniformity, which is the uniformity of the head of the camera only. The influence of scattering and the collimator is not included in the intrinsic uniformity.

To fulfill the higher QC standards suitable for SPECT, we additionally have to include the influence of scattering and the collimator. We then talk of the system's uniformity. But this also means that each collimator has, together with the camera, its own system uniformity. For the QC protocol this means we have to use a flat source of activity that overlaps the whole FOV of the camera.

Spectrum and Scattering

For QC of a gamma camera with a collimator, flat sources of ^{57}Co activity are available. Before using ^{57}Co sources for SPECT QC, there are two major topics to be discussed: the spectrum of ^{57}Co and the lack of scattering using flat sources. The shape of the ^{99m}Tc and ^{57}Co photo peaks look somewhat different. The only gamma energy of interest emitted by ^{99m}Tc has an energy of 140.5 keV. There are neither other gamma energies surrounding the 140.5 keV energy nor are there gammas with higher energies that might scatter into the photo peak. With ^{57}Co the situation is a little bit different. Here the predominant energy is 122 keV, but there is another energy at 137 keV and an abundance of about 15 % of the 122 keV-line. Due to the limited energy resolution of NaI (Tl) they cannot be separated from each other. Thus with ^{57}Co we get a different shape for the photo peak compared to the one for ^{99m}Tc. This, on the other hand, means that the results of the uniformity control performed with ^{57}Co and ^{99m}Tc are different.

Spectrum and Scattering

The second problem we have with ^{57}Co for uniformity control is that, as ^{57}Co flat sources have a thickness of only several millimeters, they don't include scattering. As this lack of scattering again deforms the shape of the ^{57}Co spectrum, QC for SPECT has to be performed with "thick" sources. German standards demand sources filled with ^{99m}Tc have a minimum thickness of 8 cm. This guarantees spectra that are similar to the situation in the clinical routine with ^{99m}Tc.

Threshold Values

It is our experience that the values of inhomogeneity for a "good camera" vary from camera to camera. We always have to take into account that values for inhomogeneity are calculated by programs that follow different protocols, procedures and even different laws in different countries. To calculate the inhomogeneity, the programs have to perform different steps: they have to define the FOV of the camera, and the values have to be smoothed. We have already seen cameras with excellent homogeneity whose values for inhomogeneity would not have been acceptable for another camera. The only statement we can make is that very often for the integral inhomogeneity of a well-adjusted camera we have values of 1.7 to 2.3. In these cases there is no visual evidence of inhomogeneity. From 3 to 4.5%, at our institution we acquire new correction maps for the inhomogeneity. From 4.5%, inhomogeneities can clearly be detected visually. Cameras thus inhomogeneous have to be newly adjusted or repaired by the camera service. But, as said before, we also had cameras, where a homogeneous camera with no evidence of an inhomogeneity had an integral inhomogeneity of 4.5%. Therefore it's impossible to give general thresholds for the inhomogeneity of a camera. The thresholds have to be given by the manufacturers on delivery of the camera.

Measurement Procedure and Setup for System Uniformity

The goal of our QC is to obtain a camera with an inhomogeneity of about 2%. The QC setup has to take this into account.

Generally speaking, the setup for QC of the system uniformity of a camera used for SPECT has to include an activity-filled phantom "at least 8 cm thick". This guarantees that scattering is included and that the mechanical homogeneity of the phantom is better than 1%. Phantoms of only a few cm thickness are like "water filled plastic bags" and may have inhomogeneities of up to 30%, which is totally unsuitable for QC (even for planar imaging).

It is obvious that low counting statistics gives us statistically unreliable values for the parameters MAX and MIN used to calculate inhomogeneity. To obtain values with an error less than 1%, it is mandatory to have at least 5000 counts per cm^2. For a FOV of about 55 x 40 cm, this means that we need at least 11 Mio counts (at our institution 22 Mio counts are used).

In the standards, usually a maximum count rate of 20,000 cts/s is allowed. It is our experience that this very old number isn't always true for "modern" cameras. Unpublished internal experiments performed in the early 90s showed us there is essentially no influence of the count rate on the QC up to about 45,000 cts/s. We therefore perform our QC with count rates up to 40,000 cts/s. In a Nuclear Medicine facility with some double headed cameras this gain in time might be very welcome.

Spatial Resolution and Linearity

If the parameters energy window, sensitivity and especially inhomogeneity are well within their operating ranges, then usually resolution shows good values.

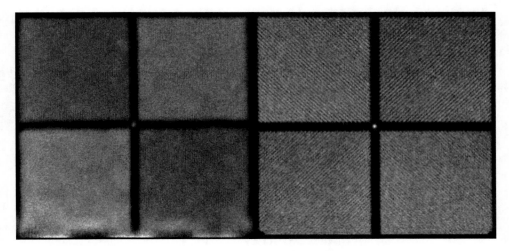

Figure 1.31. Spatial resolution of a defective (left) and the repaired (right) camera.

Therefore, if there is no obvious error, resolution needs to be tested only every six months. This may be done with bar phantoms (Figure 1.31). A typical result of these tests is: "The bars in section D (Figure 1.6a) are well visible / just visible / not visible". The reference for what's good or not is the delivery protocol. As there is no button or adjustment procedure for resolution, then if something goes wrong it's a matter for technical support.

The definition of linearity is that the image of a straight line has to be an undistorted straight line. If it's not, we get two problems:

-   pincushion and barrel shaped distortions accompany the structure of the photomultipliers, which leads to inhomogeneities where "the PMs can be seen".
-   distortion means to give the image an incorrect location. As distorted projections mean an incorrect set of data for tomographic reconstruction in SPECT, linearity needs to be tested routinely every six months.

In contrast to resolution, a slightly incorrect linearity may be corrected by "linearity maps", which are generated by the technical service with appropriate phantoms. But generally, if something goes wrong with linearity, like with resolution, a camera setup has to be performed.

Center of Rotation (COR)

There are two "centers of rotation": the mechanical of the camera and the mathematical in the tomographic reconstruction matrix. If they don't match, artifacts will be generated in the resulting tomograms, especially in the center. This parameter is usually tested for correctness monthly or at least every six months.

Imaging Scale

The scale of a matrix probably isn't crucial for qualitative diagnostics. If distances, areas or volumes are important for clinical investigation or research, then errors in the size of the pixels/voxels result in erroneous quantification. This, for example, is the case with dosimetry calculations, where the deposited energy (Gray, Gy) is defined by the energy deposited per kilogram of tissue (Joule/kg). To prevent quantitative errors, the imaging scale has to be controlled every 6 months.

References

[1]   Cherry S, Sorenson J, Phelps M, eds. Physics in Nuclear Medicine: Expert Consult Fourth ed: Saunders 2004.

[2]   Valk P, Bailey D, Townsend D, Maisey M, eds. Positron Emission Tomography: Clinical Practice 1st ed: *Springer, 2006.*

[3]   Doria D, Singh M. Comparison of Reconstruction Algorithms for an Electronically Collimated Gamma Camera *IEEE Trans Nucl. Sci.*, 1982; 29: 447-51.

[4]   Çonka-Nurdan T, Nurdan K, Walenta A, Chiosa I, Freisleben B et al. First Results on Compton Camera Coincidences With the Silicon Drift Detector. *IEEE Trans Nucl. Sci.,* 2005: 1381 - 5.

[5]   Anger H. The scintillation camera for radioisotope localization. In: Hoffmann G, Scheer K, eds. *Radioisotope in der Lokalisations-diagnostik*: Schattauer 1966.

[6]   Anger H. Radioisotope cameras. In: Hine G, ed. Instrumentation in Nuclear Medicine: Academic Press, New York and London 1967.

[7]   Hine G, Erickson J. Advances in scintigraphic instrumentation. In: Hine G, Sorenson J, eds. Instrumentation in Nuclear Medicine: Academic Press, New York and London 1974.

[8]   Nyquist–Shannon sampling theorem. [cited; Available from: http://www.princeton.edu /achaney/tmve/wiki100k/docs/Nyquist%E2%80%93Shannon_sampling_theorem.html.

[9]   Jaszczak RJ, Li J, Wang H, Zalutsky MR, Coleman RE. Pinhole collimation for ultra-high-resolution, small-field-of-view SPECT. *Physics in medicine and biology,* 1994; 39: 425-37.

[10] Browne E, Firestone R, Lederer C, VS S. Table of Isotopes John Wiley & Sons Inc 1979.

[11] Zhu X. Recovery coefficient in PET as a function of object size and respiratory motion trajectory. Nuclear Science Symposium Conference Record, *2005 IEEE,* 2005:2170 - 2.

[12] Glynn E. USAF 1951 and Microcopy Resolution Test Charts and Pixel Profiles. 2002 [cited; Available from: www.efg2.com/Lab/ImageProcessing/TestTargets/.

[13] Budinger TF, Derenzo SE, Greenberg WL, Gullberg GT, Huesman RH. Quantitative potentials of dynamic emission computed tomography. *Journal of nuclear medicine : official publication, Society of Nuclear Medicine,* 1978; 19: 309-15.

[14] Kuwert T, Grünwald F, Haberkorn U, Krause T, eds. Nuklearmedizin. 4 ed: Thieme, Stuttgart 2007.

[15] Radon J. On the Determination of Functions from Their Integral Values along Certain Manifolds. *IEEE transactions on medical imaging,* 1986; 5: 170-6.

[16] Gopi P. Reconstruction of an Image Using the Filtered Back Projection Method. 2004.

[17] De Witte Y, Vlassenbroeck J, Van Hoorebeke L. A multiresolution approach to iterative reconstruction algorithms in X-ray computed tomography. *IEEE transactions on image processing : a publication of the IEEE Signal Processing Society,* 2010; 19: 2419-27.

[18] Radon J. Über die Bestimmung von Funktionen durch ihre Integralwerte längs gewisser Mannigfaltigkeiten. Berichte über die Verhandlungen der Königlich Sächsischen Gesellschaft der Wissenschaften zu Leipzig. *Mathematisch-Physische Klasse,* 1917; 69: 262-77.

[19] Chang L. A Method for Attenuation Correction in Radionuclide Computed Tomography. *IEEE Trans Nuc. Sci.,* 1978: 638-43.

[20] He ZX, Scarlett MD, Mahmarian JJ, Verani MS. Enhanced accuracy of defect detection by myocardial single-photon emission computed tomography with attenuation correction with gadolinium 153 line sources: evaluation with a cardiac phantom. *Journal of nuclear cardiology : official publication of the American Society of Nuclear Cardiology,* 1997; 4: 202-10.

[21] Patton JA, Turkington TG. SPECT/CT physical principles and attenuation correction. *Journal of nuclear medicine technology,* 2008; 36: 1-10.

In: SPECT   ISBN: 978-1-62808-344-6
Editors: Hojjat Ahmadzadehfar and Elham Habibi   © 2013 Nova Science Publishers, Inc.

Chapter II

The Impact of SPECT on Medical Internal Dosimetry

*Michael G. Stabin**

Associate Professor of Radiology and Radiological Sciences,
Department of Radiology and Radiological Sciences, Vanderbilt University, Nashville

Introduction

Internal dose calculations are an essential element of the safety evaluation of any radiopharmaceutical. For both diagnostic and therapeutic radiopharmaceuticals, dosimetric calculations are an integral part of the new drug approval process, overseen by the US Food and Drug Administration (FDA). For diagnostic pharmaceuticals, the dosimetric information obtained becomes part of the drug's package insert material and is used infrequently. Radiation doses are usually not of interest for every routine administration, but become important when misadministrations occur, for example, when pregnant women are given the drug (whether intentionally or accidentally) and in other limited situations. For therapeutic agents, dosimetry should ideally be evaluated in all patients, as is done for external beam radiotherapy, but unfortunately this is not often the case. A limited dosimetric evaluation is normally performed for the therapeutic use of ^{131}I-labeled Tositumomab ('Bexxar'). Its activity in whole body is obtained at three time points, and the dose to a unit-density ellipsoid of the subject's mass is used as a surrogate for marrow dose. For other agents, activity is generally prescribed on the basis of patient body weight or body surface area, with no dosimetric evaluation. This results in a suboptimal therapeutic regime, as will be briefly discussed below. Nuclear medicine physicians simply do not have the same mindset as radiation oncologists, who evaluate each patient's normal tissue and tumor doses, and attempt to optimize each individual's therapy plan. Nuclear medicine physicians think in terms of 'unit dosing', in which activity administered to all patients is basically similar, with minor adjustments applied using a few simple individualized considerations. There are a number of reasons for the current mindset of nuclear medicine physicians, one of which often cited is the accuracy

* Phone (615) 343-4628, Fax (615) 322-6119, Email michael.g.stabin@vanderbilt.edu, internet www.doseinfo-radar.com

of dose calculations. Most dose calculations are based on standardized individual body sizes (i.e., 'reference' individuals) and thus, are poorly applicable to individual patients. Adjustments can be made, but the quality is still considerably poorer than that of external beam dosimetric workups. The use of quantitative single photon emission computed tomography (SPECT) imaging, coupled to computed tomography (CT) imaging of individual patients, has created the possibility of significantly improving the quality of internal dosimetry for the therapeutic use of radiopharmaceuticals, as well as of dosimetry becoming part of routine practice in nuclear medicine therapy. It remains to be seen if this will be sufficient to change the mindset of the nuclear medicine community.

Current Dosimetric Practice

Before discussing the use of SPECT in radiopharmaceutical dosimetry, a brief overview of general dosimetric practice will be given. Radiopharmaceutical dose estimates for standardized applications may be calculated using the methodology developed by the RAdiation Dose Assessment Resource (RADAR) Task Group of the Society of Nuclear Medicine [1]. This method uses a simple equation for internal doses in nuclear medicine patients:

$$D_T = \sum_S N_S \times DF(T \leftarrow S) \tag{1}$$

where D_T is the dose to the target region T, N_S the number of nuclear transitions that occur in the source region S, and $DF(T \leftarrow S)$ the "dose factor" for the source region S irradiating the target region T. Dose factors are usually precalculated, using human body models as 'reference' individuals, e.g., a reference adult male has a body weight of around 70 kg and an adult female around 57 kg, with references also existing for individuals of younger ages [2]. For a new radiopharmaceutical, the values of N_S for organs that have a significant accumulation of the agent ('source organs') must be calculated. This is done by taking serial images of a number of subjects and making a quantitative assessment of the activity in the source organs. The most common method used is the 'conjugate view' approach, which uses combined anterior/posterior projection images, with regions of interest (ROIs) drawn over identified anatomical structures. Data taken from ROIs for individual organs (such as the liver or spleen) must be expressed as a percentage or fraction of the initial activity administered. The number of counts in an ROI must therefore be related to activity by a calibration constant, but corrections for attenuation and scatter counts in the photopeak must also be made. Corrections for body 'background' (activity in blood and other tissues possibly superimposed over an organ's ROI) must also be made [3]. For a projection image, the actual depth of the objects containing activity within the patient is not known. This geometric mean of the anterior and posterior counts, when corrected for attenuation, is theoretically independent of depth and is used to make a quantitative estimate of activity within the organ [4]. Corrections for scattered radiations in the photopeak window can be addressed with various methods; one popular approach is the Double or Triple Energy Window method [5], which involves establishing small windows just below and/or above the photopeak window.

After scatter correction has been performed by subtracting the appropriate number of counts from the ROI photopeak, the activity within an organ's ROI is calculated as:

$$A_{ROI} = \sqrt{\frac{I_A I_P}{e^{-\mu_e t}}} \frac{f_j}{C}$$

(2)

where I_A and I_P are the anterior and posterior counts in the region, μ_e is the effective attenuation coefficient for the radionuclide imaged, t is the average patient thickness over the ROI (often evaluated using a 'sheet' ^{57}Co source with the defined ROIs superimposed over images with and without the patient in the field), f_j is the source's 'self-attenuation coefficient' (given as $[(\mu_e t/2)/\sinh(\mu_e t/2)]$, but is rarely of much use in the calculation and is therefore usually neglected), and C is the source's calibration factor (counts/sec per Bq), obtained by counting a source of known activity in air [6].

When multiple values of organ activity are obtained at different imaging times, the N_S values are obtained by integrating the source activity over time and normalizing to the total activity initially administered. The most common fitted function is in the form of one or more exponentials [7]. Dose factors (DF) may then be applied, such as those available in the OLINDA/EXM software code [8].This is the most common and standard approach, but other methods may be equally adequate. Doses provided using standard DFs, as noted above, apply to people similar to the defined 'reference' individuals from which they were calculated. The liver of the reference adult male, for example, is 1910 g; in a given patient, this value may vary considerably depending on body type. Estimates of patient-specific organ masses may be readily obtained from the subject's CT images. For alpha and beta emissions, the DF alters inversely with changes in the mass of the organ:

$$DF_2 = DF_1 \frac{m_1}{m_2}$$

(3)

where DF_1 and DF_2 are the dose factors appropriate for use with organ masses m_1 and m_2, respectively.

For photons, Snyder [9] showed that the photon absorbed fractions (a key component of the DF) vary directly with the cube root of the mass for self-irradiation (i.e., the source organ is the target organ) if the photon mean path length is large compared to the organ diameter, and vary directly with the mass for cross-irradiation (i.e., when the source and target organs are different). Thus, for self-irradiation, the absorbed fraction increases with the cube root of the mass of the organ:

$$\phi_2 = \phi_1 \left(\frac{m_2}{m_1}\right)^{1/3}$$

(4)

This relationship is useful, but not exactly true for all body regions and radionuclides [10]. Using good quality quantitative estimates of organ uptakes (making proper corrections for attenuation and scatter) and scaling DFs for individual patient organ masses, doses for many organs can probably be estimated with an accuracy of 10 to 20% [11].

SPECT Imaging for Dosimetry

Most quantitative dosimetry for patients is performed using the conjugate view technique described above. Positron emission tomography (PET) agents are routinely imaged using quantitative PET, drawing volumes of interest (VOIs) over identified source organ regions on multiple slices of the 3D rendered activity distributions. These image data are quantitative, as PET scanners are calibrated regularly to obtain quantitative data about organ uptakes for diagnostic purposes. SPECT is generally performed in a qualitative way to provide the physician information about the distribution of the pharmaceuticals, but mostly without knowing the absolute values of activity in any region or organ. However, SPECT data certainly can be obtained in a quantitative way and used for dosimetric analysis. The fusion of patient-individualized quantitative SPECT data with patient-individualized CT results creates the possibility of developing three-dimensional dose 'maps' for each subject, and not just calculating average doses for whole organs and tumors. Activity distributions are often non-uniform within organs or tumors, and average doses do not account for such non-uniformities. Even when these distributions are uniform, organ doses are somewhat non-uniform [12]. Such 3D dose calculations have been realized in several research centers, however the routine use of such data in clinical nuclear medicine has not been implemented, for the reasons cited above about the 'mindset' of the nuclear medicine community One commercial product implementing this technology was on the market at the time of writing; it remains to be seen if this or other software products will be used routinely in the clinical use of therapeutic radiopharmaceuticals.

An overview of many important aspects of quantitative SPECT imaging was presented by Dewaraja et al. [13]. They note that the spatial resolution of current SPECT cameras is around 5 to 25 mm, which is the best resolution that can be expected in any dose calculation using SPECT. Nonetheless, use of quantitative SPECT to obtain 3D dosimetric maps is a significant step forward from calculating organ and tumor average doses. They also highlight the observations of O'Donoghue [14] that if tumor activity distributions are non-uniform, use of tumor-average dose calculations may mischaracterize treatment success, as parts of the tumor may receive excessive doses during treatment and others will receive suboptimal doses.

Attenuation corrections in hybrid SPECT/CT imaging are facilitated by the application of CT attenuation maps. Hybrid imaging on the same machine also eliminates many problems formerly associated with image registration of SPECT and CT images taken on separate machines at different times. Corrections for photon scatter may be implemented on most imaging systems using a similar multiple energy window approach, as is used in the conjugate view method. Ljungberg et al. [15], using a computer code simulating the response of gamma cameras to incident radiations, showed the contributions of scattered radiation to the photopeak window of various radionuclides.

The accuracy of quantitative SPECT has been evaluated by a number of authors employing physical phantoms. Due to the inherent resolution of existing systems, the accuracy of quantitative measurements of activity within objects is affected when the objects are small. Dewajara et al. [13] summarized the findings of several of these studies and gave a general accuracy of 5 to 20%. Ljungberg et al. [16] estimated ^{111}In and ^{90}Y activity in simulated SPECT projections. Their results displayed good accuracy, but there was some over- and underestimation of activity (up to30–50%) in some cases due to count spillover into and out of the defined organ regions. El Fakhri et al. [17] measured levels of ^{99m}Tc in a cardiac (left ventricle) and liver phantom. They suggested the following factors in order of importance for quantification accuracy: (1) attenuation; (2) partial volume; (3) scatter; and (4) collimator response. Pereira et al. [3] assessed quantitative accuracy in both conjugate view planar and SPECT imaging of several radiopharmaceuticals with more and less complex decay schemes in phantoms with spheres, cardiac and liver compartments (with simulated tumors), varying the background activity and levels of activity concentration in the source regions. Recovery was excellent in larger objects and at high concentrations, even for nuclides with a complex decay scheme, but was degraded for smaller objects, lower concentrations and higher levels of background. Dewaraja et al. [13] also discussed other details of SPECT quantitative imaging, including acquisition modes, collimators, reconstruction methods, corrections for dead time (where needed), partial volume effects, and the particular difficulty of time-integration of SPECT data, as images at different times involve patients in different positions, and linking voxels defined for a source at one time to the voxels in images at other times is difficult.

Software Implementations

Several groups have successfully coupled quantitative SPECT imaging with patient CT or magnetic resonance imaging data to provide patient-individualized 3D dose calculations, including the 3D-ID and 3D-RD codes [18, 19], the SIMDOS code from the University of Lund [20], the RTDS code from the City of Hope Medical Center [21], the RMDP code from the Royal Marsden Hospital [22], the DOSE3D code [23] and the PEREGRINE code [24]. One commercial product is available on the market [25], details about its technical basis are unclear at the moment.

Present and Future Clinical Utility of SPECT-Based Dosimetry

Several authors have provided evidence that the use of quantitative dose estimates can improve the quality of nuclear medical care provided to patients. Dorn et al. [26] revealed that targeting lesion doses of 100 Gy or more improved the level of complete responses (CRs), in a population of more than 120 subjects treated for differentiated thyroid cancer. Transient marrow toxicity was observed in some patients, but these reactions were explained by marrow dose calculations, with marrow mass adjusted for the estimated marrow mass of individual subjects. Jonsson and Mattsson [27] compared retrospectively the theoretical levels of activity that could have been given to nearly 200 patients administered radioiodine to treat Graves' disease if patient-specific dose calculations had been applied instead of a 'unit dosing' approach. They showed that "most of the patients were treated with an unnecessarily high activity, as a mean factor of 2.5 times too high and in individual patients up to eight times too high, leading to an unnecessary radiation exposure both for the patient, the family and the public." Kobe et al. [28] evaluated the success of treating Graves' disease in 571 subjects, targeting a dose to the thyroid of 250 Gy. They demonstrated significantly higher success rates of the first treatment, compared to a fixed activity administration approach. Stabin [1] addressed every major argument against performing patient-individualized dosimetry in nuclear medicine, including the difficulty and cost of making this extra effort, the lack of standardized dosimetric models, observation of clear dose/response relationships, and the need for objective evidence that the use of dosimetry will produce better clinical outcomes. A substantial amount of data from the literature and objective answers were given to address each of these issues.

As shown in this chapter, the science and tools are available for the routine use of SPECT/CT data in producing individualized dosimetric plans for patients receiving radiopharmaceuticals for therapy. The only element still lacking is the collective will of the nuclear medicine community to accept and implement these procedures. It is impossible to develop and improve our understanding of dose/response relationships with the use of these agents if no one is willing to calculate the doses. Currently, the impact that SPECT *has had* on clinical dosimetry is purely theoretical, relegated to the realm of research. The impact that it *should have* is much greater.

References

[1] Stabin MG, Siegel JA. Physical models and dose factors for use in internal dose assessment. *Health Phys.,* 2003; 85: 294-310.

[2] Stabin MG, Xu XG, Emmons MA, Segars WP, Shi C et al. RADAR reference adult, pediatric, and pregnant female phantom series for internal and external dosimetry. *J. Nucl. Med.,* 2012; 53: 1807-13.

[3] Pereira JM, Stabin MG, Lima FR, Guimaraes MI, Forrester JW. Image quantification for radiation dose calculations--limitations and uncertainties. *Health Phys.,* 2010; 99: 688-701.

[4] King M, Farncombe T. An overview of attenuation and scatter correction of planar and SPECT data for dosimetry studies. *Cancer Biother Radiopharm,* 2003; 18: 181-90.

[5] Ichihara T, Ogawa K, Motomura N, Kubo A, Hashimoto S. Compton scatter compensation using the triple-energy window method for single- and dual-isotope SPECT. *J. Nucl. Med.,* 1993; 34: 2216-21.

[6] Siegel JA, Thomas SR, Stubbs JB, Stabin MG, Hays MT et al. MIRD pamphlet no. 16: Techniques for quantitative radiopharmaceutical biodistribution data acquisition and analysis for use in human radiation dose estimates. *J. Nucl. Med.,* 1999; 40: 37S-61S.

[7] Stabin M. Fundamentals of Nuclear Medicine Dosimetry. New York, NY: Springer 2008.

[8] Stabin MG, Sparks RB, Crowe E. OLINDA/EXM: the second-generation personal computer software for internal dose assessment in nuclear medicine. *J. Nucl. Med.,* 2005; 46: 1023-7.

[9] Snyder W. Estimation of absorbed fraction of energy from photon sources in body organs. In: Cloutier R, Edwards C, Snyder W, eds. Medical Radionuclides: Radiation Dose and Effects: USAEC Division of Technical Information Extension 1970:33-49.

[10] Siegel JA, Stabin MG. Mass scaling of S values for blood-based estimation of red marrow absorbed dose: the quest for an appropriate method. *J. Nucl. Med.,* 2007; 48: 253-6.

[11] Stabin MG. Uncertainties in internal dose calculations for radiopharmaceuticals. *J. Nucl. Med.,* 2008; 49: 853-60.

[12] Yoriyaz H, Stabin MG, dos Santos A. Monte Carlo MCNP-4B-based absorbed dose distribution estimates for patient-specific dosimetry. *J. Nucl. Med.,* 2001; 42: 662-9.

[13] Dewaraja YK, Frey EC, Sgouros G, Brill AB, Roberson P et al. MIRD pamphlet No. 23: quantitative SPECT for patient-specific 3-dimensional dosimetry in internal radionuclide therapy. *J. Nucl. Med.,* 2012; 53: 1310-25.

[14] O'Donoghue JA. Implications of nonuniform tumor doses for radioimmunotherapy. *J. Nucl. Med.,* 1999; 40: 1337-41.

[15] Ljungberg M, Strand SE. A Monte Carlo program for the simulation of scintillation camera characteristics. *Computer methods and programs in biomedicine,* 1989; 29: 257-72.

[16] Ljungberg M, Frey E, Sjogreen K, Liu X, Dewaraja Y et al. 3D absorbed dose calculations based on SPECT: evaluation for 111-In/90-Y therapy using Monte Carlo simulations. *Cancer Biother Radiopharm.,* 2003; 18: 99-107.

[17] el Fakhri GN, Buvat I, Pelegrini M, Benali H, Almeida P et al. Respective roles of scatter, attenuation, depth-dependent collimator response and finite spatial resolution in cardiac single-photon emission tomography quantitation: a Monte Carlo study. *Eur. J. Nucl. Med.,* 1999; 26: 437-46.

[18] Kolbert KS, Sgouros G, Scott AM, Bronstein JE, Malane RA et al. Implementation and evaluation of patient-specific three-dimensional internal dosimetry. *J. Nucl. Med.,* 1997; 38: 301-8.

[19] Prideaux AR, Song H, Hobbs RF, He B, Frey EC et al. Three-dimensional radiobiologic dosimetry: application of radiobiologic modeling to patient-specific 3-dimensional imaging-based internal dosimetry. *J. Nucl. Med.,* 2007; 48: 1008-16.

[20] Dewaraja YK, Wilderman SJ, Ljungberg M, Koral KF, Zasadny K et al. Accurate dosimetry in 131I radionuclide therapy using patient-specific, 3-dimensional methods for SPECT reconstruction and absorbed dose calculation. *J. Nucl. Med.,* 2005; 46: 840-9.

[21] Liu A, Williams LE, Lopatin G, Yamauchi DM, Wong JY et al. A radionuclide therapy treatment planning and dose estimation system. *J. Nucl. Med.,* 1999; 40: 1151-3.

[22] Guy MJ, Flux GD, Papavasileiou P, Flower MA, Ott RJ. RMDP: a dedicated package for 131I SPECT quantification, registration and patient-specific dosimetry. *Cancer Biother Radiopharm.,* 2003; 18: 61-9.

[23] Clairand I, Ricard M, Gouriou J, Di Paola M, Aubert B. DOSE3D: EGS4 Monte Carlo code-based software for internal radionuclide dosimetry. *J. Nucl. Med.,* 1999; 40: 1517-23.

[24] Lehmann J, Hartmann Siantar C, Wessol DE, Wemple CA, Nigg D et al. Monte Carlo treatment planning for molecular targeted radiotherapy within the MINERVA system. *Phys. Med. Biol.,* 2005; 50: 947-58.

[25] Research Dosimetry Solution - STRATOS and STRATOS+. [cited; Available from: http://www.imalytics.philips.com/sites/philipsimalytics/products/dosimetry/dosimetry.p age.

[26] Dorn R, Kopp J, Vogt H, Heidenreich P, Carroll RG et al. Dosimetry-guided radioactive iodine treatment in patients with metastatic differentiated thyroid cancer: largest safe dose using a risk-adapted approach. *J. Nucl. Med.,,* 2003; 44: 451-6.

[27] Jonsson H, Mattsson S. Excess radiation absorbed doses from non-optimised radioiodine treatment of hyperthyroidism. *Radiat. Prot. Dosimetry,* 2004; 108: 107-14.

[28] Kobe C, Eschner W, Sudbrock F, Weber I, Marx K et al. Graves' disease and radioiodine therapy. Is success of ablation dependent on the achieved dose above 200 Gy? *Nuklearmedizin,* 2008; 47: 13-7.

In: SPECT
Editors: Hojjat Ahmadzadehfar and Elham Habibi

ISBN: 978-1-62808-344-6
© 2013 Nova Science Publishers, Inc.

Chapter III

SPECT in Primary Hyperparathyroidism

*Paloma García-Talavera San Miguel**

Department of Nuclear Medicine, University Hospital of Valladolid, Spain

Introduction

Hyperparathyroidism (HPT) is one of the most common endocrine disorders. Diagnosis is clinical and biochemical. Pre-operative imaging tests are not in themselves a means of diagnosis, but rather facilitate surgical intervention insofar as they assist surgeons in locating the pathological parathyroid gland [1].

Currently, non-invasive examinations are initially carried out, such as scintigraphy, ultrasonography (US), computed tomography (CT) or magnetic resonance imaging (MRI). The use of one particular technique or another mainly depends on its availability, cost and the physician's experience. Although an increasing number of surgeons support its routine use before an initial surgical intervention, there remains an element of controversy. Very often the decision is related to the type of operation to be carried out. Some surgeons favor systematic bilateral neck exploration and consequently consider pre-operative imaging tests unnecessary. Others opt for a more selective exploration requiring the exact localization of the lesion prior to surgery [2]. This type of intervention has the advantages of shortening the surgery time and reducing morbidity. In spite of this, some centers [3] advocate the use of pre-operative localization, above all scintigraphy with ^{99m}Tc-metoxiisobutilisonitrile (Tc-MIBI), even in cases of bilateral surgery, with a view to localizing the adenoma, reducing the length of the intervention and minimizing surgical trauma.

Certain situations exist in which there is general agreement on the need to perform pre-surgical localization, for instance, on patients undergoing further intervention (either as a result of persistent or recurrent illness, or because of previous neck surgery for another reason), patients with a high surgical risk (severe hypercalcemia, cardiopathy, etc.) or those

---

* Department of Nuclear Medicine, University Hospital of Valladolid, Avd. Ramón y Cajal, 3, 47003 [Valladolid], Spain. Email: palomagtalavera@gmail.com.

with characteristics hindering intervention (thyroid pathology, columnar disorders, etc.) [4, 5].

Despite the perfecting of imaging techniques in the last few years, there are certain aspects of parathyroid pathology that make localization difficult and therefore sometimes result in surgical failure. Among such aspects are the occasionally small sizes of pathological glands: parathyroid glands under 5 mm and weighing less than 500 mg are not easy to identify. Other aspects include the possible existence of multi-glandular disease (showing low sensitivity in imaging tests), the ectopic condition of the hyper-functioning tissue, and associated thyroid nodule pathology, which can hinder differentiation between diseased parathyroid glands and thyroid nodules [2].

1.1. Anatomy and Physiology of Parathyroid Glands

There are four parathyroid glands, 5×3×3 mm in size, located in the posterior-lateral capsule of the thyroid gland; however, they may be found inside the thyroid or elsewhere ectopically. On occasion the number of parathyroid glands may vary from 3 to 8. The weight of a parathyroid gland is usually less than 30 mg, with a maximum of 70 mg [6, 7].

The most important parathyroid gland cells are the chief cells, responsible for synthesizing and secreting parathyroid hormone (PTH). Other types of cells include oxyphils, which do not secrete PTH under normal conditions and are rich in mitochondria, and clear cells, which are derived from the chief cells and are capable of secreting PTH.

PTH is a hypercalcemic hormone that acts via cyclic AMP. It stimulates osseous reabsorption in bones, liberating calcium and phosphorous, by activating osteoclastic osteolysis. In the kidney it activates the reabsorption of calcium and inhibits that of phosphorous in the renal tubules. It also stimulates the renal enzyme that hydroxylates 25-hydroxycholecalciferol (25-OH-D) on carbon 1, transforming it into 1-25-dihydroxy-cholecalciferol (1-25 $(OH)_2$-D). This active metabolite of vitamin D promotes intestinal absorption of calcium and phosphorous. Hypercalcemia and hypocalcemia inhibit and stimulate PTH secretion, respectively. In addition, PTH secretion is halted by 1-25 $(OH)_2$-D. [8].

1.2. Physiopathology of the Primary Hyperparathyroid Glands

Primary hyperparathyroidism (PHPT) represents the third most common endocrine disorder (an incidence of 1/500–1000), after thyroid diseases and diabetes mellitus, and is 2–3 times more frequent in women than men. Together with a tumoral osteopathy, PHPT is the most common cause of hypercalcemia [7, 9].

PHPT is characterized by uncontrolled hyper-secretion of PTH by the parathyroid glands, which persists despite the presence of hypercalcemia. This hyper-secretion of PTH may be produced by an adenoma (90%), a double adenoma (4%), a hyperplasia of multiple glands (6%), or by a carcinoma (<1%) [10].

A parathyroid adenoma is a benign neoplasia composed of chief and/or mixed cells. It usually appears during the decades of middle age. Adenomas vary in size, normally weighing between 0.5–5.0 g; however, they may occasionally weigh 10–100 g [7, 9].

The first symptoms of a PHPT are largely non-specific, and half of patients are asymptomatic at the time of diagnosis. Hypercalcemia is most commonly detected when a laboratory study is carried out. Frequent PHPT complications are nephro- or urolithiasis, which are encountered in ¾ of patients during diagnosis. Diagnosis is fundamentally biochemical, by means of PTH determinations in plasma, hypercalcemia, hypophosphatemia, calciuria, and phosphaturia [7, 9].

1.3. PHPT Surgery

Surgery is the only curative treatment for PHPT. Patients who have overt signs and symptoms of HPT benefit from parathyroidectomy in almost all cases [11]. The indications for surgery in asymptomatic patients with HPT are listed in Table 3.1 [11-15].

The traditional approach is a bilateral neck exploration. Although using this approach is becoming less frequent, it is compulsory when there is a suspicion of multiglandular disease (MGD). In the case of a minimally invasive surgery, the patient should be evaluated by an imaging test for precise localization of the pathological gland/s. In addition, in order to ensure success of the surgery, there are other complementary tools, such as the gammaprobe or the intraoperative intact PTH (iPTH) determination [16, 17].

2. Imaging Tests

2.1. Planar Scintigraphy

2.1.1. ^{201}Tl-Chloride and ^{99m}Tc-Pertechnetate Subtraction

The generalized use of scintigraphy techniques with radionuclides in HPT began with using ^{201}Tl-chloride and ^{99m}Tc-pertechnetate (^{99m}TcO$_4$) subtraction. Thallium is a potassium analogue. It reaches tissues proportional to the blood flow and is actively taken up by cells via Na-K ATPase pumps into the cytoplasm.

Since the first studies by Ferlin et al. [18], which showed a sensitivity of 92% in the detection of adenomas, many authors have employed this method, with quite variable results (62%–92%) [18-20]. Gimlette et al. [21] obtained a sensitivity of 64% in the case of glands and 73% in the case of patients, concluding that the technique is useful despite its sensitivity being limited by the size of the glands, particularly those under 0.5 grams.

The main reason for false positive results is concomitant thyroid pathology. Cold thyroid nodules in ^{99m}TcO$_4$ scintigraphy with ^{201}Tl uptake can lead to a misidentification of pathological parathyroid glands.

Scintigraphy with ^{201}Tl also has certain pitfalls, since ^{201}Tl is a radioisotope emitting energy predominantly in the form of 80 keV X-rays, which are easily absorbed by super-imposed tissues; this makes it difficult to identify ectopic adenomas localized in the mediastinum. Due to the long physical half-life of ^{201}Tl (73 hours), in order to keep radiation exposure within permissible levels the amount of radioisotope allowed is low (74 MBq), which impairs the quality of the image and prolongs acquisition time, making the study uncomfortable for patients. Moreover, ^{201}Tl is taken up by both the normal thyroid and the hyper-functioning parathyroid tissue and therefore concomitant scintigraphy with ^{123}I or [99m]TcO$_4$ must be performed. Digital subtraction of the thyroid image makes it possible to detect the pathological parathyroid tissue.

2.1.2. Scintigraphy with ^{99m}Tc-MIBI

Tc-MIBI was initially employed as an agent for myocardial perfusion. It is a lipophilic cationic complex that passively traverses the cellular membrane and, due to electrical attraction from the negative potential of the mitochondrial membrane, enters this organelle [22, 23].

Coakley et al. [24] suggested the clinical use of Tc-MIBI in parathyroid scintigraphy, obtaining very favorable results. The exact mechanism of Tc-MIBI uptake in the context of parathyroid lesions is unknown. However, it is likely that there are various factors that intervene concomitantly. Some of these factors are the biochemical properties of Tc-MIBI, the degree of local vascularization, trans-capillary exchange, interstitial transport and the negative intra-cellular charge across the cellular and mitochondrial membranes [4].

Table 3.1. Indications for PHPT surgery [11-15]

Serum calcium: 1 mg/dl above normal
24 hour urine calcium > 400 mg (used by some physicians but not indicated in the 2008 guidelines)
Creatinine clearance reduced to 60 ml/min
Bone density: T-score ≤ -2.5 at any site (Lumbar spine, total hip, femoral neck, or 33% radius) and/or previous fracture fragility
Age < 50 years
Patients for whom medical surveillance was either not desirable or not possible
Nephrolithiasis
Osteitis fibrosa cystic
Neuromuscular symptoms: documented proximal weakness, athrophy, hyper-reflexia, and gait disturbance
History of an episode of life threatening hypercalcemia

Planar Scintigraphy with Tc-MIBI has limited spatial resolution and some glands may be too small to be detected [23, 25-28]. Nevertheless, there are tiny adenomas that may be seen, whilst other large ones may not. It depends on the capacity of the pathological gland to accumulate the radiotracer, which may be dependent on the number of oxyphil cells [22, 23, 29], in spite of the fact that this has not been confirmed by other authors [30]. In addition, it has been known that p-glycoprotein, a membrane protein encoded by the multi-drug resistance (MDR) gene, has an effect on the uptake and extraction of Tc-MIBI from cells, which would explain certain false negatives in delayed images, as elevated expression of P-glycoprotein increases the ratio of parathyroid washout [25, 31, 32].

Further reasons for unsuccessful detection of an adenoma are interference with surrounding structures (mediastinal structures or a multi-nodular thyroid) [33] and the presence of cystic or necrotic areas inside the gland [34, 35]. There is a positive correlation between the values of calcium [28] as well as pre-surgical iPTH and the sensitivity of scintigraphy [24, 28, 36, 37].

Unlike ^{201}Tl, MIBI is labeled with ^{99m}Tc, a radionuclide with a short physical half-life (6 hours) and energy of 140 keV, which allows a high dose to be administered without subjecting the patient to high doses of radiation. In this way it is possible to obtain images with better quality and less absorption by other tissues, thereby facilitating detection of ectopic adenomas. As with ^{201}Tl, Tc-MIBI is taken up by the hyper-functioning parathyroid as well as by normal thyroid tissue. However, unlike with ^{201}Tl, there is a different washout rate between the two glands; washout is more rapid in the thyroid and as a consequence performing delayed imaging is of importance.

Coakley et al. [24] reported sensitivities of 92 % and 97.5 % for ^{201}Tl and Tc-MIBI, respectively, for localizing parathyroid adenomas. In this study, sensitivity dropped to 53.3% in the case of hyperplastic lesions.

Taillefer et al. [38] studied the behavior of Tc-MIBI as a single radiopharmaceutical agent compared to ^{201}Tl/^{99m}TcO$_4$ and found a sensitivity of 90% for Tc-MIBI against 75% for ^{201}Tl/^{99m}TcO$_4$.

O'Doherty et al. [39] reported the results of Tc-MIBI/^{123}I subtraction scintigraphy versus the ^{201}Tl/^{99m}TcO$_4$ subtraction technique in a series of 57 patients with HPT. The sensitivity was 98% versus 90% in patients with adenoma, and 55% versus 47.5% in patients with glandular hyperplasia. The greater effectiveness of Tc-MIBI was due to its higher lesion to background ratio and more favorable physical characteristics.

2.1.2.1. Dual-phase Technique

The "dual-phase" scintigraphy protocol consists of using Tc-MIBI as a single radiotracer. After application of approximately 740 MBq Tc-MIBI, two planar scintigraphies should be obtained after 10 minutes (early scan) and 2–3 hours (late scan). The parathyroid adenoma can be diagnosed based on the different "washout" times of the radiotracer in the thyroid and parathyroid glands. Generally, pathological parathyroid tissue is defined as a focal accumulation of the tracer in the thyroid region, surrounding areas or the mediastinum, which persists or increases in the delayed image. This is unlike the uptake in normal thyroid tissue, which decreases over time (washout or differential washout).

Although, as mentioned previously, there is disagreement in terms of performing routine pre-operative localization tests, using sequential scintigraphy with Tc-MIBI is completely justified in patients with persistent or recurrent PHPT, in those with suspected ectopic or mediastinal adenoma, and in patients having previously undergone neck surgery.

Sensitivity prior to the first surgical experience is around 82% (78–100%) for the detection of adenomas and between 44% and 78% in the case of MGD. In patients undergoing further surgery for persisting PHPT, there is 70–86% sensitivity, with 90–95% specificity for the detection of ectopic lesions [4].

Among patients with PHPT, the most common source of false positive results is the co-existence of benign thyroid disease. In a dual-phase study, solitary adenomas and hyper-functioning thyroid nodules, as well as multi-nodular goiter, very often take up and retain Tc-MIBI, resulting in images that may be very similar to parathyroid adenoma. This is an important issue because in over a third of PHPT cases a benign thyroid disease is also present. To avoid such misinterpretations, performing a conventional thyroid scintigraphy and US prior to interpreting a parathyroid scintigraphy is of importance. Other less frequent causes of false positives may be brown tumors of hyperparathyroidism, thymoma, carcinoid tumor, thyroid carcinoma, lymphoma and other causes of lymphoadenopathy (metastatic disease, inflammation and even sarcoidosis) [31, 40].

False negative results can be due to the presence of necrotic or cystic tissue associated with the parathyroid lesion, the small size of a lesion (less than 1 cm or 500 mg) or low metabolic activity in the parathyroid lesion [23, 31].

Rapid tracer washout from parathyroid adenomas due to lack of oxyphilic cells has been reported as an important issue for false negative results [41]. Therefore, it is not always possible to find the typical pattern of a visible focus of activity with delayed washout. Rapid tracer washout of parathyroid glands being common ones and, in addition, described in up to 39% of adenomas [42].

2.1.2.2. ^{99m}Tc-MIBI and ^{99m}Tc-Pertechnetate or ^{123}I-Iodide Subtraction Technique

In order to get around these problems, different dual radiotracer subtraction techniques were examined. Subtraction techniques classically used ^{123}I, but subtraction with ^{99m}TcO$_4$ is favored because ^{123}I has a higher cost, is less available and delivers about a 3-fold higher radiation dose.

The principal limitation of this method is image co-registration. To minimize this problem Rubello et al. [43] recommended the following steps:

1) 150 MBq technetium injection; wait 20 minutes.
2) Oral administration of 400 mg of potassium perchlorate (KClO$_4$) in order to force ^{99m}TcO$_4$ to exit the thyroid gland.
3) Neck immobilization;
4) Acquisition of a 5-minute technetium thyroid scan;
5) Subsequent administration, beneath the gamma camera and without changing the position of the patient, of 500 MBq of Tc-MIBI;
6) Acquisition of a sequence of seven MIBI images, each lasting 5 minutes; during the protocol and following initial imaging, the exit of ^{99m}TcO$_4$ from the thyroid gland can be observed and, at the same time, a constant increase in activity in the parathyroid adenoma.
7) Processing: image realignment when necessary, background subtraction, normalization of MIBI images to the maximum pixel count of the technetium image, and subtraction of the technetium image from the MIBI images.

These authors showed that KClO$_4$ can cause a rapid and nearly complete technetium washout from the thyroid. Furthermore, the KClO$_4$ effect becomes evident only 10 minutes after its oral administration; this period is sufficient to position the patient under the gamma camera and obtain a technetium thyroid image before Tc-MIBI injection.

Another protocol has been described by Hindiè et al. [44] using dual-tracer Tc-MIBI/^{123}I scintigraphy, with 94% sensitivity. They resolved the difficulties of motion artifacts and prolonged immobilization, employing simultaneous acquisition of the two isotopes by a non-super-imposable double window rather than successive images.

Its main advantage is minimizing false positive results due to thyroid nodules, since thyroid scintigraphy allows for the evaluation of hyperactive nodules that could otherwise be equivocally interpreted as a parathyroid adenoma. The technique of Rubello et al. is recommended among populations with a high prevalence of thyroid nodule pathology, together with US evaluation [43].

2.1.2.3. Scintigraphy with ^{99m}Tc-MIBI Using a Pinhole Collimator

Imaging with a pinhole collimator may enhance the detection of diseased parathyroid glands. Arverschoug et al. [45] demonstrated that adding images with a pinhole collimator to dual-phase parathyroid scintigraphy increased the sensitivity from 54% to 88%, diminishing the number of equivocal localizations with regard to the sides, albeit with a loss of specificity from 89% to 77%. In another study [46] the same authors, adding oblique images with a pinhole at an early stage, obtained an enhanced level of inter-observer concordance and a greater number of correct localizations, in terms of the sides, in patients with rapid washout of Tc-MIBI.

The benefit of viewing oblique images at an early stage has been confirmed by Ho Son et al. [47], raising the sensitivity to 88%. Its routine use in both early and delayed scintigraphies represents a clear advantage over previous parallel-hole collimator projection, as it provides information concerning the depth of the adenoma, which is very useful when surgery is undertaken.

Yoon et al. [48] described the usefulness of pinhole images in evaluating foci with high uptake completely separated from the inferior thyroid pole, which in all probability indicate an intra-thymus adenoma.

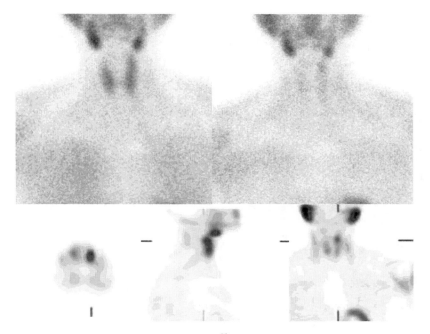

Figure 3.1. Top: Double phase planar scintigraphy with ^{99m}Tc-MIBI. In the delayed phase (top right) there is a doubtful focus of very mild increased uptake in the localization of the left upper pole of the thyroid gland. Bottom: Axial, sagital and coronal slices of an early SPECT acquisition: A focus of increased uptake is confirmed in the left upper pole of the thyroid gland, compatible with a solitary adenoma with a rapid washout.

2.1.3. Scintigraphy with ^{99m}Tc-Tetrofosmin

Parathyroid scintigraphy is also possible with ^{99m}Tc-tetrofosmin (555–740 MBq). Like MIBI, tetrofosmin images are taken at 15 and 120 minutes. However, tetrofosmin washes out more slowly from thyroid tissue than Tc-MIBI [49, 50]. Thus, it necessarily requires an imaging subtraction protocol. Therefore there is no advantage over Tc-MIBI, especially for perioperative studies [1, 49].

Arbab et al. [51] showed that only a small fraction of ^{99m}Tc-tetrofosmin accumulates inside mitochondria, while most Tc-MIBI accumulates inside the mitochondria. This difference in accumulation sites might explain differences in washout kinetics.

2.2. SPECT and SPECT-CT

SPECT and SPECT-CT have proven to be useful and to provide more accurate anatomical localization, above all in the case of ectopic lesions. In particular, in the mediastinum a more precise localization may help to select the most suitable surgical procedure. It has also been described how useful it is to review a maximum-intensity projection because it may be helpful in reviewing images with referring physicians, as it permits a rapid estimation of the anterior or posterior situation of both neck and mediastinum lesions [52].

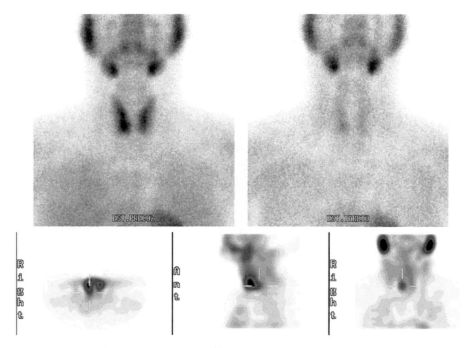

Figure 3.2. Top: Double phase scintigraphy with ^{99m}Tc-MIBI. In the delayed phase there is a doubtful focus of very mild increased uptake in the localization of the right lower pole of the thyroid gland. Bottom: In the early tomographic images (axial, sagital and coronal slices) there is an asymmetric bulging of the thyroid contour in the posterior surface of the right lower pole, compatible with a solitary adenoma with a rapid washout.

2.2.1. ^{99m}Tc-MIBI SPECT

2.2.1.1. Usefulness of the SPECT Technique

The most common reasons for persisting PHPT following surgical intervention are: non-identification of an adenoma (principally due to an ectopic parathyroid), the presence of an unexpected MGD or insufficient extent of surgery in the case of a known MGD. Using SPECT can enhance the detection of pathological parathyroid glands [1, 53].

SPECT compared to planar imaging enhances contrast and resolution, increases sensitivity in certain cases, and offers a better presurgical anatomical localization [31, 54-56].

Therefore, the routine use of SPECT in conjunction with planar imaging has been supported [53]. Using multiplicative iterative SPECT reconstruction (MISR) rather than filtered back projection (FBP) is recommended, since with the former a clear improvement in image quality can be achieved. By using planar Tc-MIBI scans, correct localization of the side of the adenoma was possible in 81% of cases. Sensitivity increased to 94% using SPECT with FBP, while with MISR it rose still further, to 97%. In patients with adenomas weighing less than 500 mg, the sensitivity of planar imaging was 58%; however, SPECT showed a sensitivity of 81% with FBP and 88% with MISR [53].

In another study by this group, they reported a sensitivity of up to 95 % for detection of small adenomas ($\leq$ 1g) with SPECT versus 87% with planar scintigraphy [57]. Likewise, other authors [23, 58] have acknowledged higher levels of sensitivity with SPECT (95–96%) when comparing it with planar scintigraphy (68-79%). In addition, Slater et al. [59] advocated the use of SPECT as a pre-operative protocol in all patients.

Additional values of SPECT are in confirming a doubtful diagnosis [60] (Figure 3.1), helping to better localize adenomas [60, 61] or even changing the diagnosis [61]. In a recently published review, Prats et al. [62] recommended that SPECT should be included in the imaging protocol in all patients, particularly in the following circumstances: ectopic adenomas, associated thyroid pathology, pre-surgical studies (especially if radioguided surgery is planned), patients having previously undergone neck surgery, persistent or recurrent hyperparathyroidism, or in explorations with normal static images.

Regarding its usefulness in patients with concomitant thyroid disease, SPECT could visualize parathyroid glands situated behind a thyroid lesion that were not differentiated with planar imaging [31, 36, 55, 59, 60]. Loberboym et al. [63] give support to the employment of pre-operative SPECT for parathyroid adenomas in patients with multinodular goiter when selecting those suitable for surgery and may also be a source of important information concerning thyroid nodules which might be malignant.

Additionally, using SPECT is recommended prior to minimally invasive HPTP surgery. The parathyroid to background index should be calculated so as to predict measures with the gamma detector probe. Calculation of this index is more accurate when using SPECT than by planar scintigraphy, as radiation may be partially attenuated by the depth of the adenoma or because of its position behind the sternum [64]. In addition, a negative SPECT is associated with an increased risk of surgery failure [65].

SPECT can also improve the detection of double adenomas [55]; however, like planar scintigraphy, SPECT also suffers from false negative results in patients with small-sized hyperplasias [66, 67]. Regarding localization, SPECT with Tc-MIBI displayed less sensitivity in identifying pathological glands in superior neck quadrants than in inferior quadrants.

Pathological parathyroid glands over 1.5 cm in diameter tended to be more accurately localized by SPECT than those under 1.5 cm in diameter [67].

2.2.1.2. Type of Protocol

In dual-phase scintigraphy the time of SPECT imaging is controversial. Some recommend performing SPECT after a delayed scan [57, 67] and even at a very late stage in certain cases [68]; however, most centers perform SPECT after an early scan [5, 36, 54, 55, 61] because at this time better localization of diseased parathyroid glands regarding thyroid gland situation is possible. The most commonly accepted reason for performing SPECT at an early stage is the existence of a rapid tracer washout, which is the case in up to 40% of adenomas [54, 55, 61, 69].

Pérez-Monte et al. [70] compared the results of early SPECT (15–30 minutes) with those of late SPECT (2–4 hours) in a series of 47 patients with HPT; early SPECT sensitivity was 91% versus 74% in the case of late SPECT.

Certain authors have performed early and late SPECT subtraction in small series of patients with secondary HPT, with 90.9% sensitivity and 92.8% accuracy [71]. In addition, studies have been undertaken whereby SPECT with ^{123}I and with ^{99m}Tc-MIBI are subtracted, yet here sensitivity (71%) and specificity (48%) are low [72].

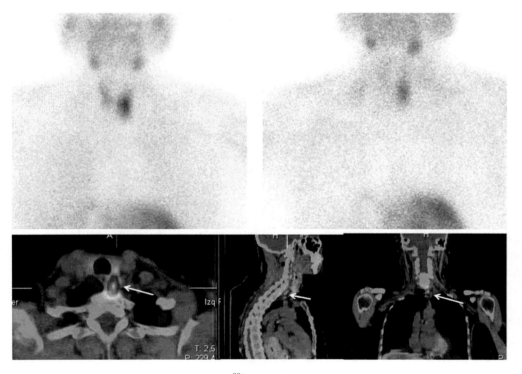

Figure 3.3. Top: Double phase scintigraphy with ^{99m}Tc-MIBI. In both images there is a focus of increased uptake in the localization of the left lower pole of the thyroid gland. Bottom: SPECT-CT fusion (axial, sagital and coronal slices). The focus of increased uptake is localized in the left paraesophageal space. It corresponds to a solitary ectopic adenoma.

2.2.1.3. Interpreting the Images

Maximum-intensity projection images are particularly useful for initially detecting parathyroid uptake or asymmetric thyroid contours which may be secondary to a parathyroid adenoma [73]. The scintigraphy patterns observed in early-phase SPECT images depend on radiotracer uptake by the parathyroid and thyroid glands and their relative anatomical positions. Anatomically, the parathyroid gland may either be contiguous with or separate from the thyroid gland. In the early phase an adenoma that is separated from the thyroid may be distinguished as a focus of radiotracer accumulation.

A parathyroid adenoma contiguous to the thyroid gland can be detected in the early phase only if its own uptake is greater than that of the thyroid, or if it produces an asymmetric bulging of the thyroid contour, typically in the inferior pole or on the posterior surface [73, 74] (Figure 3.2).

On early phase images, intrathyroidal parathyroid adenomas may accumulate more radiotracer than the thyroid gland, and in such cases might be detected as an asymmetric uptake focused inside the thyroid [74]. Delayed washout images may be helpful when the proximity of the adenoma to the thyroid gland makes differentiation between the two structures difficult.

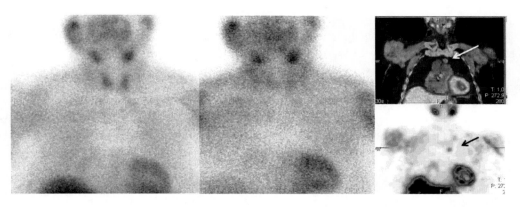

Figure 3.4. Left and middle: Double phase planar scintigraphy with ^{99m}Tc-MIBI showing no evidence of pathological parathyroid glands. Right: Coronal slices of a SPECT and SPECT-CT acquisition. In the SPECT image a focus of increased uptake is visualized in the mediastinum. In the SPECT-CT image it is localized in the superior mediastinum, in the prevascular space.

2.2.2. SPECT with a Pinhole Collimator

Some favor the use of SPECT with a pinhole collimator, complementing planar images and ultrasonography [75]. SPECT with a pinhole collimator enhances the sensitivity of parallel-hole SPECT, especially in small and none-too-active parathyroid adenomas [66].

Pinhole collimator SPECT has a higher spatial resolution compared with parallel collimation, therefore irregularities in dystrophic thyroid lobes and thyroid nodules that could be falsely interpreted as parathyroid lesions, especially in case of heterogeneous and faint thyroid uptake, were easily detected due to the better definition of thyroid contours. However, SPECT with a pinhole may result in false negative results in ectopic localization as the adenoma is not found within the field of view. It is helpful to combine it with US or thyroid scintigraphy in order to minimize this error.

2.2.3. SPECT-CT

SPECT-CT contributes to the localization of parathyroid adenomas by providing an anatomical context to scintigraphic images and correcting for attenuation effects. Initially, SPECT and CT studies were acquired independently [56] and later fused together; however, a successful fusion of SPECT and CT is not always possible because of the different positioning of the patients. This is not the case when using hybrid SPECT-CT cameras, offering the advantage of acquiring SPECT and CT images sequentially, with the patient in the same position and on the same scanning bed. There is some debate concerning whether SPECT-CT constitutes an advantage over other scintigraphy techniques, most fundamentally SPECT, in terms of both sensitivity and pre-surgical localization.

Imaging with SPECT-CT may provide an accurate localization of supernumerary diseased glands, in ectopic conditions (Figure 3.3), in cases of persistent or recurrent HPT, or previous neck surgery [56, 62, 76-79]. In comparison with SPECT, SPECT-CT offers anatomical information that permits localization of the adenoma and shows its relationship with nearby structures. Moreover, SPECT-CT can reduce the morbidity, radiation exposure, time and cost of evaluation by avoiding multiple diagnostic explorations and making possible a minimally invasive surgery [77]. SPECT-CT would be recommended in the following situations: ectopic adenomas, patients undergoing a neck intervention and pre-surgical analyses (especially in radioguided surgery) [62].

SPECT-CT of the neck region facilitates the planning of the surgery in cases in which the neck is distorted following exploration or when the thyroid gland is not visualized after an intervention [78]. Moreover, SPECT-CT had a positive impact on the localization of all ectopic adenomas (28%) and, in addition, is useful in surgery management, above all in adenomas with atypical localization, such as in the retro-tracheal and retro-esophageal spaces, avoiding sternotomy in the case of an ectopic adenoma situated in the superior mediastinum. Using SPECT-CT makes a reduction in the extent and length of surgery possible [78]. Moreover, in the case of planning minimally invasive parathyroidectomy (MIP), it increases the confidence and precision in localization of adenomas (Figure 3.4).

SPECT-CT can reduce the false positive results of planar scintigraphy, for instance, in the case of brown fat tissue [81, 82] or costal uptake due to a costal brown tumor [83]. This benefit has also been reported by Neuman et al. [84]. They demonstrated the superiority of SPECT-CT versus ^{99m}Tc-MIBI/^{123}I SPECT subtraction in localizing pathological parathyroid glands. SPECT-CT has significantly better specificity versus SPECT (96% vs. 48%, respectively) with a similar level of sensitivity (71% for SPECT and 70% for SPECT-CT).

As with SPECT, there is a lack of consensus on the imaging timing with SPECT-CT. Lavely et al. [85] reported that performing an early SPECT-CT acquisition combined with any delayed method (SPECT-CT, SPECT or planar images) was statistically superior to single- or dual-phase planar imaging, or to dual-phase SPECT. In their study, for any of the three modalities (planar imaging, SPECT or SPECT-CT), dual-phase was better than single-phase. In contrast, Ciappuccini et al. [28] performed a planar scintigraphy with dual-phase ^{99m}Tc-MIBI and delayed SPECT-CT. This protocol had the capacity to identify a parathyroid adenoma in approximately two-thirds of patients and allowed the surgeon to plan an appropriate intervention. In this study they acquired a sensitivity of 92% and a specificity of 83%.

SPECT-CT is more precise than SPECT and planar imaging for pre-operative identification of parathyroid lesions in patients with nodular thyroid disease [86], with a sensitivity and specificity of about 77.6% and 96.8%, respectively, versus 67.3% and 87.1% for SPECT.

The combined use of SPECT and MR is less common, but as with the combination of SPECT and CT it provides a better localization of scintigraphic foci and facilitates the evaluation of non-conclusive MR findings [87].

2.3. Comparison of Different Scintigraphic Techniques

Table 3.2 summarizes a list of proposed protocols for the different scintigraphic techniques. The dual-phase method has fundamental benefits in terms of the efficiency and simplicity of the protocol. The dual-radiotracer method has a better diagnostic value; however, it is complicated to use. Therefore, in regions where goiter is not endemic, the dual-phase method is the most recommended. In other regions a subtraction technique should be carried out or the method should be accompanied by US or thyroid scintigraphy [88].

Hindiè et al. [44] compared the dual-phase and Tc-MIBI/^{123}I subtraction methods, acquiring sensitivity levels of 79% and 94% and rates of false positives of 10% and 3%, respectively. In this series the subtraction techniques were more rapid and sensitive than those relying on the dual phase method. Using the dual-radiotracer method has been recommended except in the following circumstances: patients in whom the thyroid may not be seen on account of previous surgery, thyroiditis, the administering of iodinated contrast agent or thyroxin [5, 89, 90].

Caveny et al. [90] compared Tc-MIBI dual-phase single tracer (pinhole and parallel-hole collimator image), Tc-MIBI/^{123}I dual-tracer single phase, and ^{99m}Tc-MIBI/^{123}I dual-tracer dual-phase, obtaining successful localization rates of 66%, 94% and 90%, respectively. They concluded that dual-tracer scintigraphy is considerably better than dual phase (p< 0.01) and preferred the dual-tracer, single-phase with Tc-MIBI/^{123}I technique, as the additional delayed phase did not produce any statistically significant differences. Using dual-tracer scintigraphy has been favored by EANM guidelines [5], arguing that it is more sensitive for MGD and it can visualize thyroid nodules which can be extirpated in initial surgery.

Regarding pinhole images, Tomas et al. [91] performed a dual-phase Tc-MIBI scintigraphy and compared acquisition with a pinhole collimator and a parallel-hole collimator; they obtained better sensitivity with the first, 89% vs. 56% (p=0.0003), and similar specificities, 93% vs. 96% (p=0.29), respectively. The limitation of pinhole collimators is their small field of view. Ho Son et al. (92) have compared anterior and oblique parathyroid images with pinhole and an anterior thyroid image with pinhole, with that of early SPECT and dual-phase planar scintigraphy, acquiring better sensitivity in the first combination.

Öksüz et al. [29] made a comparative study of the accuracy of dual-phase planar scintigraphy with Tc-MIBI SPECT and SPECT-CT. In this study SPECT was superior to planar imaging. SPECT-CT had exactly the same sensitivity as SPECT, but the latter provides additional topographical information that was particularly helpful in localizing ectopic adenomas.

Chen et al. [93] assert that delayed imaging, digital subtraction and SPECT are unnecessary as these methods contribute merely marginal benefits to a visual comparison of early Tc-MIBI with ^{99m}TcO$_4$ images. Prats et al. [62] suggested thyroid scintigraphy may be of use as a complement to parathyroid scintigraphy, especially in patients with thyroid nodules, slow washout of thyroid activity, an asymmetric thyroid, following neck surgery and prior to radio-guided surgery.

Table 3.2. Modified proposed protocol of the SNM guideline [52]

	Dual-phase protocol	Dual radiotracer protocol
Dosage and route of administration	Tc-MIBI: 740-1110 MBq e.v.	$^{99m}TcO_4$: 74-370 MBq e.v. or ^{123}I: 12 MBq ^{99m}Tc-MIBI: 740-1110 MBq e.v.
Time to imaging	Planar: Early 10-30 minutes Delayed 1.5-2.5 hours SPECT: variable	Option 1: $^{99m}TcO_4$: 30 min + Tc-MIBI: 10 min Option 2: ^{123}I: 4h +Tc-MIBI: 10 min
Time of imaging	Planar: 10 minutes SPECT: 25 minutes	10 minutes
Planar acquisition protocol	Anterior projection images Right or left oblique images (optional) Matrix 256x256 Pinhole or LEHR parallel-hole collimator	Anterior projection images Right or left oblique images (optional) Matrix 256x256 Pinhole or LEHR parallel-hole collimator
SPECT-CT acquisition protocol	**SPECT:** LEHR 20% energy window centered at 140KeV 360° arc Body- contoured elliptic orbit Step and shoot protocol 120 steps, 15-25 s/step Matrix 128x128 **CT:** 100-200 mAs 120 KVp (ranging from 100-140KVp)	
Reconstruction	**SPECT**: 2-dimensional ordered-subset expectation maximization iterative technique (e.g.10 subsets and 2 iterations). A 3-dimensional post-processing filter (e.g. Hanning post-processing filter with a cut-off frequency of 0.85 cycles/cm).	

In Table 3.3 the results of planar scintigraphy versus SPECT or SPECT-CT in diagnosing PHPT are summarized. It is believed that the optimum solution is to combine different scintigraphic techniques in order to enhance localization of diseased parathyroid glands [66, 94]. Koranda et al. share this view [95]. They propose the addition of early SPECT, with a protocol similar to that of Rubello et al. [43], employing, first of all, scintigraphy of the thyroid, followed by early phase parathyroid planar scintigraphy, early SPECT, and finally, delayed phase parathyroid planar scintigraphy. Obviously, this would imply longer exploration time under the gamma camera.

2.4. Other Imaging Modalities

2.4.1. Ultrasonography

The sensitivity of US is between 51% to 80% in patients without previous neck surgery. False negative results are more commonly encountered in small-sized glands, ectopic lesions, intrathyroidal localization and in the presence of co-existing thyroid disease [34, 66]. False positive results are due to posterior exophytic thyroid nodules and neck adenopathies.

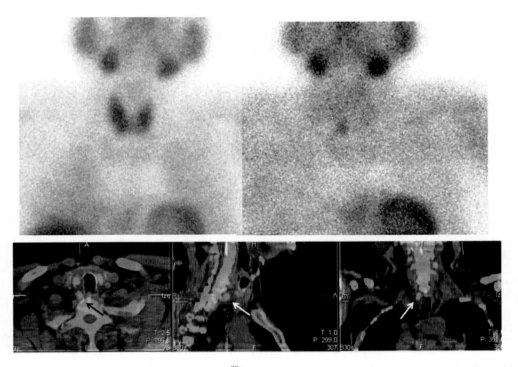

Figure 3.5. Top: Double phase scintigraphy with ^{99m}Tc-MIBI. In the delayed planar image there is a focus of increased uptake in the position of the right lower pole of the thyroid gland. Bottom: SPECT-CT fusion images (axial, sagital and coronal slices). The focus of increased uptake, in the right paraesophageal localization, corresponds to a solitary ectopic adenoma.

2.4.2. CT and MRI

Both CT and MRI are helpful for diagnosis. When US and ^{99m}Tc-MIBI scintigraphy either do not detect an adenoma or do not concur, CT may provide useful pre-operative localization before surgery for hyperparathyroidism, particularly in patients with recurrent or persistent disease [96]. Furthermore, MRI and CT are indicated in the pre-operative stage of localizing ectopic parathyroids detected by scintigraphy.

CT is preferable to US for localizing retro-esophageal, retro-tracheal and mediastinal parathyroid lesions. It allows a combined puncture-biopsy procedure. Its sensitivity for localizing anomalous parathyroidal tissue has varied in different series from 43% to 92%, and its sensitivity is greater in initial surgery than in re-interventions [89, 96, 97].

For MRI, sensitivity varies from 40% to 93%, and is greater in the first intervention and less in further surgery and hyperplasias. MRI allows excellent assessment of the mediastinum and the only source of error is the existence of adenopathies or multiple ectopic lesions [40].

Table 3.3. Sensitivity of planar scintigraphy versus SPECT or SPECT-CT in diagnosis of HPT

Authors	# Cases	Planar scintigraphy		SPECT or SPECT-CT	
		Technique	Results	Technique	Results
Ansquer [60]	49 pt 49 gs	MIBI DP + $^{99m}TcO_4$	S= 86%	SPECT	S= 80%
				MIBI DP + SPECT	S= 92%
Lorberboym [59]	41 pt	MIBI DP + $^{99m}TcO_4$	S= 78%	SPECT	S= 96%
Moka [53]	62 pt	MIBI DP + MIBI/$^{99m}TcO_4$ Sub	S= 81%	Delay SPECT	S= 97%
Moka [57]	92 pt	MIBI/$^{99m}TcO_4$ Sub	S= 87%	Delay SPECT	S= 95%
Oudoux [75]	51 pt 55 gs	MIBI DP + MIBI/$^{99m}TcO_4$ Sub	S^*= 76%	SPECT	S^*= 82%
				PH SPECT	S^*= 87%
Schachter [55]	82 pt	MIBI DP + MIBI/$^{99m}TcO_4$ Sub	S= 78%	SPECT	S= 96%
Öksüz [29]	60 pt	MIBI DP (25 pt)	S= 76%	MIBI SPECT or SPECT-CT (35 pt)	S= 97%
Kim [80]	24 pt 35 gs	MIBI DP	S^*= 68%	Delay SPECT	S^*= 76%
				Delay SPECT-CT	S^*= 100%
Carlier [66]	51 pt 55 gs	MIBI/$^{99m}TcO_4$ Sub	S^*= 76%	SPECT	S^*= 82%
				SPECT + Sub	S^*= 84%
				PH SPECT	S^*= 87%
				PH SPECT + Sub	S*= 93%
Taïeb [94]	35 pt 36 gs	MIBI/^{123}I PH Sub	S^*= 86	SPECT	S^*= 78%
Gayed [61]	48 pt	MIBI DP	S= 89%	SPECT-CT	S= 89%
Slater [58]	37 pt	MIBI DP	S= 62%	SPECT	S= 73%
Krausz [78]	36 pt	MIBI DP	S= 92%	SPECT-CT	S= 92%
Loberboym [36]	52 pt	MIBI DP	S= 60%	SPECT	S= 96%
		MIBI DP + Sub	S= 79%		

Pt: patients; gs: glands; DP: Double phase; Sub: subtraction; PH: pinhole S: Sensitivity; S^*: Sensitivity per gland; MIBI: Tc-MIBI.

2.4.3. Positron Emission Tomography (PET)

Performing PET or PET-CT with ^{11}C-methionine as a highly precise technique for identifying the location of adenomas is recommended for patients in whom other imaging protocols were unsuccessful [29, 98, 99].

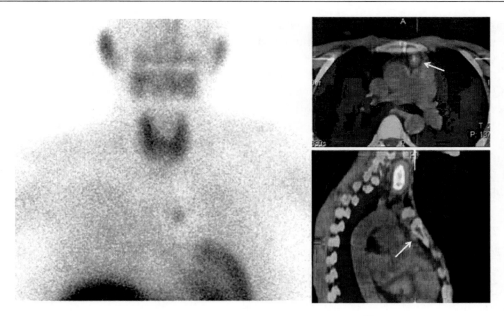

Figure 3.6. Left: Early phase planar image of a double phase scintigraphy with ^{99m}Tc-MIBI shows a focus of increased uptake in the mediastinum. Right: SPECT/CT (axial and sagital slices). In the SPECT-CT images this focus of increased uptake is localized in the prevascular space, retrosternal.

2.5. A Single Imaging Technique or a Combination of Techniques

According to certain authors [100], scintigraphy is the most sensitive, specific and accurate protocol for the diagnosis of parathyroid adenoma and is an improvement on the other diagnostic methods for localizing parathyroid glands in cases of hyperplasia. Ruda et al. [101] consider scintigraphy a first option for minimally invasive surgery, but they argue that if this technique is negative, then US is more cost-effective than SPECT or bilateral neck exploration.

However, some authors recommend US as a sole pre-operative localization test prior to unilateral neck exploration, because US is less complicated, less expensive and non-invasive [102-103]. In their view, scintigraphy should be undertaken when US is negative or equivocal. However, a combination of both techniques, especially high-resolution US and scintigraphy [34, 104-108], significantly improves the sensitivity, specificity and predictive value of the diagnostic; this is because scintigraphy is based on the functional activity of the parathyroid glands, and therefore it is possible to characterize non-typified nodules in the US and detect ectopic lesions, whilst US supplies a high-resolution image with an accurate description of anatomical position, permitting lesions to be identified which, due to their small size, low metabolic activity and/or the presence of necrotic or cystic areas, are not visualized by scintigraphy. Additionally, it could augment the detection of MGD and improve information concerning accompanying thyroid pathology.

This combined use of scintigraphy and US is also of importance in patients with accompanying thyroid disease. Rubello et al. [109] propose the combined use of Tc-MIBI/^{99m}TcO$_4$ scintigraphy subtraction and US. Likewise, Lumachi et al. [110] are of the opinion that this combination represents the most reliable non-invasive localization tool. If both techniques are negative or not in agreement, the patient should undergo bilateral neck exploration.

The EANM guidelines [5] states that imaging tests prior to a reoperation are mandatory and that scintigraphy must be confirmed with a second imaging technique, generally US for a focal uptake in the neck and CT or MRI in the case of the mediastinum. Lumachi et al. (97) have assessed the association of CT and Tc-MIBI/^{99m}TcO$_4$ subtraction scintigraphy, and found a sensitivity and PPV of 86% and 97.4% for scintigraphy, 88.1% and 94.9% for CT, and 100% and 97.4% for their combination, respectively. Whilst Kim et al. [80] emphasize the role played by SPECT-CT versus US or CT in evaluating peri-thyroidal lesions in order to make a distinction between parathyroid glands or lymph nodes.

In Tables 3.4 and 3.5 the results of scintigraphy versus US, CT, MR and PET-CT in diverse series of patients are presented.

Table 3.4. Scintigraphy versus US in the localization diagnosis of HPT

Authors	# Cases	Technique	Results	Technique	Results
Lumachi [110]	253 pt 258 gs	^{99m}Tc-MIBI/^{99m}TcO$_4$ Sub (90 pt)	S= 85% Sp= 96%	US (191 pt)	S= 83% Sp= 94%
Chapuis [102]	70 pt	^{99m}Tc-MIBI DP	S= 94%	US	S= 80%
Hajioff [104]	48 pt 48 gs	^{99m}Tc-MIBI DP	S= 83% PPV= 87%	US	S= 64% PPV= 100%
Carlier [66]	51 pt 55 gs	^{99m}Tc-MIBI/^{99m}TcO$_4$ Sub + SPECT	S= 84% Sp= 95%	US	S= 51% Sp= 91%
Taïeb [95]	35 pt 36 gs	^{99m}Tc-MIBI/^{123}I PH Sub	S= 86%	US	S= 77%
		SPECT	S= 78%		
Gawabde [111]	569 pt	^{99m}Tc-MIBI DP + SPECT	S= 63% Sp= 92% PPV= 89%	US	S= 63% Sp= 90% PPV= 89%
Alexandrides [105]	55 pt (59 % MND)	^{99m}Tc-MIBI or Tetrofosmin DP	S= 89%	US (44 pt)	S= 70%
Ansquer [60]	49 pt 49 gs	^{99m}Tc-MIBI DP + SPECT	S= 92%	US	S= 57%
				US + DP + SPECT	S= 96%
Oudoux [75]	51 pt 55 gs	^{99m}Tc-MIBI/^{99m}TcO$_4$ Sub + ^{99m}Tc-MIBI DP	S= 76%	US	S= 51%
				US + Sub + DP + PH SPECT	S= 94.5%
		PH SPECT	S= 87%		
de Feo [34]	16 pt 24 gs	^{99m}Tc-MIBI DP	S=71% Sp= 89%	US	S=67%
				US + DP	S=96% Sp=83%

Pt: patients; gs: glands; DP: Double phase; Sub: subtraction; Tetrof: ^{99m}Tc-Tetrofosmin; US: Ultrasonography; PH: pinhole; S: Sensitivity; Sp: Specificity; PPV: Positive Predictive Value; MIBI: Tc-MIBI.

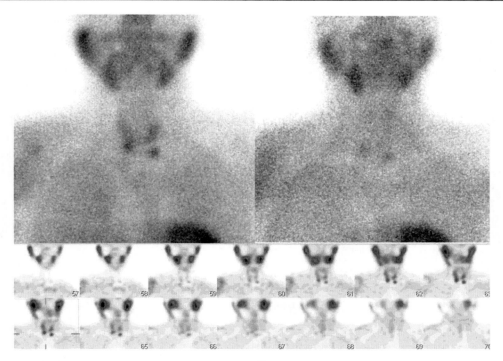

Figure 3.7. Top: Double phase planar scintigraphy with ^{99m}Tc-MIBI. In both phases two foci of increased uptake are seen in both lower poles of the thyroid gland. Bottom: coronal slices of a SPECT acquisition. Four foci with increased uptake, two in both lower and upper poles, compatible with multiglandular disease.

2.6. Special Situations

Two of the most frequent causes of unsuccessful surgery are the existence of ectopic parathyroid glands and unsuspected MGD.

2.6.1. Ectopy

Between 11% and 20% of pathological parathyroid glands [28, 36, 79] are ectopic, with neck ectopies being more common (80%) than those related to the mediastinum (20%). Superior or inferior parathyroid glands located above or below the level of the thyroid gland in the neck or mediastinum or posterior to the pharynx or esophagus are considered ectopic. Superior parathyroid glands at the level of the inferior third of the thyroid lobe, in the tracheoesophageal groove, are also considered ectopic [73, 112-114].

Parathyroidal scintigraphy has proven to be highly sensitive in identifying these adenomas, basically due to its wide field of view (unlike US) and adequate specificity (compared with CT). Nowadays, with enhanced scintigraphy protocols, for example, with the addition of SPECT and SPECT-CT, there has been definite improvement in detecting and localizing these glands. For instance, in the case of a descended superior parathyroid, it has an inferior-posterior localization, in the posterior mediastinum; for this reason it might appear in anterior planar scintigraphy imaging as an inferior parathyroid (Figure 3.5). This could cause the surgeon to misinterpret the situation, resulting in a rise in morbidity with more extensive exploration or surgical failure. Consequently, the more posterior the abnormal focus of activity is found to be in the SPECT, the greater the chance that it is a descended superior parathyroid [73, 115].

For Tardin et al. [116] the most common ectopic localizations were paraesophageal, posterior cervical-mediastinal and cervical-thymic. According to these authors, planar images consider 45% of ectopic adenomas to be eutopic, whilst SPECT was successful in correctly localizing 18 of the 20 adenomas studied. What is more, the attenuated correction provided by CT could heighten sensitivity when detecting parathyroid glands localized in the mediastinum, particularly in obese patients or in glands with only mildly increased uptake (Figure 3.4). Also, CT supplies more anatomical information concerning their relation to proximate structures for accurate localization during surgery (Figure 3.6).

Numerous examples have been recorded in which both SPECT and SPECT-CT have been very helpful in localizing ectopic glands in diverse positions such as para-hyoidal [117], retropharingeal [118], and the aortopulmonary window [119], especially in cases of persistent HPT [118, 119].

Table 3.5. Scintigraphy and other imaging modalities (CT, MR, PET-CT) in the localization diagnosis of HPT

Author	#Cases	Technique	Results	Technique	Results
de Feo [34]	16 pt	Tc-MIBI DP	S= 71%	MR	S=50%
	24 gs		Sp= 89%	MR + DP	S= 75% PPV= 62% Ac= 59%
Gotway [40]	98 pt 130 gs (persistent or recurrent HPT)	Tc-MIBI DP (Conv + PH)	S= 85% PPV= 89%	MR	S= 82% PPV= 89%
				MR + DP	S= 94% PPV= 98%
Pino [96]	29 pt			MR (9 pt)	S= 89%
				CT (20 pt)	S= 65%
Lumachi [97]	44 pt	TcMIBI/ $^{99m}TcO_4$ Sub	S= 86% PPV= 97%	CT	S= 88% PPV= 95%
				CT + Sub	S= 100% PPV= 97%
Ösküz [29]	60 pt	Tc-MIBI DP (25 pt)	S=76%	^{11}C-metionine PET or PET-CT (8 pt)	S= 100%
		^{99m}Tc-MIBI SPECT or SPECT-CT (35 pt)	S= 97%		

Pt: patients; gs: glands; DP: Double phase; Sub: subtraction; PH: pinhole; Conv: LEHR. S: Sensitivity; Sp:Specificity; PPV: Positive Predictive Value; MIBI: Tc-MIBI.

2.6.2. Multi-glandular Disease

One of the main problems when performing minimally invasive surgery is predicting the existence of MGD (Figure 3.7). There is a higher false negative rate in patients with double adenomas and hyperplasia in 4 glands compared to patients with solitary adenomas [10, 120]. This could result in an unsuccessful minimally invasive intervention [121]. Siperstein et al. [122] publish a large series of patients that in 22 % of cases there were unsuspected MGD that had not been diagnosed with US or scintigraphy. Incorporating an intra-operative iPTH determination, this diminished to 16%.

The problem of MGD is difficult to overcome with any imaging technique. Chiu et al. [123] claimed that the prevalence of MGD among those for whom localization by ^{99m}Tc-MIBI scintigraphy was successful was 4%, compared with 24% among those for whom localization failed. Yip et al. [65] added that PHPT patients with equivocal ^{99m}Tc-MIBI SPECT scans have a higher rate of MGD and a higher rate of operative failure. Other authors have encountered limitations, not only with planar scintigraphy but also with the combined use of SPECT [61].

Nonetheless, Gordon et al. [125] argued that dual-phase scintigraphy has a sensitivity of 96% and specificity of 88% in localizing hyperplastic glands prior to surgery. They employed a thyroid ratio between immediate and delayed images, which assisted them in differentiating between parathyroid hyperplasia, parathyroid adenoma and normal parathyroid tissue.

Conclusion

The applications of SPECT and SPECT-CT in the field of Nuclear Medicine are constantly increasing. Due to the wide diversity of techniques and protocols used in the management of HPT, it is difficult to perform fair comparisons. Nevertheless, both techniques have been proven to increase the sensitivity of planar imaging and improve the localization of foci visualized in planar images, which is highly beneficial for surgery, especially in unilateral or minimally invasive approaches. Although hybrid imaging does not significantly increase the sensitivity of SPECT, it can improve the localization of pathological glands and offering anatomical information. Furthermore, SPECT-CT can increase the specificity of the scintigraphic technique, specifically in patients with concomitant thyroid nodular pathology and in patients with distorted anatomy because of a previous cervical surgery. Although most centers use early SPECT or SPECT-CT, especially to detect rapid washout adenomas, they have also been performed in the delay phase with good results. SPECT is usually performed with parallel collimators. A pinhole collimator can be used instead, but this requires specific software to process the images and is not useful in ectopic localizations outside the cervical region.

References

[1]   Coakley, A. J. Symposium on parathyroid localization. Editorial. *Nucl Med Commun*, 2003, 24: 111-3.

[2]   Ferrer, M. J., Arroyo, M., López, C., Plá, A., Hernández, A., López, R. Análisis descriptivo y resultados quirúrgicos del hiperparatiroidismo primario. *Acta ORL Esp,* 2002, 53: 773-80.

[3]   Roka, R., Pramhas, M., Roka, S. Primary hyperparathyroidism: is there a role for imaging? (Pro). *Eur J Nucl Med Mol Imaging.* 2004, 3: 1322-4.

[4]   Lobato, L. A. La gammagrafia como técnica diagnóstica en el hiperparatiroidismo primario. *Radiobiología,* 2001, 1: 12-14.

[5]   Hindié, E., Ugur, O., Fuster, D. et al. 2009 EANM parathyroid guidelines. *Eur J Nucl Med Mol Imaging.* 2009, 36: 1201-16.

[6]   Sadler, T. W. Langman Embriología médica con orientación clínica. 8ª edición. México DF: Panamericana; 2002; pp. 343-5.

[7]   Cotran, R. S., Kumar, V., Collins, T. Robbins Patología estructural y funcional. 6ª ed. Madrid: Mc Graw-Hill Interamericana; 1999; pp. 1194-6.

[8]   Castro, S. de. *Manual de Patología general.* 5ª ed. Barcelona: Masson, 1993; p. 383-9.

[9]   Potes, J. T. *Enfermedades de las glándulas paratiroides y otros procesos hiper-calcémicos e hipocalcémicos.* In: Braunwald, Fauci, Kasper, Hauser, Longo, Jameson (eds). Harrison Principios de Medicina Interna. 15ª edición. Vol. III. Madrid: Mc Graw-Hill Interamericana.; p. 2586-8.

[10]   Ruda, J. M., Hollenbeak, C., Stack, B. C Jr. A systematic review of the diagnosis and treatment of primary hyperparathyroidism from 1995 to 2003. *Otolaryngol Head and Neck Surg.* 2005, 132: 359-372.

[11]   Uldesman, R., Pasieka, J. L., Sturgeon, C., Young, J. E. M., Clark, O. H. Surgery for asymptomatic primary hyperparathyroidism: proceeding of the third international workshop. *J Clin Endocrinol Metab,* 2009, 94: 366-72.

[12]   Consens Statement. Diagnosis and management of asymptomatic primary hyper-parathyroidism. *National Institutes of Health Consensus Development Conference.* 1990, 8: 1-18.

[13]   Bilezikian, J. P., Potts, J. T. Jr., Fuleihan G. E.-H. et al. Summary statement from a workshop on asymptomatic primary hyperparathyroidism: a Perspective for the 21st century. *J Clin Endocrinol Met,* 2002, 87: 5353-61.

[14]   Bilezikian, J. P., Khan, A. A., Potts, J. T. Jr. Guidelines for the Management of Asymptomatic Primary Hyperparathyroidism: Summary Statement from the Third International Workshop. *J Clin Endocrinol Metab,* 2009, 94: 335–339.

[15]   Jódar, E. Consensos y guías de práctica clínica en hiperparatiroidismo primario. *Endocrinol Nutr,* 2009, 56 (Supl 1): 41-7.

[16]   García-Talavera, P., García-Talavera, J. R., González, C., Martín, E., Martín, M., Gómez, A. Efficacy of in-vivo counting in parathyroid radioguided surgery and usefulness of its association with scintigraphy and intraoperative iPTH. *Nucl Med Commun,* 2011, 32: 847-52.

[17]   García-Talavera, P., González, C., García-Talavera, J. R., Martín, E., Martín M., Gómez A. Radioguided surgery of primary hyperparathyroidism in a population with a high prevalence of thyroid pathology. *Eur J Nucl Med Mol Imaging,* 2010, 37: 2060-7.

[18]   Ferlin, G., Borsato, N., Camerani, M., Conte, N., Zotti, D. New Perspectives in localizing enlarged parathyroids by technetium-thallium subtraction scan. *J Nucl Med,* 1983, 24: 438-41.

[19] Simón, I., Simó, R., Mesa, J., Aguadé, S., Boada, L., Sureda, D. G. Subtraction scintigraphy with thallium-201 chloride and technetium-99mpertechnetate versus high resolution ultrasonography in the localization of the parathyroid glands in primary hyperparathyroidism. *Med Clin* (Barc), 1992, 99: 774-7.

[20] Mazzeo, S., Caramella, D., Lencioni, R. et al. Comparison among sonography, double-tracer subtraction scintigraphy, and double-phase scintigraphy in the detection of parathyroid lesions. *AJR,* 1996, 166: 1465-70.

[21] Gimlette, T. M., Taylor, W. H. Localization of enlarged parathyroid glands by thallium-201 y technetium-99m subtraction imaging. Gland mass and parathormone levels in primary hyperparathyroidism. *Clin Nucl Med,* 1985, 10: 235-9.

[22] Bernard, F., Lefebvre, B., Beuvon, F., Langlois, M. F., Bisson, G. Rapid washout of technetium-99m-MIBI from a large parathyroid adenoma. *J Nucl Med,* 1995, 36: 241-3.

[23] Melloul, M., Paz, A., Koren, R., Cytron, S., Feinmesser, R., Gal, R. 99mTc MIBI scintigraphy of parathyroid adenomas and its relation to tumour size and oxyphyl cell abundance. *Eur J Nucl Med,* 2001, 28: 209-13.

[24] Coakley, A. J., Kettle, A. G., Wells, C. P., O´Doherty, M. J., Collins, R. E. 99mTc sestamibi: a new agent for parathyroid imaging. *Nucl Med Commun.* 1989, 10: 791-4.

[25] Bhatnagar, A., Vezza, P. R., Bryan, J. A., Atkins, F. B., Ziessman, H. A. Technetium-99m-sestamibi parathyroid scintigraphy: Effect of P-glycoprotein, histology and tumor size on detectability. *J Nucl Med.* 1998, 39: 1617-20.

[26] Erbil, Y., Barnaros, U., Yanik, B. T. et al. Impact of gland morphology and concomitant thyroid nodules on preoperative localization of parathyroid adenomas. *Laringoscope,* 2006, 116: 580-5.

[27] Ugur, O., Bozkurt, M. F., Hamaloglu, E. et al. Clinicopathologic and radiopharmaco-kinetic factors affecting gamma probe-guided parathyroidectomy. *Arch Surg,* 2004, 139: 1175-9.

[28] Ciappuccini, R., Morera, J., Pascal, P. et al. Dual-Phase 99mTc Sestamibi Scintigraphy With Neck and Thorax SPECT/CT in Primary Hyperparathyroidism. A Single-Institution Experience. *Clin Nucl Med,* 2012, 37: 223–228.

[29] Öksüz, M. O., Dittmann, H., Wicke, C. et al. Accuracy of parathyroid imaging: a comparison of planar scintigraphy, SPECT, SPECT-CT, and C-11 methionine PET for the detection of parathyroid adenomas and glandular hyperplasia. *Diagn Interv Radiol,* 2011, 17: 297–307.

[30] Westerdahl, J., Bergenfelz, A. Sestamibi scan-directed parathyroid surgery: potentially high failure rate without measurement of intraoperative parathyroid hormone. *World J Sug,* 2004, 28: 1132-38.

[31] Palestro, C. J., Tomas, M. B., Tronco, G. G. Radionuclide imaging of the parathyroid glands. *Semin Nucl Med,* 2005, 35: 266-76.

[32] Yamaguchi, S., Yachiku, S., Hashimoto, H. et al. Relation between technetium 99mTc-methoxyisobutilisonitrile accumulation and multidrug resistance protein in the parathyroid glands. *World J Surg,* 2002, 26: 29-34.

[33] Dackiw, A. P. B., Sussman, J. J., Fritsche. H. A et al. Relative contributions of technetium Tc 99m Sestamibi scintighaphy, Intraoperative gamma probe detection, and the rapid parathyroid hormona assay to the surgical management of hyperpara-thyroidism. *Arch Surg,* 2000, 135: 550-7.

[34] de Feo, M. L. Colagrande, S; Biagini et al. Parathyroid Glands: Combination of 99mTc MIBI scintigraphy and US for demostration of parathyroid glands and nodules. *Radiology,* 2000, 214: 393-402.

[35] Rubello, D., Casara, D., Pelizzo, M. R. Symposium on parathyroid localization. Optimization of peroperative procedures. *Nucl Med Commun,* 2003, 24: 133-140.

[36] Lorberboym, M., Minski, I., Macadziob, S., Nikolov, G., Schachter, P. Incremental diagnostic value of preoperative 99mTc-MIBI SPECT in patients with a parathyroid adenoma. *J Nucl Med.* 2003, 44: 904-8.

[37] Siegel, A., Alvarado, M., Barth, R. J., Brady, M., Lewis, J. Parameters in the Prediction of the sensitivity of parathyroid Scanning. *Clin Nucl Med,* 2006, 31: 679-82.

[38] Taillefer, R., Boucher, Y., Potvin, C., Lambert, R. Detection and localization of parathyroid adenomas in patients with hyperparathyroidism using a single radionuclide imaging procedure with technetium-99m-sestamibi (double-phase study). *J Nucl Med,* 1992, 33: 1801-7.

[39] O´Doherty, M. J., Kettle, A. G., Wells, F., Collins, R. E., Coakley, A. J. Parathyroid imaging with technetium-99m-sestamibi: preoperative localization and tissue uptake studies. *J Nucl Med,* 1992, 33: 313-8.

[40] Gotway, M. B., Reddy, G. P., Webb, W. R., Morita, E. T., Clark, O. H., Higgins, C. B. Comparison between MR imaging and 99mTc MIBI scintigraphy in the evaluation of recurrent of persistent hyperparathyroidism. *Radiology.* 2001, 218: 783-90.

[41] Bénard, F., Lefebvre, B., Beuvon, F., Langlois, M. F., Bisson, G. Rapid washout of technetium-99m-MIBI from a large parathyroid adenoma. *J Nucl Med.* 1995, 36: 241-3.

[42] Siegel, A., Mancuso, M., Seltzer M. The spectrum of positive scan patterns in parathyroid scintigraphy. *Clin Nucl Med,* 2007, 32: 770-4.

[43] Rubello, D., Saladini, G., Casara, D. et al. Parathtroid imaging with pertechnetate plus perclorate/MIBI subtraction scintighapy: a fast and effective technique. *Clin Nucl Med,* 2000, 25: 527-31.

[44] Hindiè, E., Melliere, D., Jeanguillaume, C., Perlemuter, L., Chehade, F., Galle P. Parathyroid imaging using simultaneous double-window recording of technetium-99m-sestamibi and iodine-123I. *J Nucl Med,* 1998, 39: 1100-5.

[45] Arveschoug, A. K., Bertelsen, H., Vammen, B. Presurgical localization of abnormal parathyroid glands using a single injection of 99mTc sestamibi; comparison of high-resolution parallel-hole and pinhole collimators, and interobserver and intraobserver variation. *Clin Nucl Med,* 2002, 27: 249-54.

[46] Arveschoug, A. K., Bertelsen, H., Vammen, B., Brochner-Mortensen, J. Preoperative Dual-Phase parathyroid imaging with 99mTc-sestamibi. Accuracy and reproducibility of the pinhole collimator with and without oblicue images. *Clin Nucl Med,* 2007, 32: 9-12.

[47] Ho Shon, I. A., Bernard, E. J., Roach, P. J., Delbridge, L. W. The value of oblique pinhole images in preoperative localization with 99mTc-MIBI for primary hyperparathyroidism. *Eur J Nucl Med,* 2001, 28: 736-42.

[48] Yoon, S., Kim, S., Eskandar, Y. et al. Appearance of intrathymic parathyroid adenomas on pinhole sestamibi parathyroid imaging. *Clin Nucl Med,* 2006, 31: 325-7.

[49] Fröberg, A. C., Valkema, R., Bonjer, H. J., Krenning, E. P. 99mTc-Tetrofosmin or 99mTc-sestamibi for double-phase parathyroid scintigraphy? *Eur J Nucl Med,* 2003, 30: 193-6.

[50] Vallejos, V., Martin-Comín, J., González, M. T. et al. The usefulness of Tc-99m tetrofosmin scintigraphy in the diagnosis and localization of hyperfunctioning parathyroid glands. *Clin Nucl Med,* 1999, 24: 959-64.

[51] Arbab, A. S., Koizumi, K., Toyama, K., Araki, T. Uptake of technetium-99m-tetrofosmin, technetium-99m-MIBI, and thallium-201 in tumor cell lines. *J Nucl Med,* 1996, 37: 1551-6.

[52] Greenspan B. S., Dillehay G., Intenzo C. et al. SNM Practice Guideline for Parathyroid Scintigraphy 4.0. *J Nucl Med Technol,* 2012, 40: 111-8.

[53] Moka, D., Eschner, W., Voth, E., Dietlein, M., Larena-Avellaneda, A., Schicha H. Iterative reconstruction: an improvement of technetium-99m MIBI SPET for the detection of parathyroid adenomas? *Eur J Nucl Med,* 2000, 27: 485-9.

[54] González, V. G., Orellana, B. P., López, M. J. M., Jiménez, M. M., Quintana, Y. J. C. Early parathyroid MIBI SPECT imaging in the diagnosis of persistent hyper-parathyroidism. *Clin Nucl Med,* 2008, 33: 475-8.

[55] Schachter, P. P., Issa, N., Schimonov, M., Czerniak, A., Lorberboym, M. Early postinjection MIBI SPECT as the only preoperative localizing study for minimally invasive parathyroidectomy. *Arch Surg,* 2004, 139: 433-7.

[56] Profanter, C., Wetscher, G. J., Gabriel, M. et al. CT-MIBI image fusion: a new preoperative localization technique for primary, recurrent, and persistent hyper-parathyroidism. *Surgery,* 2004, 135: 157-62.

[57] Moka, D., Voth, E., Dietlein, M., Larena-Avellaneda, A., Schicha, H. Technetium 99m-MIBI-SPECT: A highly sensitive diagnostic tool for localization of parathyroid adenomas. *Surgery,* 2000, 128: 29-35.

[58] Lorberboym, M., Ezri, T., Schachter, P. P. Preoperative technetium Tc-99m-sestamibi SPECT imaging in the management of primary hyperparathyroidism in patients with concomitant multinodular goiter. *Arch Surg,* 2005, 140: 656-60.

[59] Slater, A., Gleeson, F. V. Increased sensitivity and confidence of SPECT over planar imaging in dual-phase sestamibi for parathyrois adenoma detection. *Clin Nucl Med,* 2005, 30: 1-3.

[60] Ansquer, C., Mirallié, E., Carlier, T., Abbey-Huguenin, H., Aubron, F., Kraeber-Bodéré, F. Preoperative localization of parathyroid lesions. Value of 99mTc-MIBI tomography and factors influencing detection. *Nuklearmedizin.* 2008; 47: 158-62.

[61] Gayed, I. W., Kim, E. E., Broussard, W. F. et al. The value of 99mTc-sestamibi SPECT/CT over convencional SPECT in the evaluation of parathyroid adenomas or hyperplasia. *J Nucl Med,* 2005, 46: 248-52.

[62] Prats, E., Razola, P., Tardín, L. et al. Gammagrafía de paratiroides y cirugía radiodirigida en el hiperparatiroidismo primario. *Rev Esp Med Nucl,* 2007, 26: 310-30.

[63] Loberboym, M., Erzi, T., Schachter, P. P. Preoperative technetium Tc99m sestamibi SPECT imaging in the management of primary hyperparathyroidism in patients with concomitant multinodular goiter. *Arch Surg,* 2005, 140: 656-60.

[64] Rubello, D., Massaro, A., Cittadin, S. et al. Role of 99mTcsestamibi SPECT in accurate selection of primary hyperparathyroid patients for minimally invasive radio-guided surgery. *Eur J Nucl Med Mol Imaging.* 2006, 33: 1091-4.

[65] Yip, L., Pryma, D. A., Yim, J. H., Carty, S. E., Ogilvie, J. B. Sestamibi SPECT intensity scoring system in sporadic primary hyperparathyroidism. *World J Surg,* 2009, 33: 426-33.

[66] Carlier, T., Oudoux, A., Mirallié, E. et al. 99mTc-MIBI pinhole SPECT in primary hyperparathyroidism: comparison with conventional SPECT, planar scintigraphy and ultrasonography. *Eur J Nucl Med Mol Imaging,* 2008, 35: 637–4.

[67] Witteveen, J. E., Kievit, J., Stokkel, M. P. M., Morreau, H., Romijn, J. A., Hamdy, N. A. T. Limitations of Tc99m-MIBI-SPECT Imaging Scans in Persistent Primary Hyperparathyroidism. *World J Surg,* 2011, 35: 128–39.

[68] Kullkarni, K., Kim, S. M., Weigel, R. J. Utility of very delayed parathyroid MIBI SPECT for localization of parathyroid adenoma. *Clin Nucl Med,* 2004, 29: 727-9.

[69] Khan, M. S., Khan, S., Vereb, M. et al. Ectopic Parathyroid Adenoma with Tc99m MIBI washout. Role of SPECT. *Clin Nucl Med,* 2006, 31: 713-5.

[70] Pérez-Monte, J. E., Brown, M. L., Shah, A. N, et al. Parathyroid adenomas: accurate detection and localization with Tc-99m sestamibi SPECT. *Radiology,* 1996, 201: 85-91.

[71] Hara, N., Takayama, T., Onoguchi, M, et al. Subtraction SPECT for parathyroid scintigraphy based on maximization of mutual information. *J Nucl Med Technol,* 2007, 35: 84-90.

[72] Neumann, D. R., Obuchowski, N. A., DiFilippo F. P. Preoperative 123I/99mTc Sestamibi Subtraction SPECT and SPECT/CT in Primary Hyperparathyroidism. *J Nucl Med,* 2008, 49: 2012–7.

[73] Eslamy, H. K., Ziessman, H. A. Parathyroid scintigraphy in patients with primary hyperparathyroidism: 99mTc-sestamibi SPECT and SPECT/CT. *Radiographics,* 2008, 28: 1461-76.

[74] Bajoghli, M., Muthukrishnan, A., Mountz, J. Posterior bulge sign for parathyroid adenoma on 99mTc-MIBI SPECT. *Clin Nucl Med,* 2006, 31: 470-1.

[75] Oudoux, A., Carlier, T., Mirallié, E. et al. 99mTc-MIBI pinhole SPECT in primary hyperparathyroidism. *Médecine Nucléaire,* 2007, 31: 553-61.

[76] Papathanassiou, D., Flament, J. B., Pochart, J. M. et al. SPECT/CT in localization of parathyroid adenoma or hyperplasia in patients with previous neck surgery. *Clin Nucl Med,* 2008, 33: 394-7.

[77] Kaczirek, K., Prager, G., Kienast, O. et al. Combined transmisión and 99mTc-sestamibi emisión tomography for localization of mediastinal parathyroid glands. *Nuklearmedizin,* 2003, 42: 220-3.

[78] Krausz, Y., Bettman, L., Guralnik, L. et al. Technetium-99m-MIBI SPECT/CT in primary hyperparathyroidism. *World J Surg,* 2006, 30: 76-83.

[79] Serra, A., Bolasco, P., Satta, L., Nicolosi, A., Uccheddu, A., Piga, M. *Role of SPECT/CT in the preoperative assessment of hyperparathyroid patients,* 2006, 111: 999-1008.

[80] Kim, Y. I., Jung, Y. H., Hwang, K. T., Lee, H. Y. Efficacy of 99mTc-sestamibi SPECT/CT for minimally invasive parathyroidectomy: comparative study with 99mTc-sestamibi scintigraphy, SPECT, US and CT. *Ann Nucl Med,* 2012, 26: 804-10.

[81] Goetze S., Lavely W. C., Ziessman H. A., Wahl R. L. Visualization of brown adipose tissue with 99mTc methoxiisobutylisonitrile on SPECT/CT. *J Nucl Med.* 2008; 49: 752-6.

[82] Wong, K. K., Brown, R. K., Avram, A. M. Potential false positive Tc99m sestamibi parathyroid study due to uptake in brown adipose tissue. *Clin Nucl Med,* 2008, 33: 346-8.

[83] Treglia, G., Dambra, D. P., Bruno, I., Mulé, A., Giordano, A. Costal Brown tumor detected by dualphase parathyroid imaging and SPECT-CT in primary hyperparathyroidism. *Clin Nucl Med,* 2008, 33: 193-5.

[84] Neuman, D. R., Opuchowski, N. A., DiFilippo F. P. Preoperative 123I/99mTc-sestamibi subtraction SPECT and SPECT/CT in primary hyperparathyroidism. *J Nucl Med,* 2008, 49: 2012-7.

[85] Lavely, W. C., Goetze, S., Friedman, K. P. et al. Comparison of SPECT/CT, SPECT, and planar imaging with single- and dual-phase 99mTc-sestamibi parathyroid scintigraphy. *J Nucl Med,* 2007, 48: 1084-9.

[86] Shafiei, B., Hoseinzadeh, S., Fotouhi, F. et al. Preoperative 99mTc-sestamibi scintigraphy in patients with primary hyperparathyroidism and concomitant nodular goiter: comparison of SPECT-CT, SPECT, and planar imaging. *Nucl Med Commun,* 2012, 33: 1070-6.

[87] Ruf, J., López-Aniñen, E., Steinmuller, T. et al. Preoperative localization of parathyroid glands. Use of MRI, scintigraphy, and image fusion. *Nuklearmedizin,* 2004, 43: 85-90.

[88] Menzel, C. Paratiroides. In Castro-Beiras J. M., Oliva-González J. P. *Oncología Nuclear.* Madrid: MT, 2006, p. 421-31.

[89] O´Doherty, M. J., Kettle, A. G. Symposium on parathyroid localization. *Nucl Med Commun,* 2003, 24: 125-31.

[90] Caveny, S. A., Klingensmith III, W. C., Martin, W. E. et al. Parathyroid Imaging: The importance of dual-radiopharmaceutical simultaneous acquisition with 99mTc-sestamibi and 123I. *J Nucl Med Technol,* 2012, 40: 104-10.

[91] Tomas, M. B., Pugliese, P. V., Tronco, G. G., Love, C., Palestro, J., Nichols, K. J. Pinhole versus parallel-hole collimators for parathyroid imaging: an intraindividual comparison. *J Nucl Technol,* 2008, 36: 189-94.

[92] Ho Shon, I. A., Yan, W., Roach, P. J. et al. Comparison of pinhole and SPECT 99mTc-MIBI imaging in primary hyperparathyroidism. *Nucl Med Commun,* 2008, 29: 949-55.

[93] Chen, C. C., Holder, L. E., Scovill, W. A., Tehan, A. M., Gann, D. S. Comparison of parathyroid imaging with technetium-99m-pertechnetate/sestamibi subtraction, double phase technetium-99m-sestamibi and technetium-99m-sestamibi SPECT. *J Nucl Med,* 1997, 38: 834-9.

[94] Taïeb, D., Hassad, R., Sebag, F. et al. Tomoscintigraphy Improves the Determination of the Embryologic Origin of Parathyroid Adenomas, Especially in Apparently Inferior Glands: Imaging Features and Surgical Implications. *J Nucl Med Technol,* 2007, 35: 135–9.

[95] Koranda, P., Halenka, M., Myslivecek, M., Kaminek, M. Localization of parathyroid enlargement: dualtracer subtraction technique and double-phase 99mTc-MIBI scintigraphy are complementary procedures. *Eur J Nucl Med Mol Imaging,* 2008, 35: 219-20.

[96] Pino, V., Pantoja, C. G., Gonzalez, A. T. et al. Usefulness of computed tomography and magnetic resonance in the preoperative diagnosis for hyperparathyroidism. *An Otorrinolaringol Ibero Am,* 2005, 32: 491-8.

[97] Lumachi, F., Tregnaghi, A., Zucchetta, P. et al. Technetium-99m sestamibi scintigraphy and helical CT together in patients with primary hyperparathyroidism: a prospective clinical study. *Br J Radiol,* 2004, 77: 100-3.

[98]   Beggs, A. D., Hain, S. F. Localization of parathyroid adenomas using 11C-methionine positron emission tomography. *Nucl Med Commun,* 2005, 26: 133-6.

[99]   Schmidt, M. C., Kahraman, D., Neumaier, B., Ortmann, M., Stippel, D. Tc-99m-MIBI-Negative Parathyroid Adenoma in Primary Hyperparathyroidism Detected by C-11-Methionine PET/CT After Previous Thyroid Surgery. *Clin Nucl Med,* 2011, 36: 1153–5.

[100] Phitayakorn, R., McHenry, C. R. Incidence and location of ectopic abnormal parathyroid glands. *Am J Surg,* 2006, 191: 418-23.

[101] Ruda, J. M., Snack, B. C. Jr., Hollenbeak, C. S. The cost-effectiveness of additional preoperative ultrasonography or sestamibi-SPECT in patients with primary hyperparathyroidism and negative findings on sestamibi scans. *Arch Otolaryngol Head Surg,* 2006, 132: 46-53.

[102] Chapius, Y., Fulla, Y., Bonnichon, P. et al. Values of ultrasonography, sestamibi scintigraphy, and intraoperative measurement of 1-84 PTH for unilateral neck exploration of primary hiperparathyroidism. *World J Surg,* 1996, 20: 835-40.

[103] Solorzano, C. C., Carneiro-Pla, D. M., Irvin, G. L. 3rd. Surgeon-performed ultrasonography as the initial and only localizing study in sporadic primary hyperparathyroidism. *J Am Coll Surg,* 2006, 202: 18-24.

[104] Hajioff, D., Iyngkaran, T., Panagamuwa, C., Hill, D., Stearns M. P. Preoperative localization of parathyroid adenomas: ultrasonography, sestamibi scintigraphy, or both? *Clin Otolaryngol,* 2004, 29: 549-52.

[105] Alexandrides, T. K., Kouloubi, K., Vagenakis, A. G. et al. The value of scintigraphy and ultrasonography in the preoperative localization of parathyroidism and concomitant thyroid disease. *Hormones* (Athens), 2006, 5: 42-51.

[106] Berri, R. N., Lloyd, L. R. Detection of parathyroid adenoma in patients with primary hyperparathyroidism: the use of office-based ultrasound in preoperative localization. *Am J Surg,* 2006, 191: 311-4.

[107] Casara, D., Rubello, D., Pelizo, M. R., Shapiro, B. Clinical role of 99mTcO4/MIBI scan, ultrasound and intraoperative gamma probe in the performance of unilateral and minimally invasive surgery in primary hiperparathyroidism. *Eur J Nucl Med,* 2001, 28: 1351-9.

[108] Lumachi, F., Zuccheta, P., Marzola, M. C. et al. Advantages of combined technetium-99m-sestamibi scintigraphy and high-resolution ultrasonography in parathyroid localization: comparative study in 91 patients with primary hyperparathyroidism. *Eur J Endocrinol,* 2000, 143: 755-60.

[109] Rubello, D., Toniato, A., Pellizzo, M. R., Casara, D. Papillary Thyroid Carcinoma Associated with parathyroid adenoma detected by pertechnetate-MIBI substraction scintigraphy. *Clin Nucl Med,* 2000, 25: 898-900.

[110] Lumachi, F., Ermani, M., Basso, S. et al. Localization of parathyroid tumours in the minimally invasive era: wich technique should be chosen? Population based analysis of 253 patients undergoing parathyroidectomy and factors affecting parathyroid gland detection. *Endocr Relat Cancer,* 2001, 8: 63-9.

[111] Gawande, A. A., Monchick, J. M., Abbruzzese, T. A., Ianuccilli, J. D., Ibrahim, S. I., Moore, F. D. Jr. Reassessment of parathyroid hormona monitoring during parathyroidectomy for primary hyperparathyroidism after 2 preoperative localization studies. *Arch Surg,* 2006, 141: 381-4.

[112] Phytayakorn, R., McHenry, C. R. Incidence or localization of ectopic abnormal parathyroid glands. *Am J Surg,* 2006, 191: 418-23.

[113] Lal, G., Clark, O. H. *Endocrine surgery.* In: Greenspan, F. S., Gardner, D. G. editors. Basic and clinical endocrinology. 7th ed. New York: Mc Graw-Hill Medical, 2003, p. 902-19.

[114] Pelliteri, P. K., Sofferman, R. A., Randoph, G. W. *Surgical management of parathyroid disorders.* In: Cummings, C. W., Haughey, B. H., Thomas, J. R., Harker, L. A., Flint, P. W. editors. Cummings otolaryngology: head and neck surgery. 4th ed. Philadelphia, Pa: Mosby, 2005.

[115] Chul Kim, S., Kim S., Inabnet, W. B., Krynyckyi, B. R., Machac J; Kim, CK. Appearance of descended superior parathyroid adenoma on SPECT parathyroid imaging. *Clin Nucl Med,* 2007, 32: 90-3.

[116] Tardin, L., Prats, E., Andrés, A. et al. Adenoma ectópico de paratiroides: detección gammagráfica y cirugía radioguiada. *Rev Esp Med Nucl,* 2011, 30: 19-23.

[117] Rajagopalam, M., Narla, V. V., Kanderi, T., Muthukrishnan, A. Parahyoid ectopic parathyroid adenoma localized by 99mTc-MIBI SPECT. *Clin Nucl Med,* 2008, 33: 880-1.

[118] García-Talavera, P., González, M. L., Aís, G. et al. SPECT-CT in the localization of an ectopic retropharyngeal parathyroid adenoma as a cause for persistent primary hyperparathyroidism. *Rev Esp Med Nucl Imagen Mol,* 2012, 31: 275-7.

[119] Gouveia, S., Rodrigues, D., Barros, L. et al. Persistent primary hyperparathyroidism: an uncommon location for an ectopic gland – Case report and review. *Arq Bras Endocrinol Metab,* 2012, 56: 6.

[120] Heller, K. S., Attie, N., Dubner S. Parathyroid localization: inability to predict multiple gland involvement. *Am J Surg,* 1993, 166: 357-9.

[121] Katz, S. C., Wang, G. J., Kramer, E. L., Roses, D. F. Limitations of technetium 99mTc sestamibi scintigraphic localization for primary hyperparathyroidism associated with multiglandular disease. *Am Surg,* 2003, 69: 170-5.

[122] Siperstein, A., Berber, E., Barbosa, G. F. et al. Predicting the success of limited exploration for primary hyperparathyroidism using ultrasound, sestamibi and intra-operative parathyroid hormone: analysis of 1158 cases. *Ann Surg,* 2008, 248: 420-8.

[123] Chiu, B., Sturgeon, C., Angelos, P. What is the link between non localizing sestamibi scans, multigland disease, and persistent hypercalcemia? A study of 401 consecutive patients undergoing parathyroidectomy. *Surgery,* 2006, 140: 418-22.

[124] Gordon, L., Burkhalter, W., Mah, E. Dual-phase 99mTc-sestamibi imaging: its utility in parathyroid hiperplasia and use of immediate/delay image ratios to improve diagnosis. *J Nucl Med Technol,* 2002, 30: 179-84.

In: SPECT ISBN: 978-1-62808-344-6
Editors: Hojjat Ahmadzadehfar and Elham Habibi © 2013 Nova Science Publishers, Inc.

Chapter IV

SPECT in Malignant Bone Diseases

Ali Gholamrezanezhad[1,2,], Edward Pinkus[3] and Rathan Subramaniam[4]*

[1]Yale New Haven Hospital-Saint Raphael Campus, Yale School of Medicine, New Haven, CT, US
[2]Research Center for Nuclear Medicine, Tehran University of Medical Sciences, Tehran, Iran
[3]Lahey Clinic, Tuft Medical School, Burlington, MA, US
[4]Johns Hopkins University, Baltimore, MD, US

Introduction

Although anatomical imaging, most typically computed tomography (CT), has been the conventional imaging modality in oncologic applications, well-known limitations of CT have led to the frequent application of physiologic/metabolic imaging techniques, e.g. nuclear medicine studies. Bone scintigraphy, including planar scintigraphy, single photon emission computed tomography (SPECT), and integrated imaging techniques that allow SPECT and CT to be performed in the same setting and their images to be fused, are the most commonly used modalities for detection of bone metastases. The extensive application of these imaging approaches is due to their wide availability and provision of an entire skeletal visualization within a reasonable amount of time and cost and a high degree of sensitivity [1-3]. Scintigraphic approaches are also of paramount importance in the work-up of patients with primary bone malignancies, partly because of their high sensitivity in the early detection of osseous tumors. This explains why bone imaging continues to be the second greatest-volume procedure of nuclear imaging (after myocardial perfusion studies) and the most commonly performed hospital-based procedure [4], with more than 3,450,000 bone scintigraphies

---
* Corresponding author: Ali Gholamrezanezhad, MD, FEBNM, Research Center for Nuclear Medicine, Tehran University of Medical Sciences, Tehran, Iran. Email: a.gholamrezanezhad@yahoo.com or ali.gholamrezanezhad@ynhh.org.

performed in the United States in 2005 [5]. Currently, almost all bone scans are performed as a planar study (whole-body, 3-phase or regional), with the radiologist often adding SPECT or SPECT-CT imaging to visualize more details or to enhance the local sensitivity of imaging [4]. In fact, SPECT or SPECT-CT imaging is usually ordered to provide a detailed view of the area of interest on the basis of patients' symptomatology or planar bone findings [4]. Specifically, SPECT-CT appears to be extremely useful because it combines the advantages of both SPECT and CT techniques, particularly due to adding the structural information by CT [6].

Biological Mechanism of Imaging

The power of bone scintigraphy rests in the physiological uptake and pathophysiological behavior of ^{99m}Tc-diphosphonates (e.g. ^{99m}Tc-methylene diphosphonate (^{99m}Tc-MDP)) [4] and they are the most commonly used tracer for skeletal imaging in general nuclear medicine [7]. Bone is constantly remodeling, with an ongoing level of osteoblastic bone formation and osteoclastic bone resorption [4]. The osteoid matrix which is formed by osteoblasts is later mineralized with hydroxyapatite crystals. ^{99m}Tc-diphosphonates are believed to be chemisorbed onto hydroxyapatite crystals, and its uptake is reflective of osteoblastic activity and local blood flow [2, 3, 8]. Most sites of malignant bone involvement show reactive increased osteoblastic activity and, therefore, increased ^{99m}Tc-MDP uptake [6]. They quickly localize to bone and clear from the background, making a high target to background ratio; so that even a 5% change in bone turnover can be detected on bone scintigraphy [9], which makes them favorable for imaging. In fact, bone scintigraphy can often detect bone abnormalities sooner than anatomic changes [4]. On anatomical imaging of conventional radiography and CT, 40%-50% of mineral loss is needed before the detection of bone lucency [10-12]. ^{99m}Tc-MDP scintigraphy detects abnormalities of bone metabolism as early as 24 to 48 hours after the commencement of pathology and is almost always positive by 8 days [11].

The most common finding in bone scintigraphy is increased osteoblastic activity; even destructive bone lesions cause an intensely osteoblastic healing process that surrounds the lytic area, so they present as areas of increased radiotracer uptake in bone scintigraphy. However, sometimes aggressive processes (e.g., bone metastasis) or indolent processes that induce little healing reaction (indolent bony metastases like plasmacytoma/neuroblastoma), or the disruption of blood flow lead to pathologic bone image findings characterized by "cold" areas [4]. In such scenarios, SPECT imaging has a remarkable advantage over planar imaging, as detection of such cold lesions is much easier on three-dimensional SPECT imaging.

Scintigraphic imaging of bones might also be useful when using other radiopharmaceuticals that specifically localize bone lesions (e.g., [111]In- or ^{99m}Tc-labeled leukocytes or granulocytes as the gold standard to diagnose bone infections, ^{131}I in skeletal metastases of differentiated thyroid carcinoma, ^{123}I-MIBG/^{111}In-octreotide in skeletal metastases of neuroendocrine tumors or neuroblastoma), and FDG in tumor imaging. Table 4-1 summarizes some of the most commonly used radiopharmaceuticals in primary and secondary bone tumors.

Table 4.1. Radiopharmaceuticals used in bone scintigraphy

Radiopharmaceutical	Trade Name
^{99m}Tc-Medronate (MDP)	Bracco
	Osteolite - CIS
	Draximage
	Mallinckrodt
	Amersham
^{99m}TcOxidronate (HDP)	Mallinckrodt HDP
^{99m}Tc Sestamibi	Cardiolite
	Miraluma
	Draximage
Thallium-201	DuPont
	Mallinckrodt
	Amersham
Gallium-67	Neoscan (GE)
	DuPont Ga-67
	Mallinckrodt Ga-67
Indium-111 pentetreotide	Octreoscan
WBC (White Blood Cells) labeled with Indium-111 oxyquinoline (oxine)	Indium-111 oxine

Sensitivity of Bone Scintigraphy

In contrast with plain radiographic images, as little as a 5%–10% change in the ratio of lesion to normal bone is sufficient to unmask an abnormality on bone scintigraphy [2, 6]. It has been estimated that bone scintigraphy is able to detect malignant bone diseases 2–18 months earlier than conventional radiologic imaging [6]. Therefore, it is generally accepted that CT and magnetic resonance imaging (MRI) may supplement, but cannot replace, scintigraphic bone imaging, which often detects pathologic changes before anatomic changes [4]. Although the supplemental value of anatomical imaging to scintigraphy is widely appreciated, the importance of dose reduction by avoiding unnecessary CT acquisitions as well as reducing the dose of ^{99m}Tc-diphosphonates has been stressed [4].

Although plain radiography is the initial imaging modality in patients suspected of primary osseous tumors, for patients with a known non-osseous malignancy (e.g. advanced-stage breast or prostate cancer) who are at high risk for bone metastases, bone scintigraphy is the primary modality of screening for bone metastases, with sensitivity rates varying between 62% and 100% and specificity rates of 78%–100% [1].

Specificity of Bone Scintigraphy

Despite its high sensitivity, ^{99m}Tc-diphosphonates are not tumor-specific tracers and increased accumulation of these radiopharmaceuticals might also be noticed in benign bone pathologies. For this limited specificity of bone scintigraphy, there are some major exceptions:

1. Specifically in the spine, different disease processes have a tendency to involve special components of the vertebra. Accurate localization of a scintigraphic lesion within the spine by SPECT has been reported to improve the specificity of bone scintigraphy, assisting in the differentiation between benign and malignant etiologies [4, 13-15]. It is the location of the vertebral venous network which provides the route for hematogenous spread of tumor cells into the spine that explains the predilection of metastatic disease to the posterior part of the vertebral body and pedicle [4, 16]. Accordingly, the differentiation between benign and malignant diseases of vertebrae on SPECT and anatomical modalities of CT, and MRI often depends on the pattern of involvement of the spine and appearance of the posterior part of the vertebral body and pedicle [4, 13, 17].

2. The detection of multiple randomly distributed bone lesions on bone scintigraphy in a patient with a known malignancy is most likely suggestive of a metastatic etiology. Although this pattern of scan findings increases the specificity of the bone scintigram in the diagnosis of malignant pathology with metastatic spread, it should be kept in mind that there are a number of benign conditions, such as trauma, osteoporotic fractures, metabolic bone disease, osteomyelitis, etc, which may also manifest multifocally [4].

On the other hand, the detection of solitary or a few bone lesions on bone scintigraphy often warrants further assessment of the lesions by other imaging modalities, which indicates the poor specificity of the bone scintigraphy with these study findings. Focally increased radiotracer uptake in a bone scan has a wide differential diagnosis, including several benign conditions, e.g. degenerative joint disease. This applies to the vertebrae in particular, as degenerative joint disease of the spine is found in at least 50% of women older than 50 years, coinciding with the peak incidence of breast cancer (Figures 4-1 – 4-3) [18]. To overcome the limited specificity of bone scintigraphy and to reduce the rate of non-diagnostic bone lesions in scintigraphy, correlation with CT is commonly performed, which often leads to the sequential ordering of different diagnostic procedures in daily routine, causing an unnecessary loss of time and sometimes money, if redundant information is obtained without establishing a final diagnosis [1, 3, 4, 19]. In this regard, integrated SPECT-CT machines have an advantage over the SPECT only machines. Therefore, false-positive benign lesions which show increased tracer uptake and, thus, need a correlation with CT for accurate diagnosis, can be optimally detected by the CT part of the study. The potential to immediately report a benign etiology of a scintigraphic finding avoids unnecessary diagnostic work ups, reduces medical expenses, and obviates unnecessary worry on the part of the patient [7]. In the study of Romer et al., SPECT-CT camera equipped with a two-slice spiral-CT was employed to classify 52 lesions defined as indeterminate on SPECT imaging. SPECT-CT allowed the correct classification of SPECT findings as either benign or malignant in 92% of patients [20]. In another study by Horger et al., SPECT-CT was also able to correctly classify 85% of unclear uptake foci versus 36% by SPECT alone [21]. The sensitivity was in a similar range for both SPECT and SPECT-CT (>90%), while specificity was significantly higher for SPECT-CT (81% versus 19%).

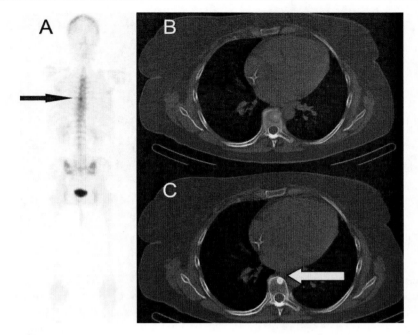

Figure 4.1. Whole body bone scintigraphy (A) of a patient with breast cancer shows an indeterminate finding involving T6, proved to be an osteoblastic bone metastasis on SPECT-CT (B & C) (courtesy of Dr. Elham Habibi, Department of Nuclear Medicine, University Hospital Bonn, Germany).

SPECT and SPECT-CT

Numerous studies have demonstrated the superiority of SPECT-CT over stand-alone SPECT in terms of diagnostic accuracy [18]. These integrated imaging systems have led medical imaging to new horizons, and present the potential for simultaneous acquisition of morphologic, functional, and molecular information [18]. The limitation of anatomic localization on planar imaging by tissue superimposition is overcome by SPECT and particularly SPECT-CT [7]. Even in SPECT imaging, it may be difficult to precisely localize a lesion with non–bone-specific tracers (e.g. [131]I, ^{111}In-somatostatin, and ^{67}Ga-citrate) [4, 22]. Physiological variations in biodistribution, leading to foci of radiotracer activity unrelated to the underlying pathology, can also be partly overcome by SPECT-CT integration [23].

The CT part of the integrated SPECT-CT machine could be low-dose CT, integrated mainly with a SPECT gamma camera, or single-slice or multi-slice diagnostic CT. Although the data acquired by reduced-dose CT have been reported to be non-diagnostic, but mainly valuable for attenuation correction and as anatomical landmarks of the scintigraphic findings [22], the contrast between lesion and normal bone is clear on low-dose CT images, obviating the need for separate full-dose CT to correlate with scintigraphic findings [6]. However, data obtained by diagnostic full-dose CT provide detailed morphologic information of the lesions, adequate for diagnostic purposes [7, 24]. Although proven to be diagnostically valuable, the major shortcoming of SPECT acquisition is that images are obtained for only a limited body region; therefore, in the daily clinical practice of nuclear medicine it is practically impossible to perform several SPECT acquisitions to tomographically assess the entire skeleton [7].

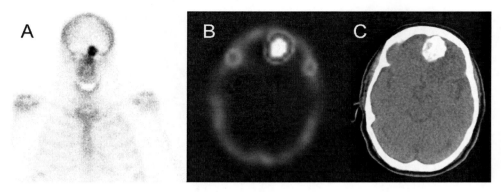

Figure 4.2. Planar bone scintigraphy showed a suspicious area of focally increased uptake in the left supraorbital region (A). SPECT imaging revealed the radiotracer accumulation to be an extraosseous uptake (B). Further evaluation by a CT scan (C) showed a calcified brain lesion, which was found to be a Meningioma (courtesy of Dr. Elham Habibi, Department of Nuclear Medicine, University Hospital Bonn, Germany).

Zhao et al. compared the diagnostic efficacy of SPECT-CT fusion imaging with that of SPECT alone and with SPECT + CT for the diagnosis of bone metastasis in patients with known cancer [25]. The sensitivity of SPECT, SPECT + CT, and SPECT-CT fusion imaging for malignant lesions was reported to be 82.5%, 93.7%, and 98.4%, respectively. The respective specificity values were 66.7%, 80.8%, and 93.6% and accuracy rates were 73.8%, 86.5%, and 95.7%, respectively. Among equivocal lesions revealed with SPECT, the accuracy of SPECT + CT was 45.9% and SPECT-CT fusion imaging was 81.1%. The number of equivocal lesions was significantly lower in SPECT + CT, and SPECT-CT fusion imaging than SPECT alone. The authors concluded that SPECT-CT is particularly valuable for the diagnosis of bone metastasis in patients with known cancer by providing precise anatomic localization and detailed morphologic characteristics [25].

The incremental diagnostic values of integrated SPECT-CT images compared with SPECT alone, or SPECT correlated with a CT obtained at a different time have been noted to include the following: (a) improvement in the localization of radiotracer activity resulting in improved differentiation of physiological from pathologic uptake, (b) remarkable lesion detection improvement on both CT and SPECT images, (c) accurate localization of the lesion (e.g. in the skeleton versus soft tissue), (d) confirmation of tiny, subtle, or atypical lesions, and [5] characterization of serendipitous findings [23], and (e) improved diagnostic confidence with the potential to influence medical practice with newer imaging algorithms [26]. A major contribution of the CT to bone scintigraphy is its ability to detect soft-tissue involvement and to guide biopsies of skeletal lesions [7, 24, 27]. These advantages of integrated SPECT-CT technique are important in all steps of clinical assessment, including at the time of initial diagnosis, assessment of early response to treatment, at the conclusion of therapy, and in follow-up of patients [23] and affect the clinical management in a significant proportion of patients by (a) guiding additional diagnostic studies, (b) avoiding unnecessary studies, and (c) changing both inter- and intra-modality therapy, including soon after treatment has been initiated [23].

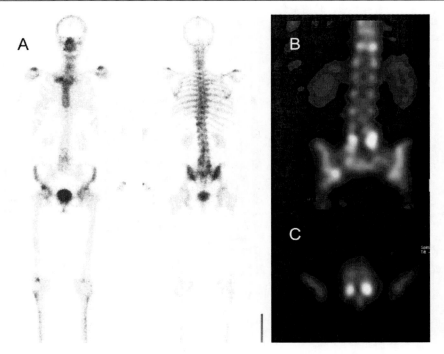

Figure 4.3. Whole body bone scintigraphy of a patient with breast cancer shows multiple focal areas of increased uptake involving the spine (A). SPECT shows typical uptake in the facet joints (facet joint arthritis) and also in the left sacroiliac joint (B & C) (courtesy of Dr. Elham Habibi, Department of Nuclear Medicine, University Hospital Bonn, Germany).

Tumoral Bone Lesions

In oncology, whole-body bone scintigraphy is the standard procedure for: (a) detection of metastases or local invasion for pre-therapeutic staging of tumor, (b) detection of pathologic fractures, (c) assessment of abnormal laboratory findings indicating bone involvement (e.g. elevated prostatic specific antigen in a patient with prostate cancer), (d) differential diagnosis of new-onset musculoskeletal symptoms, and (e) evaluation of treatment response. Regarding the high sensitivity of bone scan, in case of a negative study, no further imaging is usually needed [19]. However, additional SPECT scans of the body area in question should be considered to increase diagnostic sensitivity of the study.

Primary Bone Tumors

Primary bone tumors are uncommon and account for 0.2% of all malignancies with the 5-year survival rate of 67.9% [28]. Bone scans have a sensitivity of 92%, specificity of 71%, and accuracy of 88% for osteogenic sarcoma, compared with 68%, 87%, and 82%, respectively for Ewing's sarcoma [29]. Sensitivity partly depends on the size of the lesion and location of the tumor: planar images may detect lesions as small as 2 cm, while SPECT images are able to detect lesions as small as 1 cm. It is also not uncommon to unmask soft tissue metastases of primary bone tumors in bone scintigraphy, in which case SPECT and SPECT-CT are superior to planar imaging for anatomic localization of the metastatic lesions [30].

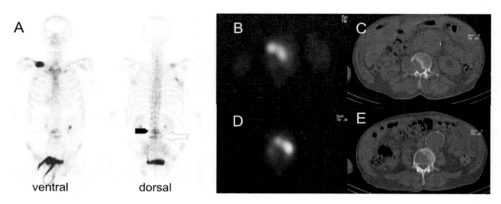

Figure 4.4. Whole body scintigraphy of a patient with ovarian cancer with known pathologic fracture of the right clavicle shows foci of focally increased radiotracer uptake involving the lumbar spine (L3 and L4). SPECT and SPECT/CT images (B-D) show that the L3 uptake is due to a lytic lesion and L4 uptake is caused by degenerative changes (courtesy of Dr. Elham Habibi, Department of Nuclear Medicine, University Hospital Bonn, Germany).

Osteosarcoma

Osteosarcoma is a primary malignant tumor of bone derived from primitive mesenchymal cells and characterized by formation of immature bone or osteoid tissue [31]. Bone scintigraphy is an essential part of metastatic work-up at presentation [31]. Scintigraphically, osteogenic sarcoma manifest as an area of intense radiopharmaceutical uptake; however, areas of decreased activity inside the primary lesion and non-homogenous radiotracer uptake can sometimes be seen, which can be explained by foci of necrosis inside the tumor.

Although at presentation the likelihood of bone metastasis is low, a bone scan is considered a part of initial work-up of patients with osteosarcoma, because it may change the treatment plan, even if the patient is asymptomatic. Although soft tissue metastases of osteosarcoma could theoretically uptake bone-avid radiotracers, a negative result on a bone SPECT study of the chest cannot exclude the possibility of lung metastases. However, if bone SPECT is positive, it may confirm abnormalities seen on chest CT and may also unmasks subtle lesions missed on CT scans [32]. [201]Thallium and ^{99m}Tc-MIBI, and ^{18}F-FDG PET/CT imaging have been employed for the evaluation of recurrence of disease and response to treatment [33-37]. Although in the evaluation of the tumors of the limbs, planar imaging is expected to provide satisfactory results, in the lesions of the pelvis and bones adjacent to organs that uptake ^{99m}Tc-MIBI, SPECT and SPECT-CT present a significant added value.

Due to partial volume effect, bone scans may overestimate the dimensions of the lesion, so MRI is preferred over bone scintigraphy for evaluating the size and extent of tumor in preoperative planning [38]. However, SPECT-CT could potentially be an alternative approach to provide accurate definition of the lesion boundaries [21], but it has not yet been extensively compared with MRI for preoperative planning.

Another advantage of SPECT-CT in the management of osteosarcomas is its adjunctive role to the application of unstructured finite-element discrete ordinate method (DOM) for voxel-based absorbed dose calculations for targeted radionuclide therapy (TRT) with high dose [153]Sm EDTMP. The accuracy of this method has been reported to be comparable to Monte Carlo (MC) simulations in a clinically acceptable amount of time for voxel-based TRT dosimetry. On the other hand, the SPECT-CT voxel-based dose calculation method does not have the associated statistical noise inherent in MC simulations [39]. As conventional techniques based on planar imaging overestimate the radiation dose to bone marrow, SPECT-CT can potentially optimize measurements of the effective dose to the primary bone lesions as well as to bone marrow, the former parameter not being assessable with conventional techniques [40, 41]. SPECT-CT can be employed as a post-[153]Sm EDTMP treatment screening tool for metastatic lesions in complex parts of the body like the chest [42].

Ewing's Sarcoma

Ewing's sarcoma is a rare malignant bone tumor that primarily affects children and adolescents and is considered to be the most lethal bone tumor. In bone scintigram, Ewing's sarcoma shows a focal area of increased radionuclide activity, sometimes with central necrosis (photopenia). As with osteosarcoma, CT and MRI are the primary imaging modalities for the assessment of the local extent of Ewing's sarcoma. Bone scintigraphy is part of the initial work up of patients with Ewing's sarcoma, mainly as a method to screen for metastasis. SPECT-CT has the advantage of providing the opportunity to evaluate bone and adjacent soft tissue involvement at the same time. Three-phase dynamic bone scintigraphy has been employed in the assessment of treatment effects, with a reported accuracy of 88% [43].

Giant Cell Tumor

Giant cell tumor (GCT) is a benign but locally aggressive and destructive tumor of bone, which usually develops in mature skeleton and typically involves the epiphysiometaphyseal region of long bones (particularly the distal femur, proximal tibia and distal radius). Radiographically, GCT is a lytic lesion centered in the epiphysis and extending to the metaphysis and adjacent articular cortex. No mineralized tumor matrix is seen in these lesions [44]. GCT shows increased radiotracer uptake on bone scintigraphy, with patterns that are diffuse (40%) or peripheral with little central activity (60%). The pattern of uptake extends beyond the margins of the primary lesion, which precludes accurate definition of the intramedullary extent [44, 45]. It is not infrequent that increased uptake in the bone across the adjacent joint as well as in other joints of the same extremity not involved by tumor occur [44, 46], a phenomenon which is referred to as "contiguous bone activity" or "extended pattern of uptake," and is related to increased blood flow to the affected limb [47]. Therefore, bone scintigraphy in GCT is nonspecific and unreliable in defining the extent of the tumor and its role is limited [48].

Osteoid Osteoma and Osteoblastoma

Osteoid osteomas and osteoblastomas are primary benign painful skeletal tumors arising from osteoblasts that preferentially afflict young male patients. These tumors are readily treatable and their growth is usually self-limited. Histologically, these neoplasms resemble each other, and are characterized by increased osteoid formation encircled by perilesional sclerosis and fibrous vascular stroma [49]. Therefore, differentiation is usually not histological, but based on the size and site criteria [50]: osteoblastomas are larger than osteoid osteomas with a definition of less than 2 cm for osteoid osteomas, considering larger neoplasms as osteoblastomas; osteoid osteomas most commonly develop in long bones (e.g., femur, tibia), while osteoblastomas are most frequently located in axial skeleton (e.g. vertebrae); and osteoblastomas have a higher rate of recurrence than osteoid osteomas [49].

If clinical suspicion suggests that an osteoid osteoma may still be present in spite of negative radiographic study, bone scintigraphy would be useful because it has a sensitivity of 100% [51]. Early angiographic and blood pool images (phase one and two) often, but not always, show increased activity and allow early localization of the tumor. Delayed static skeletal views (phase three) reveal focally intense radiopharmaceutical uptake at the lesion periphery (the so called double density sign), which is best visualized by a pinhole magnification technique [51]. Superiority of SPECT over planar imaging, particularly in areas with complex anatomy, such as the spine, has been emphasized by a number of case reports [52-57]. In this specific situation, SPECT-CT improves scintigraphic accuracy of osteoid osteoma diagnosis and is superior to SPECT alone study [54, 55]. This is partly because of the complex anatomic structure of the spine. Bone scintigraphic evaluation using a hand-held radiation-detecting device also may be applied preoperatively and intraoperatively to localize the tumor and to ascertain complete removal of the nidus [51].

Multiple Myeloma

Multiple myeloma (MM) is an incurable plasma cell dyscrasia involving bone marrow [58]. Multiple myeloma hardly activates osteoblastic reaction, meaning that bone scintigraphy is less sensitive than CT. Therefore; SPECT-CT is superior to SPECT alone or planar imaging in these patients, with the potential to have higher sensitivity. Also, incremental diagnostic value of SPECT-CT in precise localization of extraskeletal uptake of bone-seeking agents in multiple myeloma has been appreciated [59].

Secondary Bone Tumors

Metastatic bone tumors are much more common than primary bone tumors. Although nuclear medicine modalities generally play a limited role in the diagnosis of primary bone tumors, they are very sensitive and useful in the detection of secondary involvement of bone by tumors and metastases, gauging the response to therapy and estimating the prognosis [51]. ^{99m}Tc-diphosphonates are the main radiopharmaceuticals for this purpose, but some other radiopharmaceuticals such as ^{123}I-MIBG, [201]Thallium chloride, ^{99m}Tc-MIBI, and ^{18}F-FDG have been also employed to detect bone metastases [51].

Bone scintigraphy is a reliable tool for screening metastases from breast, prostate, lung and a number of other cancers which produce osteoblastic metastatic lesions. However, it is less sensitive for detecting tumors with predominately lytic bone lesions or only minimal osteoblastic reaction, such as multiple myeloma or aggressive metastatic lesions with rapid bone destruction. Such lytic lesions may come out "cold" on planar bone scintigraphy and are not uncommonly overlooked. In this specific situation, SPECT imaging has the remarkable advantage to more easily detect abnormalities not found in planar imaging. Although SPECT acquisition for osteoblastic metastatic lesions has the advantage of a better anatomical localization of the lesion and higher diagnostic accuracy, this advantage is much more pronounced and appreciated for osteolytic metastases [7]. On the other hand, benign conditions such as hemangioma may also present as photopenic spots, a fact which emphasizes the accurate differentiation of them from malignant disease [19]. The differentiation can often be achieved by analyzing anatomical details provided by concomitant CT imaging [19]. SPECT-CT is superior to planar imaging or SPECT alone for the evaluation of primary bone lesions: in a study of 47 patients with tumors who had 104 equivocal lesions on bone scintigraphy, with histological confirmation or long-term follow-up as the gold standard, SPECT-CT allowed the correct diagnosis in 85% of cases. The highest diagnostic gain is in the spine, rib cage, skull and pelvis, by characterizing the true nature of focal areas of increased uptake. Small osteolytic lesions were missed because of the limited resolution of transmission images [21]. In the largest study to date, with 440 lesions in 69 patients and considering a 6 month follow-up as the reference standard, SPECT-CT detected 64% more lesions than planar bone scan and correctly classified over 88% of lesions and 95% of patients [60].

In some anatomical locations, such as the spine, SPECT has been proven to be significantly superior to planar imaging in detecting bone lesions: SPECT detects 20%–50% more lesions in the spine compared with planar bone scintigraphy [14]. SPECT shows the respective sensitivity, specificity, positive predictive value, and negative predictive value of 91%, 93%, 73%, and 98% for the detection of bone metastases [15]. Increased radiotracer uptake by the pedicles or posterior vertebral body often points to a metastasis, whereas high radiotracer activity in the facet joints is usually due to a benign etiology like degenerative diseases. This improved anatomic localization of the lesions plays a major role in the increased specificity of the test [61]. Another advantage of SPECT-CT is the definition of suspicious bone lesions to guide subsequent biopsy [19]. SPECT also allows for a straightforward comparison of bone scintigraphy findings with other tomographic-based techniques, e.g. CT and MRI.

In a study of 45 oncologic patients, Utsunomiya et al. showed increased diagnostic confidence obtained with fused SPECT-CT images compared with separate sets of bone scintigraphy and CT images in differentiating malignant from benign bone lesions.

The term "SPECT-guided CT" refers to the adjustment of CT field of view based on bone metabolism as shown by bone scintigraphy [41]. Employing this method in patients with undetermined lesions, 92% of abnormal uptake foci visualized by SPECT could be correctly classified, with the highest gain for lesions in the spine column, ribs and pelvis [20]. The study of Strobel et al. validated the above-mentioned findings by classifying 100% of focal lesions of the axial skeleton, with significant advantages over both planar and SPECT alone imaging [62].

A healing "flare phenomenon" has been characterized by increased radiotracer uptake in an area of previously noted skeletal metastasis on a bone scan associated with increased sclerosis on radiographs or CT scan. Flare phenomenon is usually observed during the first 3 months after chemotherapy [51]. Although this represents a favorable response to therapy, the most important challenge is to differentiate flare phenomenon from progressive disease. In this specific situation, SPECT-CT has a remarkable advantage over SPECT and planar imaging, as CT findings of increased bone destruction in the areas of increased radiotracer uptake point toward progressive disease, while increased osteoblastic sclerosis points toward flare phenomenon.

SPECT-CT is also advantageous over SPECT alone studies, when other radiopharmaceuticals (e.g. ^{123}I-MIBG; see chapter 7) are used: SPECT-CT improves differentiation of physiological diffuse intraluminal bowel activity from pathologic uptake by the tumor, localization of lesions with abnormal uptake, and detection of bone and bone marrow involvement and tumor recurrence adjacent to organs with physiological ^{123}I-MIBG activity [23].

Conclusion and Future Directions

Nuclear medicine has come into a new era of multimodality imaging, in which scintigraphic findings are simultaneously correlated with anatomical modalities, mainly with CT. The hybrid and integrated systems that acquire SPECT and CT data at the same fused functional–anatomic images have been found to improve the diagnostic accuracy of scintigraphic studies in detecting malignant bone involvement and can also assist in identifying accompanying complications in the soft tissue from the CT component of the study. Therefore, SPECT-CT should be applied whenever planar bone imaging findings are equivocal (Figures 4-1 & 4-4). It also improves diagnostic accuracy of leukocyte scanning to diagnose osteomyelitis and to detect sites of inflammation [19]. SPECT-CT has revolutionized and optimized conventional nuclear medicine by achieving accurate diagnosis in a fast, noninvasive, comprehensive, and inexpensive approach [19]. This hybrid imaging technology will eventually grow to be the gold standard for conventional scintigraphy, including bone imaging for cancer staging [18]. However, further gamma cameras and software advances are needed to allow for the performance of whole-body SPECT bone scintigraphy in a practical acquisition and processing time [7]. The role of integrated metabolic/anatomic imaging (e.g. SPECT-CT) in changing clinical management will continue to evolve and these tools will be the basic elements of "personalized medicine" [51].

References

[1]   Hamaoka T., Madewell J. E., Podoloff D. A., Hortobagyi G. N., Ueno N. T. Bone imaging in metastatic breast cancer. *J Clin Oncol* 2004; 22: 2942-53.

[2] Blake G. M., Park-Holohan S. J., Cook G. J., Fogelman I. Quantitative studies of bone with the use of 18F-fluoride and 99mTc-methylene diphosphonate. *Semin Nucl Med* 2001; 31: 28-49.

[3] Tryciecky E. W., Gottschalk A., Ludema K. Oncologic imaging: interactions of nuclear medicine with CT and MRI using the bone scan as a model. *Semin Nucl Med* 1997; 27: 142-51.

[4] Brenner A. I., Koshy J,. Morey J., Lin C., di Poce J. The bone scan. *Semin Nucl Med* 2012; 42: 11-26.

[5] Mettler F. A., Bhargavan M., Thomadsen B. R., Gilley D. B., Lipoti J. A. et al. Nuclear medicine exposure in the United States, 2005-2007: preliminary results. *Semin Nucl Med* 2008; 38: 384-91.

[6] Padhani A. R., Husband J. E., Gueret Wardle D. Radiation induced liver injury detected by particulate reticuloendothelial contrast agent. *Br J Radiol* 1998; 71: 1089-92.

[7] Even-Sapir E. Imaging of malignant bone involvement by morphologic, scintigraphic, and hybrid modalities. *Journal of nuclear medicine : Official publication, Society of Nuclear Medicine* 2005; 46: 1356-67.

[8] Schirrmeister H., Guhlmann A., Kotzerke J., Santjohanser C., Kuhn T. et al. Early detection and accurate description of extent of metastatic bone disease in breast cancer with fluoride ion and positron emission tomography. *J Clin Oncol* 1999; 17: 2381-9.

[9] Vijayanathan S., Butt S., Gnanasegaran G., Groves A. M. Advantages and limitations of imaging the musculoskeletal system by conventional radiological, radionuclide, and hybrid modalities. *Semin Nucl Med* 2009; 39: 357-68.

[10] Ziessman H., O'Malley J. P., Thall J. H. *Nuclear Medicine:* The Requisites 3ed: St Louis, MO, Mosby 2006.

[11] Patel M. Upper extremity radionuclide bone imaging: shoulder, arm, elbow, and forearm. *Semin Nucl Med* 1998; 28: 3-13.

[12] Handmaker H., Leonards R. The bone scan in inflammatory osseous disease. *Semin Nucl Med* 1976; 6: 95-105.

[13] Even-Sapir E., Martin R. H., Barnes D. C., Pringle C. R., Iles S. E. et al. Role of SPECT in differentiating malignant from benign lesions in the lower thoracic and lumbar vertebrae. *Radiology* 1993; 187: 193-8.

[14] Gates G. F. SPECT bone scanning of the spine. *Semin Nucl Med* 1998; 28: 78-94.

[15] Savelli G., Maffioli L., Maccauro M., de Deckere E., Bombardieri E. Bone scintigraphy and the added value of SPECT (single photon emission tomography) in detecting skeletal lesions. *Q J Nucl Med* 2001; 45: 27-37.

[16] Algra P. R., Heimans J. J., Valk J., Nauta J. J., Lachniet M. et al. Do metastases in vertebrae begin in the body or the pedicles? Imaging study in 45 patients. *AJR Am J Roentgenol* 1992; 158: 1275-9.

[17] Yuh W. T., Zachar C. K., Barloon T. J., Sato Y., Sickels W. J. et al. Vertebral compression fractures: distinction between benign and malignant causes with MR imaging. *Radiology* 1989; 172: 215-8.

[18] Bockisch A., Freudenberg L. S., Schmidt D., Kuwert T. Hybrid imaging by SPECT-CT and PET/CT: proven outcomes in cancer imaging. *Semin Nucl Med* 2009; 39: 276-89.

[19] Horger M., Bares R. The role of single-photon emission computed tomography/ computed tomography in benign and malignant bone disease. *Semin Nucl Med* 2006; 36: 286-94.

[20] Romer W., Nomayr A., Uder M., Bautz W., Kuwert T. SPECT-guided CT for evaluating foci of increased bone metabolism classified as indeterminate on SPECT in cancer patients. *Journal of nuclear medicine : Official publication, Society of Nuclear Medicine* 2006; 47: 1102-6.

[21] Horger M., Eschmann S. M., Pfannenberg C., Vonthein R., Besenfelder H. et al. Evaluation of combined transmission and emission tomography for classification of skeletal lesions. *AJR Am J Roentgenol* 2004; 183: 655-61.

[22] Keidar Z., Israel O., Krausz Y. SPECT-CT in tumor imaging: technical aspects and clinical applications. *Semin Nucl Med* 2003; 33: 205-18.

[23] Delbeke D., Schoder H., Martin W. H., Wahl R. L. Hybrid imaging (SPECT-CT and PET/CT): improving therapeutic decisions. *Semin Nucl Med* 2009; 39: 308-40.

[24] Metser U., Lerman H., Blank A., Lievshitz G., Bokstein F. et al. Malignant involvement of the spine: assessment by 18F-FDG PET/CT. *Journal of nuclear medicine : official publication, Society of Nuclear Medicine* 2004; 45: 279-84.

[25] Zhao Z., Li L., Li F., Zhao L. Single photon emission computed tomography/spiral computed tomography fusion imaging for the diagnosis of bone metastasis in patients with known cancer. *Skeletal Radiol* 2010; 39: 147-53.

[26] Gnanasegaran G., Barwick T., Adamson K., Mohan H., Sharp D. et al. Multislice SPECT-CT in benign and malignant bone disease: when the ordinary turns into the extraordinary. *Semin Nucl Med* 2009; 39: 431-42.

[27] van Goethem J. W. M., van den Hauwe L., Ozsarlak O., de Schepper A. M. A., Parizel P. M. Spinal tumors. *Eur J Radiol* 2004; 50: 159-76.

[28] Franchi A. Epidemiology and classification of bone tumors. *Clin Cases Miner Bone Metab* 2012; 9: 92-5.

[29] Franzius C., Sciuk J., Daldrup-Link H. E., Jurgens H., Schober O. FDG-PET for detection of osseous metastases from malignant primary bone tumours: comparison with bone scintigraphy. *Eur J Nucl Med* 2000; 27: 1305-11.

[30] Gholamrezanezhad A., Moinian D., Mirpour S., Hajimohammadi H. Unilateral pulmonary metastases from Ewing's sarcoma shown in a technetium-99m-methylene-diphosphonate bone scan. *Hell J Nucl Med* 2006; 9: 181-3.

[31] Ritter J. G., Spille J.-H., Kaminski T., Kubitscheck U. A cylindrical zoom lens unit for adjustable optical sectioning in light sheet microscopy. *Biomed Opt Express* 2010; 2: 185-93.

[32] Pevarski D. J., Drane W. E., Scarborough M. T. The usefulness of bone scintigraphy with SPECT images for detection of pulmonary metastases from osteosarcoma. *AJR Am J Roentgenol* 1998; 170: 319-22.

[33] Huang Z. K., Lou C., Shi G. H. (2) (0) (1) TI and (99m)Tc-MIBI scintigraphy in evaluation of neoadjuvant chemotherapy for osteosarcoma]. *Zhejiang da xue xue bao Yi xue ban = Journal of Zhejiang University Medical sciences* 2012; 41: 183-7, 91.

[34] Miwa S., Shirai T., Taki J., Sumiya H., Nishida H. et al. Use of 99mTc-MIBI scintigraphy in the evaluation of the response to chemotherapy for osteosarcoma: comparison with 201Tl scintigraphy and angiography. *Int J Clin Oncol* 2011; 16: 373-8.

[35] Soderlund V., Larsson S. A., Bauer H. C., Brosjo O., Larsson O. et al. Use of 99mTc-MIBI scintigraphy in the evaluation of the response of osteosarcoma to chemotherapy. *Eur J Nucl Med* 1997; 24: 511-5.

[36] Garcia-Fernandez R., Hernandez-Hernandez D. M., Iwasaki-Otake L., Mantilla-Morales A., Ortiz-Rodriguez L. et al. [Scintigraphy with 99mTc-MIBI for assessment of tumor response to preoperative chemotherapy in patients with osteosarcoma]. *Revista de investigacion clinica; organo del Hospital de Enfermedades de la Nutricion* 2001; 53: 324-9.

[37] Bar-Sever Z., Cohen I. J., Connolly L. P., Horev G., Perri T. et al. Tc-99m MIBI to evaluate children with Ewing's sarcoma. *Clinical nuclear medicine* 2000; 25: 410-3.

[38] Enneking W. F. Is limb amputation necessary for locally advanced soft tissue sarcomas? Arbiter. *Eur J Cancer* 1997; 33: 2300-1.

[39] Mikell J., Vassiliev O., Erwin W., Wareing T., Failla G. et al. A novel SPECT-CT voxel-based dose calculation method for targeted radionuclide therapy. *J NUCL MED MEETING ABSTRACTS* 2009; 50: 271-.

[40] Vanzi E., Genovesi D., di Martino F. Evaluation of a method for activity estimation in Sm-153 EDTMP imaging. *Medical physics* 2009; 36: 1219-29.

[41] Mariani G., Bruselli L., Kuwert T., Kim E. E., Flotats A. et al. A review on the clinical uses of SPECT-CT. *European journal of nuclear medicine and molecular imaging* 2010; 37: 1959-85.

[42] Tiemann K., Stypmann J., Stymann J., Landeta F., Wiebe S. et al. Three-dimensional echocardiography and 153Sm-EDTMP SPECT-CT in extensive cardiac metastases from osteosarcoma. *European journal of nuclear medicine and molecular imaging* 2010; 37: 2406-.

[43] Ozcan Z., Burak Z., Kumanlioglu K., Sabah D., Basdemir G. et al. Assessment of chemotherapy-induced changes in bone sarcomas: clinical experience with 99Tcm-MDP three-phase dynamic bone scintigraphy. *Nuclear medicine communications* 1999; 20: 41-8.

[44] Purohit S., Pardiwala D. N. Imaging of giant cell tumor of bone. *Indian J Orthop* 2007; 41: 91-6.

[45] Hudson T. M., Schiebler M., Springfield D. S., Enneking W. F., Hawkins I. F. et al. Radiology of giant cell tumors of bone: computed tomography, arthro-tomography, and scintigraphy. *Skeletal Radiol* 1984; 11: 85-95.

[46] Gudmundsson J., Ekelund L., Pettersson H. New diagnostic modalities in the diagnosis of primary and recurrent giant-cell tumors of bone. *Radiologe* 1984; 24: 222-6.

[47] Murphey M. D., Nomikos G. C., Flemming D. J., Gannon F. H., Temple H. T. et al. From the archives of AFIP. Imaging of giant cell tumor and giant cell reparative granuloma of bone: radiologic-pathologic correlation. *Radiographics* 2001; 21: 1283-309.

[48] van Nostrand D., Madewell J. E., McNiesh L. M., Kyle R. W., Sweet D. Radionuclide bone scanning in giant cell tumor. *Journal of nuclear medicine : official publication, Society of Nuclear Medicine* 1986; 27: 329-38.

[49] Atesok K. I., Alman B. A., Schemitsch E. H., Peyser A., Mankin H. Osteoid osteoma and osteoblastoma. *J Am Acad Orthop Surg* 2011; 19: 678-89.

[50] Kirwan E. O., Hutton P. A., Pozo J. L., Ransford A. O. Osteoid osteoma and benign osteoblastoma of the spine. Clinical presentation and treatment. *J Bone Joint Surg Br* 1984; 66: 21-6.

[51] Nikpoor N. Scintigraphy of the Musculoskeletal System In: Weissman B, ed. *Imaging of Arthritis and Metabolic Bone Disease*: Elsevier 2009:17-32.

[52] Banzo I., Montero A., Uriarte I., Vallina N. K., Hernandez A. et al. [Localization by bone SPET of osteoid osteoma in the vertebral lamina]. *Rev Esp Med Nucl* 1999; 18: 47-9.

[53] Birchall J. D., Blackband K., Freeman B. J., Ganatra R. H., O'Leary M. et al. Precise localisation of osteoblastoma with SPET/CT. *European journal of nuclear medicine and molecular imaging* 2004; 31: 308-.

[54] Farid K., Meissner W. G., Samier-Foubert A., Barret O., Menegon P. et al. Normal cerebrovascular reactivity in Stroke-like Migraine Attacks after Radiation Therapy syndrome. *Clinical nuclear medicine* 2010; 35: 583-5.

[55] Hephzibah J., Theodore B., Oommen R., David K., Moses V. et al. Use of single-photon emission computed tomography/low-resolution computed tomography fusion imaging in detecting an unusually presenting osteoid osteoma of the lumbar vertebra. *Am J Orthop (Belle Mead NJ)* 2009; 38: 117-9.

[56] Murray I. P., Rossleigh M. A., van der Wall H. The use of SPECT in the diagnosis of epiphyseal osteoid osteoma. *Clinical nuclear medicine* 1989; 14: 811-3.

[57] Ryan P. J., Fogelman I. Bone SPECT in osteoid osteoma of the vertebral lamina. *Clinical nuclear medicine* 1994; 19: 144-5.

[58] Walker R. C., Brown T. L., Jones-Jackson L. B., de Blanche L., Bartel T. Imaging of multiple myeloma and related plasma cell dyscrasias. *Journal of nuclear medicine : official publication, Society of Nuclear Medicine* 2012; 53: 1091-101.

[59] Gholamrezanezhad A., Sabet A., Ezziddin S., Biersack H.-J., Ahmadzadehfar H. Incremental diagnostic value of SPET/CT in precise localization of extraskeletal uptake of bone-seeking agents in multiple myeloma. *Hell J Nucl Med* 2010; 13: 285-6.

[60] Granier P., Mourad M. Évaluation par la TEMP–TDM des lésions classées indéterminées en scintigraphie osseuse chez les patients de cancérologie. *Med Nuc* 2008; 32: 265-72.

[61] Papathanassiou D., Bruna-Muraille C., Jouannaud C., Gagneux-Lemoussu L., Eschard J.-P. et al. Single-photon emission computed tomography combined with computed tomography (SPECT-CT) in bone diseases. *Joint Bone Spine* 2009; 76: 474-80.

[62] Strobel K., Burger C., Seifert B., Husarik D. B., Soyka J. D. et al. Characterization of focal bone lesions in the axial skeleton: performance of planar bone scintigraphy compared with SPECT and SPECT fused with CT. *AJR Am J Roentgenol* 2007; 188: 467-74.

In: SPECT   ISBN: 978-1-62808-344-6
Editors: Hojjat Ahmadzadehfar and Elham Habibi   © 2013 Nova Science Publishers, Inc.

Chapter V

Ventilation/Perfusion Tomography in Diagnosis of Pulmonary Embolism and Other Pulmonary Diseases: Methodology and Clinical Implementation

Marika Bajc*
Department of Clinical Physiology,
Lund University Hospital, Lund, Sweden

Introduction

Pulmonary embolism (PE) remains a big diagnostic challenge since the clinical symptoms and signs which are frequently observed in PE are also a feature of other conditions. Accordingly, the initial clinical suspicion needs to be confirmed or negated using a conclusive imaging test. Multidetector CT (MDCT) has been suggested as the initial imaging study by many authors, although the latest evidence shows that the optimal test is ventilation/perfusion (V/P) SPECT interpreted with holistic principles according to European Guidelines [1]. Before performing imaging tests, it is recommended to estimate the clinical probability of PE [2, 3]. Usually, the Wells score is applied [4], although a more precise predictive model developed by Miniati et al. is recommended [5]. Easy-to-use software is also available for computation (palm computer) (http://www.ifc.cnr.it/pisamodel).

The measurement of D-dimer - a breakdown product of the cross-linked fibrin clot - is widely used in the investigative workup of patients with suspected venous thromboembolism [4, 6]. However, D-dimer has low specificity (40%), because a number of conditions, other than venous thromboembolism, may cause it to be elevated, e.g. acute myocardial infarction,

---

* E-mail: marika.bajc@med.lu.se.

stroke, inflammation, active cancer and pregnancy. The specificity declines even further with age and, in the elderly, may reach only 10% [6]. Due to the low predictive value, a positive quantitative D-dimer test does not modify the pretest probability. A negative quantitative D-dimer test combined with a low clinical probability is associated with a low risk of thromboembolic disease. At moderate to high pretest clinical probability, D-dimer has no incremental value.

In this chapter, the advantages of V/P SPECT in accordance with the European Guidelines for V/P SPECT are demonstrated [1, 2]. It will be emphasized that V/P SPECT gives diagnostic information in other conditions such as pneumonia, COPD and left heart failure. Moreover it fulfills the basic requirements of a diagnostic method for PE, such as low radiation dose, high diagnostic accuracy, few non-diagnostic reports, utility for selection of treatment strategy suitability for follow-up and research.

Basic Principles of PE Diagnosis with V/P SPECT

The lung circulation has a distinct construction where each bronchopulmonary segment and sub-segment is supplied by a single end-artery. Embolisms are usually multiple, occluding the arteries causing segmental or sub-segmental perfusion defects within still ventilated regions, causing so called mismatch (Figure 5-1). PE is often a recurring process giving rise to multiple emboli in various stages of resolution (Figure 5-2).

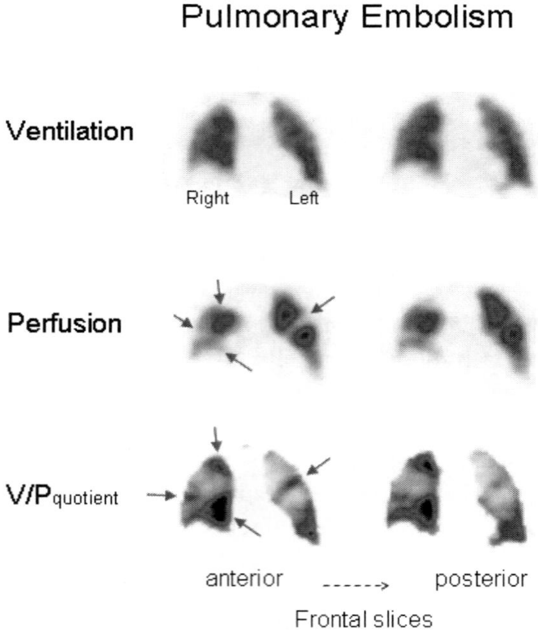

Figure 5.1. Patient with PE. Coronal slices; ventilation with corresponding perfusion images and quotient images. Multiple areas with absent perfusion (arrows) and preserved ventilation, clearly visible as mismatch on V/P quotient images.

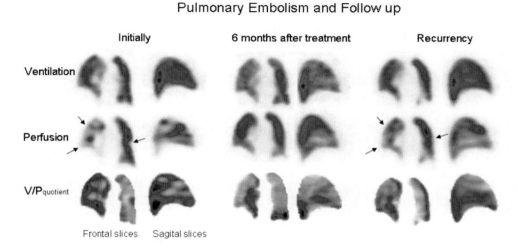

Figure 5.2. Patient with PE. Follow up, coronal and sagittal slices; ventilation with corresponding perfusion images and quotient images. Initially (left), after 6 months treatment (middle), and recurrence (right). Arrows show areas with PE with absent of perfusion and preserved ventilation.

In clinical practice, it is essential to have a procedure that is both fast and conclusive to avoid the risks associated with untreated disease. Therefore it is recommended that imaging tests for PE diagnosis should be carried out as soon as possible, preferably within 24 hours of the onset of symptoms.

Imaging Protocols

V/P SPECT Acquisition

Administration of ventilation and perfusion agents should be performed with patients in a supine position, so as to minimize gravitational gradients. During inhalation, activity over the lungs should be monitored to ensure adequacy of pulmonary deposition. The procedure starts with ventilation scintigraphy, which is usually based upon inhalation of a radio-aerosol (Table 5-1).

Large particles, > 2 μm, are deposited mainly by impaction in the large airways. Very fine particles, <1 μm, are mainly deposited in the alveoli by diffusion. In comparison with liquid aerosols, Technegas has shown significantly reduced problems with central airway deposition and peripheral hotspot formation in patients with obstructive lung disease [7]. Therefore, Technegas is recommended in COPD.

Perfusion tomography follows immediately after ventilation SPECT without changing the patient position. The nearly universally used agent for perfusion scintigraphy is technetium-labeled particles of macroaggregates of human albumin (^{99m}Tc-MAA). After i.v. injection, the particles 15-100 μm in size are lodged in the pulmonary capillaries and in the precapillary arterioles in proportion to perfusion.

Table 5.1. Ventilation/perfusion protocol for lung tomography (V/P SPECT)

Patient preparation	not needed				
Patient position	supine position				
	Administration	Radiopharmaceutica and administered activity	Particle size	Acquisition protocol	Time of Imaging
Ventilation	inhalation	Technegas ® 25-30 MBq	0.09 µm	general purpose collimator: 64 x 64 matrix, 60-64 steps for each head, 10 s/step	ca. 11 minutes
Perfusion	i.v. injection	^{99m}Tc-MAA 120-140 MBq	15-100 µm	general purpose collimator: 64 x 64 matrix, 60-64 steps for each head, 5 s/step	ca. 5 minutes
Reconstruction				iterative reconstruction - eight subsets and two iterations	

To achieve adequate imaging quality, with low radiation exposure, in a short time, the relationships between activities, acquisition times, collimators and matrices for SPECT imaging must be optimized. This problem was systematically analyzed by Palmer et al. in the context of a dual head gamma camera [8]. Doses of 25-30 MBq for ventilation studies and 120-140 MBq for perfusion studies were found to be optimal using a general purpose collimator and a 64x64 matrix. This allowed a total acquisition time of only 20 minutes. A matrix of 128x128 required higher doses and/or longer acquisition time. This is not advocated as it did not yield images of significantly higher quality.

Many centers are using much higher doses. As ethical concerns and good medical practice are crucial issues, radiation exposure should be minimized to the lowest level consistent with satisfactory image quality. For V/P SPECT, it is important to use iterative reconstruction. OSEM (ordered-subset expectation maximization) is recommended with eight subsets and two iterations. Standard software can be used for image presentation in coronal, sagittal and transversal projections as well as for presentation of rotating 3-D images. We have developed a way of calculating and displaying ventilation/perfusion quotient images. This is based upon acquisition as described above. Ventilation is normalized to perfusion counts, and then the V/P quotient images are calculated. V/P quotient images facilitate diagnosis and quantification of PE extension. Using this protocol, attenuation correction is not needed [8, 9].

For quality control and fast orientation, an overview of ventilation and perfusion in coronal and sagittal slices is useful. It is important to present the images so that ventilation and perfusion are carefully aligned to each other (Figure 5-3). This is greatly facilitated by the single session protocol with the patient in an unchanged position.

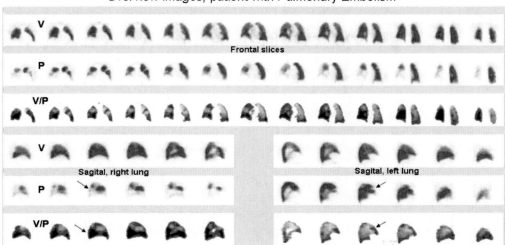

Figure 5.3. Overview image of ventilation and perfusion in coronal and sagittal slices. Ventilation and perfusion are carefully aligned to each other.

The option to triangulate between coronal, sagittal and transverse slices is valuable for the identification of matching and non-matching ventilation and perfusion changes. Proper alignment is also a prerequisite for V/P quotient images. These facilitate the interpretation and quantification of PE extension and all ventilation and perfusion defects. However, quotient images are not a prerequisite for high quality V/P SPECT.

Reporting Findings

Ventilation Perfusion Patterns

For V/P SPECT, a new holistic principle for reporting is as important as the imaging technique itself. This goal was not achieved with previous probabilistic reporting methods according to PIOPED or modified PIOPED [10, 11]. Large V/P SPECT studies have shown that interpretation of all patterns representing ventilation together with perfusion achieves this result [12-16]. Conclusive reports were given in 97 to 99% of cases.

Criteria for Acute PE

The recommended criteria for reading V/P SPECT with respect to acute PE are the following [1, 2]:

PE is reported if there is:

- V/P mismatch of at least one segment or two sub-segments that conform to the pulmonary vascular anatomy

No PE is reported if there is:
A normal perfusion pattern conforming to the anatomic boundaries of the lungs

- matched or reverse mismatched V/P defects of any size, shape or number in the absence of a mismatch
- a mismatch that does not have a lobar, segmental or sub-segmental pattern

Non-diagnostic for PE is reported if there are:

- multiple V/P abnormalities not typical of specific diseases.

It is important to report that, with PE, a mismatch has its base along the pleura and conforms to known sub-segmental and segmental vascular anatomy, as stressed in the PISAPED study [17]. Applying these principles of interpretation, recent V/P SPECT studies amounting to over 3000 cases report a negative predictive value of 97-99%, sensitivities of 96-99%, and specificities of 91-98% for PE diagnosis; rates of non-diagnostic findings were 1-3% [12, 14, 15].

An important step in the diagnostic procedure is to quantify the extent of embolism. V/P SPECT is particularly suitable for this because of its greater sensitivity compared to alternative planar scintigraphy and MDCT [12, 13, 16]. As suggested by Olsson et al., the number of segments and sub-segments indicating PE typical mismatch are counted and expressed as a percentage of the total lung parenchyma [18]. Furthermore, areas with ventilation abnormalities are recognized and this allows for the degree of total lung malfunction to be estimated. The study showed that patients with up 40% PE could be safely treated at home if ventilation abnormalities engaged no more that 20% of the lung. Since 2004, more than 1000 (50%) of patients with PE have been safely treated at home from the University Hospital of Lund.

Importance of Ventilation SPECT in the Diagnosis of Other Lung Diseases

Chronic Obstructive Pulmonary Disease (COPD)

A common alternative or additional diagnosis is COPD. The characteristic is a general unevenness of ventilation. Focal deposition may be observed in central or peripheral airways even when using Technegas [6].

A very important fact is that COPD patients are at high risk of PE. The rate of PE in patients hospitalized for acute exacerbations of COPD may be as high as 25% [19]. In contrast to the PIOPED study, with V/P SPECT, PE can be diagnosed even in the presence of COPD [1, 12, 20].

PE accounts for up to 10% of deaths in stable COPD patients [21]. The degree of unevenness of aerosol distribution is correlated with lung function tests [22]. Significantly, as there are no contraindications to V/P SPECT, even very sick and breathless patients can be studied.

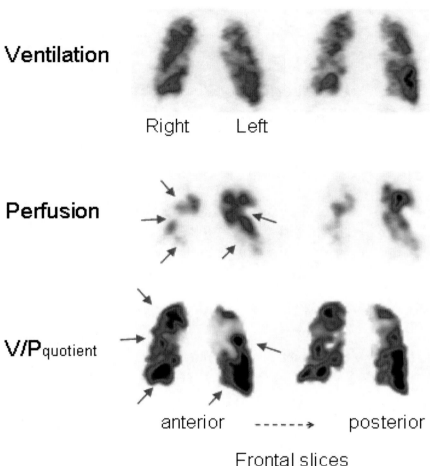

Figure 5.4. Patient with COPD and PE. Coronal slices; very uneven distribution of ventilation with deposition of aerosols in small airways (upper row). Multiple segmental and subsegmental perfusion defects (arrows) in ventilated areas well delineated on V/P quotient images.

Figure 5-4 shows coronal slices in a patient with COPD and PE. Mismatches are highlighted in V/P quotient images.

Pneumonia

Pneumonia is also frequent in patients investigated for suspected PE [10]. A typical finding is a ventilation defect in an area usually with better preserved perfusion, known as reverse mismatch [23, 24].

Pneumonia – Stripe sign

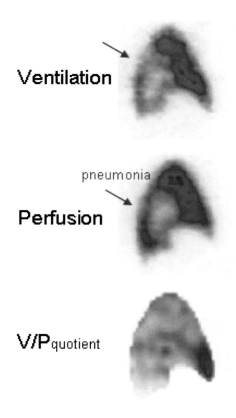

Ventilation

pneumonia

Perfusion

V/P_{quotient}

Sagital slices, left lung

Figure 5.5. Patient with pneumonia in the right lung. Sagittal slices show reduced-absent ventilation posteriorly with reduced perfusion in the same area. Preserved perfusion adjacent to the pleura known as stripe sign showed with arrow.

One of the typical patterns, which strongly support the diagnosis of pneumonia, is the "stripe sign". This refers to maintained perfusion along the pleural surface, peripheral to a central matched defect, as seen in Figure 5-5.

Left Heart Failure

Left heart failure is another diagnosis that is often observed among patients suspected of PE. The typical pattern is anti-gravitational redistribution of perfusion [25, 26]. In consecutive patients with suspected PE, V/P SPECT showed an anti-gravitational redistribution of perfusion from the posterior to anterior region in 15% of cases, indicating left heart failure [27].

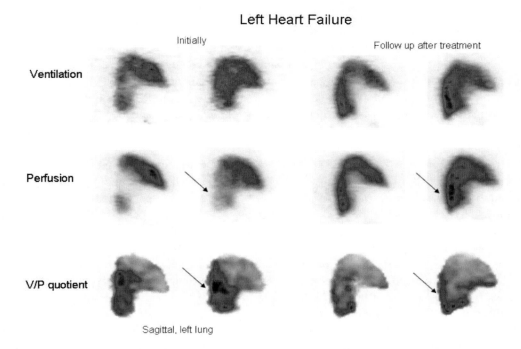

Figure 5.6. Patient with left heart failure in the initial acute stage. Sagittal slices left: Antigravitational distribution of ventilation and perfusion, causing non-segmental V/P mismatch in dorsal regions (arrows). Right: On follow up after 10 days of treatment for left heart failure normalization of distribution of ventilation and perfusion is seen.

The positive predictive value for heart failure in this study was at least 88%. As ventilation is usually less redistributed than perfusion, V/P mismatch may be observed in dorsal regions. This V/P mismatch has a non-segmental pattern and should not be misinterpreted as PE. (Figure 5-6).

V/P SPECT versus MDCT

MDCT is often recommended as the first line test for PE diagnosis [28]. However, the principal study evaluating the use of MDCT as an imaging tool for PE diagnosis shows that sensitivity is not more than 78% and that there are a high number of false positive results when the clinical probability is not high [29]. In this study, the positive predictive value for a PE within a lobar pulmonary artery was 97% but fell to 68 and 25% in segmental and subsegmental pulmonary vessels, respectively.

Advocates for MDCT stress that this method has the advantage over V/P SPECT by allowing alternative diagnoses. Nevertheless, V/P SPECT provides evidence about alternative diagnoses as well. In a V/P SPECT study comprising 1785 patients, an alternative diagnosis was reported in 39% of patients without PE, while among patients with PE, an additional pathology was reported in 22% [12]. Actually, a properly performed V/P SPECT interpreted on the basis of all patterns of ventilation and perfusion frequently allows the diagnosis of other pulmonary diseases with or without PE and a comprehensive understanding of the patient's symptoms. This added value of V/P SPECT appears at least as high as for additional diagnoses as with MDCT. Further studies are needed in order to demonstrate the clinical impact of alternative diagnoses obtained by both methods.

The lack of a satisfactory gold standard for PE diagnosis poses difficulties for the assessment of sensitivity, specificity and accuracy of all diagnostic methods for PE. The best available point of reference is adequate follow-up of the patient to identify a recurrence of PE or alternative diagnoses, as seen in Figure 5-2 and Figure 5-5, respectively.

After a negative single slice CT, PE occurred in 1.4% of patients in a meta-analysis of 4637 patients [29]. After a negative pulmonary angiography study, this was 1.6% [30], and 1.5% after a negative MDCT (n=318). After a negative ventilation/perfusion scintigraphy, the occurrence of PE during follow-up was 0.4% in a total of 1877 patients [31, 32]. Freeman stated that the results from the PIOPED II study "do not clearly support the superiority of CT angiography over ventilation/perfusion scanning for the diagnosis of PE" [33]. This conclusion was based upon the V/P planar technique and probabilistic interpretation. A direct comparison between V/P SPECT and 4-slice, and 16-slice MDCT showed higher sensitivity by V/P SPECT [13, 16]. Further prospective comparisons between up-to-date V/P SPECT and MDCT are needed. In interpreting V/P SPECT, low inter-observer variability has been shown by a kappa value of 0.92 [12]. Moreover, PIOPED II as well as the study by Gutte et al. illustrate well the limited clinical utility of MDCT [13, 29]. In 50% of eligible cases, MDCT could not be performed because of kidney failure, critical illness, recent myocardial infarction, ventilator support and allergy to the contrast agent. Furthermore, 6% of performed MDCT studies were of insufficient quality for conclusive interpretation. In about 1% of subjects, complications such as allergy, contrast extravasation and increased creatinine levels were observed [13, 29]. In contrast, V/P SPECT has no contraindications and was performed in 99% of patients referred to in a study by Bajc et al. [12]. Complications do not occur, and technically suboptimal studies are very rare. It is possible to accommodate patients who are mechanically ventilated by connecting a nebulizer to the inspiratory ventilator line. In rare cases, when V/P SPECT cannot be performed, the planar technique is the alternative.

Radiation Doses

Based upon data from ICRP reports [34], the effective dose for V/P SPECT with the recommended protocol is about 35-40% of the dose from MDCT [35]. The absorbed dose to the female breast for V/P SPECT is only 4% of the dose from MDCT with full dose-saving means according to Hurwitz[36]. This may have particular importance in pregnant women with proliferating breast tissue [37] and in the entire generative period. During the first trimester of pregnancy, the fetal dose of MDCT is greater than or equivalent to that of V/P SPECT [38]. The advantage of V/P SPECT increases after the first trimester.

Follow-Up

Follow-up of PE using imaging is essential to assess: a) the effect of therapy, b) to be able to differentiate between new and old PE where there is a suspicion of PE recurrence and

c) to explain physical incapacity after PE. Figure 5-2 shows that there was a residual perfusion defect when therapy was terminated and PE recurrence at the same locations. These demands for follow-up are only met with V/P SPECT. Obviously, the same method should be used for diagnosis and for follow-up.

Appropriateness for Research

The suitability of an imaging technique for research into PE and its treatment and clinical follow-up are, in principle, the same. However, in research, there are even stronger, ethical, grounds for the use of non-traumatic procedures associated with the lowest possible risks.

Clinical Use of Hybrid V/P SPECT-CT

The hybrid SPECT/CT system is a dual imaging modality technique whose clinical application is particularly relevant in oncological diseases, as it leads to improved sensitivity and specificity, combining the co-registration of anatomical and functional data. It may lead to improved staging and treatment monitoring. As nuclear medicine procedures have the ability to visualize early functional changes much sooner than structural changes occur, additional CT procedure may improve the correction for photon attenuation and allow co-registration of morphology and function. However, SPECT/CT acquisition of the chest constitutes a challenge due to respiratory movements, which can cause image artifacts and thus decrease diagnostic accuracy.

In our department, we use a Philips Presedence system which combines a dual head gamma camera with a Brilliance 16-slice CT.

The procedure starts with a CT overview image and continues with diagnostic low-dose CT. (120 kV, 20 mAs/slice, 16 × 1.5 collimator, 0.5 s rotation time and pitch of 0.813), not used for attenuation correction, but to exactly co-localize the morphological and functional changes visualized in either of the two modalities (Table 5-2). Thereafter, it follows the protocol for V/P SPECT as described above and according to the European Guidelines [1, 2]. Low-dose CT delivers approximately 1 mSv when used for alignment and attenuation correction. However, as a diagnostic tool in this hybrid system, it delivers 2-3 mSv and while V/P SPECT delivers 2.1 mSv.

Some authors have recently recommended V/P SPECT/low-dose CT as a first line procedure in patients with suspected PE. This was based on their prospective study performing V/P SPECT and low-dose CT and making a head-to-head comparison with MDCT [39].

Table 5.2. V/P SPECT-CT protocol

CT overview image				
	Tube potential	Tube current	Collimation/slice width	Pitch
Low dose CT	120 kV	20 mAs	16 x 1.5-0.5 s rotation	0.813

COPD and tumour

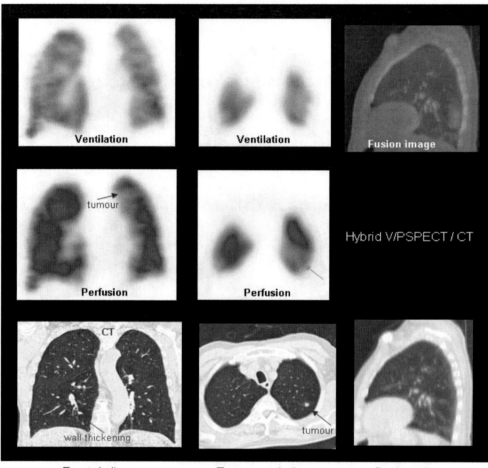

Figure 5.7. Patient with COPD; Left column: The upper images display uneven distribution of ventilation with deposition of Technegas, typical for COPD. Middle images show corresponding perfusion SPECT images presenting similar pattern as ventilation and lower images show corresponding CT images. Blue arrow on CT image shows thickening of the airway wall typical for COPD. In the middle column, transversal slices of ventilation SPECT upper row, with corresponding perfusion SPECT in the middle row. On CT image in lower row small tumor (1 cm) is visualized. Aligning both modalities small perfusion defect is observed in this area (arrow).

In a total of 81 simultaneous studies, 38% of patients had PE. They showed 97% sensitivity and 88% specificity when only V/P SPECT was used. However, adding low-dose CT, the sensitivity was unchanged but specificity increased to 100%. Interestingly, 18% of patients had a false positive PE diagnosis when V/P SPECT alone was interpreted. A reason for this may be that they were interpreting every mismatch as PE and not only mismatches that conform to segmental lung circulation as recommended by the European Guidelines [1, 2].

In our department, we use V/P SPECT as a primary tool in patients with suspected PE. Since 2003, more than 12 000 examinations have been performed. Based on our experience, we do not recommend hybrid V/P SPECT-CT as a first line procedure for all patients with suspected PE. It is not ethical to advocate the higher radiation dose (2-3mSv) for every patient with suspected PE where the prevalence of PE is about 30% at our hospital and might be as low as 10% [3]. Therefore, in our opinion, the recommendation to use the hybrid system for PE diagnosis is premature. Coco et al. [40] showed that CT utilization has increased dramatically in the evaluation of patients with suspected PE, without improving the rate of PE or other clinically significant diagnoses. Moreover, patients are exposed to the risks of radiation [41, 42]. Therefore, it is important to validate the V/P SPECT-CT system and not to adopt it too quickly, without fully assessing the benefits and risks.

We consider, however, that the dual modality will have an impact in some groups of patients. SPECT-CT may provide a significant contribution to COPD patients where architecture of the lung is changed and remodeled. COPD patients are usually also more prone to complications, such as PE, pneumonia and left heart failure. Moreover, many of these patients have a tendency to develop tumors. These tumors are usually small and can only be visualized by CT. The correlation of perfusion defects on perfusion slices with specific pulmonary arterial branches seen on CT slices and heterogeneous defects on ventilation slices caused by airway changes could be easier to understand and interpret when applying both modalities. Figure 5-7 show V/P SPECT images in a patient with COPD. An uneven distribution of ventilation and the corresponding perfusion images can be seen, typical for COPD (left column – upper and middle row). On CT, lower lobe COPD sign is seen as a thickening of the wall. In the middle column, a small tumor is delineated on the CT transversal slice in the left upper lobe. The tumor caused decreased/absent perfusion; this is clearer when aligning both modalities. Increased knowledge will improve future interpretation. Moreover, V/P SPECT-CT might help with better classifying COPD patients by improving the estimate of obstructivity [20]. A study is in progress to validate this.

Conclusion

VP SPECT should be used as a primary tool for the diagnosis of PE because it has the highest sensitivity and accuracy, and neither contraindications nor complications. In addition, it produces very few non-diagnostic reports. Furthermore, radiation doses are very low. This is particularly important for women in the reproductive period and during pregnancy.

To take full advantage of the potential of V/P SPECT, it is crucial to apply an optimal protocol for a single session of imaging for both ventilation and perfusion using low nuclide activities. Furthermore, full use should be made of display options, which are integrated into modern camera systems. Most important of all is holistic interpretation, giving a clear report with respect to PE, its extension as well as other diagnoses based on ventilation/perfusion patterns typical of various diseases.

The abovementioned advantages of V/P SPECT for studying PE imply that it may be the most suitable technique both for follow-up in patients with PE as well as for research regarding its treatment and pathophysiology.

Acknowledgments

The author thanks Kerstin Brauer for her excellent technical assistance.

References

[1]   Bajc M, Neilly JB, Miniati M, Schuemichen C, Meignan M et al. EANM guidelines for ventilation/perfusion scintigraphy: Part 1. Pulmonary imaging with ventilation/perfusion single photon emission tomography. *European journal of nuclear medicine and molecular imaging* 2009; 36: 1356-70.

[2]   Bajc M, Neilly JB, Miniati M, Schuemichen C, Meignan M et al. EANM guidelines for ventilation/perfusion scintigraphy : Part 2. Algorithms and clinical considerations for diagnosis of pulmonary emboli with V/P(SPECT) and MDCT. *European journal of nuclear medicine and molecular imaging* 2009; 36: 1528-38.

[3]   Mamlouk MD, vanSonnenberg E, Gosalia R, Drachman D, Gridley D et al. Pulmonary embolism at CT angiography: implications for appropriateness, cost, and radiation exposure in 2003 patients. *Radiology* 2010; 256: 625-32.

[4]   Wells PS, Anderson DR, Rodger M, Stiell I, Dreyer JF et al. Excluding pulmonary embolism at the bedside without diagnostic imaging: management of patients with suspected pulmonary embolism presenting to the emergency department by using a simple clinical model and d-dimer. *Ann. Intern. Med.* 2001; 135: 98-107.

[5]   Miniati M, Bottai M, Monti S, Salvadori M, Serasini L et al. Simple and accurate prediction of the clinical probability of pulmonary embolism. *Am. J. Respir. Crit. Care Med.* 2008; 178: 290-4.

[6]   Stein PD, Hull RD, Patel KC, Olson RE, Ghali WA et al. D-dimer for the exclusion of acute venous thrombosis and pulmonary embolism: a systematic review. *Ann. Intern. Med.* 2004; 140: 589-602.

[7]   Jogi J, Jonson B, Ekberg M, Bajc M. Ventilation-perfusion SPECT with 99mTc-DTPA versus Technegas: a head-to-head study in obstructive and nonobstructive disease. *Journal of nuclear medicine : official publication, Society of Nuclear Medicine* 2010; 51: 735-41.

[8]   Palmer J, Bitzen U, Jonson B, Bajc M. Comprehensive ventilation/perfusion SPECT. *Journal of nuclear medicine : official publication, Society of Nuclear Medicine* 2001; 42: 1288-94.

[9]   Bajc M, Olsson C-G, Palmer J, Jonson B. Quantitative Ventilation/Perfusion SPECT (QV/PSPECT): A primary Method for Diagnosis of Pulmonary embolism. In: Freeman LM, ed. *Nuclear Medicine Annual*: Lippincott Williams and Wilkins 2004:173-6.

[10]   Value of the ventilation/perfusion scan in acute pulmonary embolism. Results of the prospective investigation of pulmonary embolism diagnosis (PIOPED). The PIOPED Investigators. *JAMA* 1990; 263: 2753-9.

[11]   Stein PD, Hull RD, Patel KC, Olson RE, Ghali WA et al. Venous thromboembolic disease: comparison of the diagnostic process in blacks and whites. *Arch. Intern. Med.* 2003; 163: 1843-8.

[12] Bajc M, Olsson B, Palmer J, Jonson B. Ventilation/Perfusion SPECT for diagnostics of pulmonary embolism in clinical practice. *J. Intern Med.* 2008; 264: 379-87.

[13] Gutte H, Mortensen J, Jensen CV, Johnbeck CB, von der Recke P et al. Detection of pulmonary embolism with combined ventilation-perfusion SPECT and low-dose CT: head-to-head comparison with multidetector CT angiography. *Journal of nuclear medicine : official publication, Society of Nuclear Medicine* 2009; 50: 1987-92.

[14] Leblanc M, Leveillee F, Turcotte E. Prospective evaluation of the negative predictive value of V/Q SPECT using 99mTc-Technegas. *Nuclear medicine communications* 2007; 28: 667-72.

[15] Lemb M, Pohlabeln H. Pulmonary thromboembolism: a retrospective study on the examination of 991 patients by ventilation/perfusion SPECT using Technegas. *Nuklearmedizin* 2001; 40: 179-86.

[16] Reinartz P, Wildberger JE, Schaefer W, Nowak B, Mahnken AH et al. Tomographic imaging in the diagnosis of pulmonary embolism: a comparison between V/Q lung scintigraphy in SPECT technique and multislice spiral CT. *Journal of nuclear medicine : official publication, Society of Nuclear Medicine* 2004; 45: 1501-8.

[17] Miniati M, Pistolesi M, Marini C, Di Ricco G, Formichi B et al. Value of perfusion lung scan in the diagnosis of pulmonary embolism: results of the Prospective Investigative Study of Acute Pulmonary Embolism Diagnosis (PISA-PED). *Am. J. Respir. Crit. Care Med.* 1996; 154: 1387-93.

[18] Olsson C-G, Bitzen U, Olsson B, Magnusson P, Carlsson MS et al. Outpatient tinzaparin therapy in pulmonary embolism quantified with ventilation/perfusion scintigraphy. *Med. Sci. Monit.* 2006; 12: 9-13.

[19] Rizkallah J, Man SF, Sin DD. Prevalence of pulmonary embolism in acute exacerbations of COPD: a systematic review and metaanalysis. *Chest* 2009; 135: 786-93.

[20] Jogi J, Ekberg M, Jonson B, Bozovic G, Bajc M. Ventilation/perfusion SPECT in chronic obstructive pulmonary disease: an evaluation by reference to symptoms, spirometric lung function and emphysema, as assessed with HRCT. *European journal of nuclear medicine and molecular imaging* 2011; 38: 1344-52.

[21] Schonhofer B, Kohler D. Prevalence of deep-vein thrombosis of the leg in patients with acute exacerbation of chronic obstructive pulmonary disease. *Respiration* 1998; 65: 173-7.

[22] Garg A, Gopinath PG, Pande JN, Guleria JS. Role of radio-aerosol and perfusion lung imaging in early detection of chronic obstructive lung disease. *Eur. J. Nucl. Med.* 1983; 8: 167-71.

[23] Carvalho P, Lavender JP. The incidence and etiology of the ventilation/perfusion reverse mismatch defect. *Clinical nuclear medicine* 1989; 14: 571-6.

[24] Li DJ, Stewart I, Miles KA, Wraight EP. Scintigraphic appearances in patients with pulmonary infection and lung scintigrams of intermediate or low probability for pulmonary embolism. *Clinical nuclear medicine* 1994; 19: 1091-3.

[25] Friedman WF, Braunwald E. Alterations in regional pulmonary blood flow in mitral valve disease studied by radioisotope scanning. A simple nontraumatic technique for estimation of left atrial pressure. *Circulation* 1966; 34: 363-76.

[26] Pistolesi M, Miniati M, Bonsignore M, Andreotti F, Di Ricco G et al. Factors affecting regional pulmonary blood flow in chronic ischemic heart disease. *Journal of thoracic imaging* 1988; 3: 65-72.

[27] Jogi J, Palmer J, Jonson B, Bajc M. Heart failure diagnostics based on ventilation/perfusion single photon emission computed tomography pattern and quantitative perfusion gradients. *Nuclear medicine communications* 2008; 29: 666-73.

[28] British Thoracic Society guidelines for the management of suspected acute pulmonary embolism. *Thorax* 2003; 58: 470-83.

[29] Stein PD, Fowler SE, Goodman LR, Gottschalk A, Hales CA et al. Multidetector computed tomography for acute pulmonary embolism. *N. Engl. J. Med.* 2006; 354: 2317-27.

[30] Moores L, Aujesky D, Jimenez D, Diaz G, Gomez V et al. Pulmonary Embolism Severity Index and troponin testing for the selection of low-risk patients with acute symptomatic pulmonary embolism. *J. Thromb. Haemost* 2010; 8: 517-22.

[31] Henry JW, Relyea B, Stein PD. Continuing risk of thromboemboli among patients with normal pulmonary angiograms. *Chest* 1995; 107: 1375-8.

[32] van Beek EJ, Kuyer PM, Schenk BE, Brandjes DP, ten Cate JW et al. A normal perfusion lung scan in patients with clinically suspected pulmonary embolism. Frequency and clinical validity. *Chest* 1995; 108: 170-3.

[33] Freeman LM, Stein EG, Sprayregen S, Chamarthy M, Haramati LB. The current and continuing important role of ventilation-perfusion scintigraphy in evaluating patients with suspected pulmonary embolism. *Semin. Nucl. Med.* 2008; 38: 432-40.

[34] ICRP. Radiation dose to patients from radiopharmaceutical, publication 53. *ICRP*: Oxford, New York 1988:121.

[35] Valentin J. Managing patient dose in multi-detector computed tomography(MDCT). ICRP Publication 102. *Annals of the ICRP* 2007; 37: 1-79, iii.

[36] Hurwitz LM, Yoshizumi TT, Goodman PC, Nelson RC, Toncheva G et al. Radiation dose savings for adult pulmonary embolus 64-MDCT using bismuth breast shields, lower peak kilovoltage, and automatic tube current modulation. *AJR Am. J. Roentgenol.* 2009; 192: 244-53.

[37] Hurwitz LM, Yoshizumi TT, Reiman RE, Paulson EK, Frush DP et al. Radiation dose to the female breast from 16-MDCT body protocols. *AJR Am. J. Roentgenol.* 2006; 186: 1718-22.

[38] Hurwitz LM, Yoshizumi T, Reiman RE, Goodman PC, Paulson EK et al. Radiation dose to the fetus from body MDCT during early gestation. *AJR Am. J. Roentgenol.* 2006; 186: 871-6.

[39] Gutte H, Mortensen J, Jensen CV, Johnbeck CB, von der Recke P et al. Detection of pulmonary embolism with combined ventilation-perfusion SPECT and low-dose CT: head-to-head comparison with multidetector CT angiography. *Journal of nuclear medicine : official publication, Society of Nuclear Medicine* 2009; 50: 1987-92.

[40] Coco AS, O'Gurek DT. Increased emergency department computed tomography use for common chest symptoms without clear patient benefits. *J. Am. Board Fam. Med.* 2012; 25: 33-41.

[41] Einstein AJ, Henzlova MJ, Rajagopalan S. Estimating risk of cancer associated with radiation exposure from 64-slice computed tomography coronary angiography. *JAMA* 2007; 298: 317-23.

[42] Roche LM, Niu X, Pawlish KS, Henry KA. Thyroid cancer incidence in New Jersey: time trend, birth cohort and socioeconomic status analysis (1979-2006). *J. Environ. Public Health* 2011; 2011: 850105-.

In: SPECT
Editors: Hojjat Ahmadzadehfar and Elham Habibi

ISBN: 978-1-62808-344-6
© 2013 Nova Science Publishers, Inc.

Chapter VI

Imaging of Neuroendocrine Tumors with SPECT

Thorsten D. Poeppel[1],*, Ina Binse[1], Andreas Bockisch[1], James Nagarajah[1] and Christina Antke[2]

[1]University of Essen, Medical Faculty,
Department of Nuclear Medicine, Essen, Germany;
[2]University of Dusseldorf, Medical Faculty,
Department of Nuclear Medicine, Dusseldorf, Germany

Introduction

Neuroendocrine neoplasms (NEN) (e.g. neuroendocrine tumors (NET)/neuroendocrine carcinomas (NEC), pheochromocytomas/paragangliomas, medullary thyroid carcinoma, and others) are a fairly rare and heterogeneous group of neoplasms with the ability to produce various bioactive amines and polypeptide hormones [1, 2]. These secretory products are stored within characteristic granules. Proteins of these vesicles (e.g., chromogranin-A, synaptophysin) function as markers of neuroendocrine cells [2]. In order to synthesize these amines and polypeptides, neuroendocrine cells are capable of amine precursor up-take (mediated by membrane-bound transport proteins) and decarboxylation (referred to as APUD cells) [3]. The type of neuroendocrine cell from which a tumor originates determines the kind of secretory product, e.g. tumors of sympatho-adrenal lineage often produce catecholamines, usually norepinephrine/noradrenaline and to a lesser extent epinephrine/adrenaline. Hypersecretion of these bioactive amines or polypeptide hormones typically results in specific clinical syndromes. In contrast, some NET show immunohistochemical signs of hormone synthesis, whereby hormones are produced, but not secreted, or they are clinically inert, or their serum concentration is insufficient to produce symptoms. Thus, NET can be

---

* Corresponding Author: Thorsten D. Poeppel, MD, Department of Nuclear Medicine, University Hospital Essen, Hufelandstr. 55, D-45122 Essen, Phone: ++49-201-7232032, Fax: ++49-201-7235964, E-mail: Thorsten.Poeppel@uni-due.de

classified as functioning or non-functioning tumors depending on clinical symptoms. Besides the remarkable metabolic activity of specific biochemical pathways used in neuroamine/peptide synthesis, the simultaneous expression of various peptide receptors and transport proteins is another characteristic of NET [3]. Most abundant is the expression of somatostatin receptors (see below). NET typically express several subtypes of sst in a pattern related to tumor type, origin, and grade of differentiation [4, 5]. In most cases, one or two subtypes are overexpressed, with sst2 binding sites predominating in the majority of tumors [4, 5]. However, there is considerable variation in sst expression even between tumors of the same type [6].

With respect to anatomical and clinical features, NEN can be roughly assigned to the following groups [6]: i) tumors of gastrointestinal and pancreatic origin (GEP); ii) tracheo-broncho-pulmonary tumors; iii) tumors of sympatho-adrenal lineage (pheochromocytomas, paragangliomas, neuroblastomas); iv) medullary carcinomas of the thyroid gland; v) tumors within the multiple endocrine neoplasia syndrome (MEN1, MEN 2A, MEN 2B); vi) pituitary tumors. Thus, NEN can originate in almost every organ, yet gastrointestinal (56%) and bronchopulmonary (12%) primaries are most frequent [3, 7].

The unique characteristics of NET enabled the development of specific methods of nuclear medicine imaging. Positron-emitting as well as gamma-emitting radiopharmaceuticals are nowadays available for functional imaging of NET. However, the use of specific PET tracers is still more or less restricted to a limited number of PET centers, while several gamma-emitting tracers are available commercially for routine clinical use. These radiopharmaceuticals can be divided into two main categories, namely (a) tracers based on the selective expression of specific receptors, and (b) tracers based on the metabolic activity of defined biochemical pathways [3]. The APUD characteristics and secretory properties as well as the expression of peptide receptors and transporters at the cell membrane constitute the basis for this targeted imaging with radiolabelled ligands. It is thus important to understand the molecular mechanisms that drive tracer uptake or binding that eventually translates into images. Therefore, the purpose of this chapter is to describe both the techniques of imaging NET with gamma-emitting radiopharmaceuticals as well as their physiological background.

Planar Imaging, SPECT and SPECT/CT

In planar imaging, radiation emanating from all depths of the patient's body is projected onto the imaging detector. Thus, overprojection by organs or tissues with ample uptake (e.g. liver, spleen, kidneys, and intestines) may reduce lesion-to-background contrast – in some instances, to the point that a lesion may be completely obscured [8]. Manifestations of NET (primaries or metastases) are particularly prone to this kind of observational oversight as they are frequently small and preferentially located within the abdomen. Tomographic imaging eliminates, or at least minimizes contribution from activities outside the area of interest and improves image contrast and overall visualization of lesions. Another issue is that image interpretation is significantly affected by the physiological biodistribution of a radiopharmaceutical, which is related both to the molecular target (receptors or metabolic pathways) and to the elimination route via the kidneys or gastrointestinal tract.

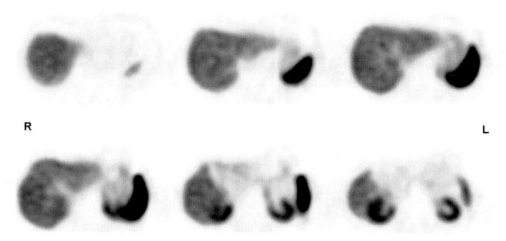

R   L

Figure 6.1. Scan with 700 MBq of ^{99m}Tc-Tektotyd at 5 h p.i. in a 53-year-old female with multifocal paraganglioma. Transaxial SPECT reconstructions demonstrate a physiological, moderately inhomogeneous uptake of ^{99m}Tc-Tektotyd in the liver. R = right, L = left.

As a consequence, it is sometimes difficult to discern physiological from pathological foci and more detailed information on the anatomical localization of tracer accumulation within the body is helpful to reach a decision. Thus, performing single photon emission computed tomography (SPECT) of appropriate regions (as indicated based on the clinical history or the planar images) is standard practice in NET. However, even with SPECT a major disadvantage is the shortage of truly detailed anatomical information. Detection or reliable localization of a lesion within part of an organ or even within a certain organ itself can be challenging. This is especially true of interpretation of hepatic findings as the liver can by nature show moderately inhomogeneous tracer uptake (Figure 6-1) [9]. These limitations can be overcome by combining nuclear medicine imaging with computed tomography (CT) or magnetic resonance imaging (MRI) scans, ideally using a hybrid SPECT/CT (or MRI) device. Hence, the main advantages of SPECT/CT are accurate localization and characterization of lesions, as well as detection of involvement of adjacent structures [10]. In addition, the CT part facilitates the identification of lesions with little or no tracer uptake. Besides, CT data can be used to generate attenuation maps to correct the SPECT images. Thus, although the reported sensitivities and specificities of imaging NET with SPECT are already quite high, there is increasing evidence that SPECT/CT dual modality imaging further improves these figures [10].

Receptor-Based Imaging

Somatostatin Receptor-Based Imaging

Somatostatin (SOM) is a small regulatory polypeptide that is produced within the hypothalamus and throughout the central nervous system, as well as in most peripheral organs/tissues by cells of the autonomous nervous, neuroendocrine, inflammatory, and immune system. SOM has a wide range of mainly inhibitory effects, such as the suppression of growth hormone release, the inhibition of pancreatic and gastrointestinal hormone secretion, as well as the induction of apoptosis. The physiological actions of SOM are mediated by its interaction with members of a family of specific membrane-bound receptors, the somatostatin receptors [11]. To date, six somatostatin receptor subtypes have been cloned and found to bind SOM with nanomolar affinity (sst1, sst2a & b, sst3, sst4, sst5) [3]. However, they show major differences in their affinity for synthetic somatostatin analogs (see below) [12]. All receptor subtypes (sst1 to sst5) are G protein coupled, mediating different biological actions of SOM via the activation of different intracellular signalling pathways, i.e., inhibition of adenyl cyclase, stimulation of phosphotyrosine phosphatase (PTP), and modulation of mitogen-activated protein kinase (MAPK). The intracellular pathway following ligand activation is similar to other G protein coupled receptors and includes receptor phosphorylation and internalization [13]. The internalized receptors are then directed to endosomes, in which they are dephosphorylated, and are either recycled back to the plasma membrane or degraded into lysosomes [13]. Down-regulation of the receptors involves lysosome degradation of internalized receptors [13]. As SOM has a rather short plasma half-life of less than 3 min, strategies to design synthetic SOM analogs incorporate a variety of cyclic or bicyclic restraints to stabilize the molecule. A number of hexa- and octapeptides have been synthesized with different binding affinities to the sst subtypes. The most important in clinical use for treatment of NET or associated syndromes are octapeptide molecules, namely Octreotide and Lanreotide, which are registered in most countries [13]. After slight structural modifications many synthetic analogs can be conjugated with chelators (e.g. DTPA, DOTA, EDDA/HYNIC) and labelled with radiometals like ^{111}In or ^{99m}Tc to visualize the sst biodistribution with gamma cameras. Moreover, labelling analogs with ^{68}Ga led to the development of several PET tracers (e.g. ^{68}Ga-DOTATOC, ^{68}Ga-DOTATATE) that provide superior imaging qualities compared to the gamma camera tracers. However, none is registered for clinical use. There are significant differences in sst subtype specific affinity even after minor structural changes in the analog molecule, the introduction of the radiometal, and the use of different radiometals and chelators [12]. However, all analogs bind with high affinity to the sst2, yet with varying affinity to the sst3, sst4, and sst5 subtype. There is virtually no analog with acceptable affinity to the sst1. Thus, receptor imaging mainly relies on a high density of sst2 in the target tissue. It is worth mentioning that somatostatin receptor imaging may be strongly positive even if immunohistology fails to demonstrate sst expression. For most ^{111}In-labelled somatostatin analogs the internalization of the radiometal–analog complex with intra-cellular residualization of the radioactive label is the most likely mechanism accounting for the good scintigraphic tumor-to-background ratio in the delayed images [3]. In contrast, internalization does not seem to be required for the imaging quality of PET tracers [3]. Somatostatin receptor imaging does not seem to depend on the functionality of a tumor in the way that metabolic imaging (see below) does [9].

^{111}In-DTPA-D-Phe1-Octreotide

^{111}In-DTPA-D-Phe1-octreotide (or ^{111}In-pentetreotide) is the most widely used radiolabelled somatostatin analog for planar scintigraphy and SPECT due to its commercial availability (OctreoScan®).

Box 6.1. Somatostatin receptor scintigraphy:
Protocol for ^{111}In-pentetreotide Octreoscan®)

Patient Preparation:

Patients should be well hydrated before and after injection.

To avoid artifacts in interpretation of abdominal images, a mild oral laxative may be administered in the evening before injection and in the evening following injection. Laxatives should be avoided in patients with active diarrhoea or in patients with insulinoma.

Uptake of radiolabelled octreotide may be reduced in the presence of high concentrations of unlabelled octreotide due to competition at the receptors. Thus, withdrawal of the standard octreotide of at least 24 hours before scintigraphy is usually performed. In patients treated with long-acting/slow release formulations, scintigraphy should be performed just before the next medication administration (usually resulting in an interval from last administration to tracer administration of about 3-6 weeks). However, this issue is still controversial.

Dosage and Route of Administration:
- 150 (120-220) MBq, 5-10 μg peptide*.
- Dosage in children according to the recommendations of the EANM Paediatric Task Group.
- Effective dose (MIRD) (mSv/MBq): Adults: 0,12, children (10 year): 0,22, children (1 year): 0,57.

Time of Imaging:
- 4, 24, 48 h p.i., up to 96 h p.i. in selected cases.
- SPECT/(CT) 4, 24, 48 h p.i.

Acquisition protocol:

Collimator:
- Medium energy, parallel hole

Energy window:
- [111]In photopeaks (172 and 245 keV) with 20 % windows summed in the acquisition frames.

Planar images:
- Both anterior and posterior of head, neck, chest, abdomen, pelvis and lower extremities
- 4 h p.i.: 7 min, 24 h p.i.: 10 min, 48 h p.i.: 15 min per view
- 128x128 or 256x265 matrix

Whole body:
- Max. scanning speed: 4 h p.i.: 10 cm/min, 24 h p.i.: 7 cm/min, 48 h p.i.: 5 cm/min
- 256x1024 matrix

(Multidetector) SPECT:
- 360° of rotation
- 4h p.i.: 3° angular sampling, 20 s per projection, 24 h p.i.: 3°, 30 s, 48 h: 6°, 60 s
- 128×128 acquisition matrix
- SPECT/CT imaging may help localise foci of abnormal tracer accumulation more accurately than planar imaging or SPECT alone and should be considered whenever indicated and available.

Image processing:

Due to the high variability of hardware and types of software of gamma camera systems recommendations are difficult. However, iterative reconstruction should be preferred (2D or 3D algorithms). Specific parameters depend on vendor recommendations and local preferences. Attenuation correction based on CT or radioactive sources should be applied if available. However, caution must be taken in CT based attenuation correction in suspected adrenal pheochromocytoma as visualisation of the adrenals is heavily affected by attenuation correction (with regard to false positive or false negative results).

Recommendations are based on the actual guidelines of the European association of Nuclear Medicine (EANM) and Society of Nuclear Medicine (SNM) [14, 15].

*Based on in vitro studies, the hormonal effect of pentetreotide is approximately 10% that of octreotide and 30 % that of natural somatostatin. The recommended dose is not expected to have a clinically significant pharmacologic effect (however, some precautions are stated in the package insert regarding insulinoma) [14, 15].

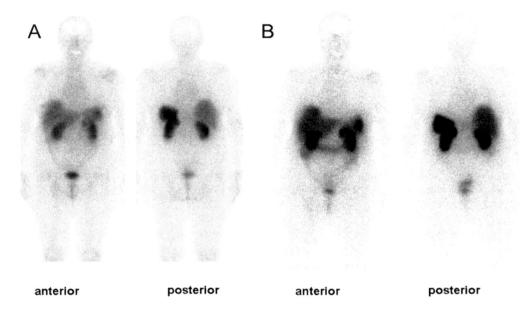

anterior   posterior   anterior   posterior

Figure 6.2. Planar images with 170 MBq of ^{111}In-Octreotide in a 72-year-old female with increasing chromogranin-A levels 8 years after resection of a typical brochopulmonary carcinoid showing a normal tracer distribution. Scan at 4 h (A), 24 h (B) p.i.

[111]In-pentetreotide is registered for the scintigraphic localization of primary and metastatic NET bearing somatostatin receptors. The radiopharmaceutical exhibits rapid plasmatic clearance: only 35% of the injected activity remains in the bloodstream after 10 minutes and the percentage falls to about 1% 24 hours after administration. Its excretion is almost entirely renal: 85% of the activity is eliminated with urine within 24 hours of administration. Hepatobiliary and fecal elimination account for less than 2%. The biological half-life is 6 h. Lesional uptake is quite slow, taking at least 4 hours [14, 15].

Imaging procedure and medications that may interfere with ^{111}In-pentetreotide binding/internalization are listed in box 6-1 [14, 15].

The normal scintigraphic pattern includes weak to moderate physiological accumulation in organs/tissues that sufficiently express sst, including the thyroid, spleen (frequently intense), liver, kidneys, and rarely the pituitary or adrenal glands (Figure 6-2). Faint diffuse breast uptake can also be seen in about 15% of female patients. Other organs are imaged at different time points as a result of tracer excretion, including the urinary tract and bladder, gallbladder, and bowel. Any sufficient non-physiological uptake indicates the presence of lesions with an increased density of sst, which is usually suspicious for malignant disease. Nevertheless, an increased density of sst may also have benign causes (see below).

Imaging with ^{111}In-pentetreotide has shown high sensitivity for NET and has sometimes shown higher accuracy than routine radiological examinations CT or MRI [6, 16]. Overall sensitivity ranges between 70 and 90%, but is related to various factors such as tumor type, origin, grade of differentiation, and localization [17]. The best results are seen in well-differentiated GEP NET (sensitivity of about 80–90%) with the exception of insulinomas (sensitivity of about 70%) due to their rather infrequent overexpression of sst2 [3, 18]. Sensitivity will decrease the less a tumour is differentiated [19]. Bronchopulmonary NET are also detected with sufficient sensitivity of about 70% [3]. Sensitivity is higher for typical than for atypical carcinoids or small cell lung cancer (sensitivity of about 60%) [3].

Somatostatin receptor scintigraphy possesses a lower sensitivity (25%) than ^{123}I-MIBG (Meta-iodobenzylguanidine) for adrenal pheochromocytomas (see chapter 7) [20], yet sensitivity for extra-adrenal paragangliomas is superior to imaging with ^{123}I-MIBG (see below) [21]. This is especially true for parasympathetic paragangliomas/head and neck paragangliomas (93% sensitivity), for which ^{123}I-MIBG scans are usually negative [22]. Furthermore, some reports indicate a higher sensitivity of ^{111}In-pentetreotide than ^{123}I-MIBG in detecting metastatic pheochromocytoma, thus it may have a complementary role in this setting [18, 20]. However, the matter is controversial [21].

In medullary thyroid cancer with only gradual progression the detection of cervical and upper mediastinal lymph node metastases may be high, yet the detection of distant metastases and of metastases in progressive disease is low [23]. Thus, overall diagnostic performance of ^{111}In-pentetreotide is poor in medullary thyroid cancer (sensitivity of about 50%) [3, 10]. The lower performance is mainly due to considerable heterogeneity in lesional receptor expression (even within patients) with rather infrequent overexpression of sst2, and in part due to dedifferentiation [10]. Moreover, metastases tend to be very small and thus might be below the limits of scintigraphic resolution.

Somatostatin receptor scintigraphy possesses an inferior sensitivity (64%) and specificity for the detection of neuroblastoma in comparison with ^{123}I-MIBG (see chapter 7) [18].

The specificity of planar imaging alone in GEP NET tends to be rather moderate (about 50%), mainly due to difficulties in interpretation caused by areas with high physiological activity or routes of elimination (Figure 6-3) [10]. Thus, SPECT imaging is routinely performed.

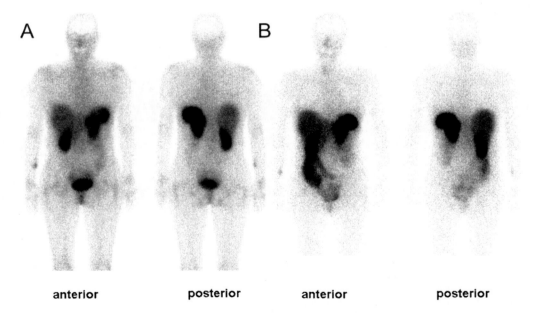

A   B

anterior   posterior   anterior   posterior

Figure 6.3. Planar images with 200 MBq of ^{111}In-Octreotide in a 51-year-old female with MEN1 showing a normal tracer distribution with intense enteral uptake. Scans at 4 h (A), 24 h (B) p.i.

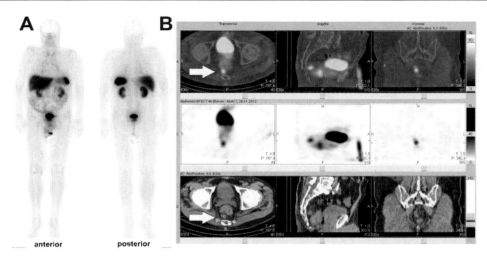

Figure 6.4. A: Planar images with 750 MBq of ^{99m}Tc-Tektotyd at 5 h p.i. in an 80-year-old male with NEC of the rectum. The tumour is obscured by activity in the bladder. B: SPECT and low-dose SPECT/CT identify the primary in the rectum and an adjacent lymph node metastasis (white arrow).

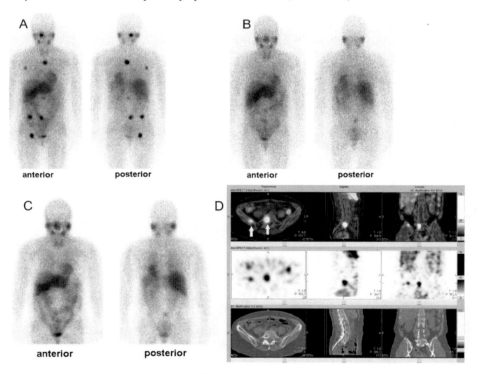

Figure 6.5. A: Planar images with 200 MBq of ^{123}I-MIBG at 24 h p.i. in a 54-year-old female who had right-sided adrenalectomy 15 years ago. Actual referral was for staging of newly diagnosed metastasised malignant pheochromocytoma. The images show intense uptake in multiple osseous metastases. B: Planar images with 190 MBq of ^{123}I-MIBG at 24 h p.i. 3 months after therapy with 11 GBq of ^{131}I-MIBG. C: Planar images with 260 MBq of ^{123}I-MIBG at 24 h p.i. and low-dose SPECT/CT (D) for restaging 8 years after ^{131}I-MIBG therapy show bone metastases (white arrows), which are not clearly identifiable on planar images (C).

However, lesion characterization and localization can be hampered by the scarcity of anatomical landmarks, a problem that persists even when employing SPECT [6]. This limitation can be overcome by fusing SPECT images with CT images, ideally using hybrid SPECT/CT (Figure 6-4 & 6-5). Dual modality SPECT/CT imaging results in a more precise anatomical localization and increases sensitivity and specificity in comparison to SPECT alone. Its accuracy was reported to be as high as 95% [24].

Although ample uptake of ^{111}In-pentetreotide is usually related to NET manifestations, uptake may also be present in tumors other than NET (e.g. lymphomas, melanomas, sarcomas, breast cancer, differentiated thyroid cancer, etc.) as well as in non-neoplastic tissues, such as (peri-tumoral) blood vessels or lymphatic tissue, or non-neoplastic lesions (inflammatory/autoimmune processes or granulomatous diseases such as sarcoidosis, rheumatoid arthritis etc.) [13].

^{99m}Tc-EDDA/HYNIC-Thr3-Octreotide

In comparison with ^{111}In-labelled compounds, ^{99m}Tc-labelled radiopharmaceuticals offer many advantages, including improved gamma camera image quality and lower radiation burden for the patient. One ^{99m}Tc-labelled compound is commercially available: ^{99m}Tc-EDDA/HYNIC-Thr3-octreotide (^{99m}Tc-TEKTROTYD®). ^{99m}Tc-EDDA/HYNIC-Thr3-octreotide is registered for the diagnosis of pathological lesions with overexpression of sst, in particular GEP-NET, pituitary adenomas, tumors of a sympatho-adrenal lineage, and medullary thyroid cancer (and some non-NET). The normal scintigraphic pattern includes moderate to high physiological uptake in the kidneys, the liver, and the spleen (Figure 6-6). Intestinal uptake is weak to moderate.

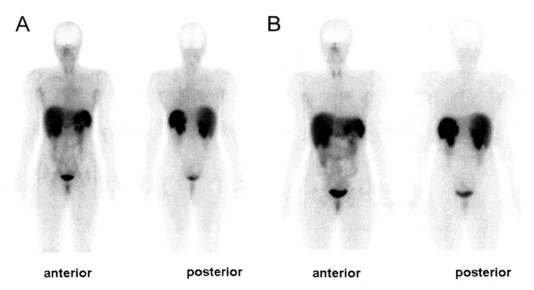

A   anterior   posterior   B   anterior   posterior

Figure 6.6. Planar images with 650 MBq of ^{99m}Tc-Tektotyd showing a normal tracer distribution in a 28-year-old female with SDH-B mutation and enlargement of cervical lymph nodes two years after resection of a cervical paraganglioma. Scans at 1 h (A), 4 h (B) p.i.

Box 6.2. Somatostatin receptor scintigraphy: Protocol for ^{99m}Tc-EDDA/HYNIC-Thr3-octreotide (^{99m}Tc-TEKTROTYD®)

Patient Preparation:
- Patients should be well hydrated before and after injection.
- If there is a need for an examination after 24 h, a mild oral laxative may be administered the evening before this scan. Laxatives should be avoided in patients with active diarrhoea or in patients with insulinoma.
- Uptake of radiolabelled octreotide may be reduced in the presence of high concentrations of unlabelled octreotide due to competition at the receptors. Thus, withdrawal of the standard octreotide of at least 24 hours before scintigraphy is usually performed. In patients treated with long-acting/slow release formulations, scintigraphy should be performed just before the next medication administration (usually resulting in an interval from last administration to tracer administration of about 3-6 weeks). However, this issue is still controversial.

Dosage and Route of Administration:
- 740 (700-925) MBq, 5-15 µg peptide* (depending on the activity used for kit preparation and the number of patients administered from one kit).
- The tracer is not recommended using in patients under 18 years of age.
- Effective dose (mSv/MBq): Adults: 0,0057, no data on children.

Time of Imaging:
- 1-2, 4 h p.i., up to 24 h p.i. in selected cases.
- SPECT/(CT) 1-2, 4 h p.i.

Acquisition protocol:
Collimator:
- Low energy, high resolution, parallel hole
Energy window:
- ^{99m}Tc photopeak (140 keV) with a 20 % window.
Planar images:
- Both anterior and posterior of head, neck, chest, abdomen, pelvis and lower extremities
- 2 h p.i.: 5 min, 4 h p.i.: 7 min, 24 h p.i.: 15 min per view
- 128x128 or 256x265 matrix
Whole body:
- Max. scanning speed: 1 to 2 h p.i.: 15 cm/min, 4 h p.i.: 10 cm/min, 24 h p.i.: 5 cm/min (predominantly only selected regions)
- 256x1024 matrix
(Multidetector) SPECT:
- 360° of rotation
- 3° angular sampling
- 2 h p.i.: 20 s per projection, 4 h p.i.: 30 s per projection
- 128×128 acquisition matrix
- SPECT/CT imaging may help localise foci of abnormal tracer accumulation more accurately than planar imaging or SPECT alone and should be considered whenever indicated and available.

Image processing:
Due to the high variability of hardware and types of software of gamma camera systems recommendations are difficult. However, iterative reconstruction should be preferred (2D or 3D algorithms). Specific parameters depend on vendor recommendations and local preferences. Attenuation correction based on CT or radioactive sources should be applied if available. However, caution must be taken in CT based attenuation correction in suspected adrenal pheochromocytoma as visualisation of the adrenals is heavily affected by attenuation correction (with regard to false positive or false negative results).

Recommendations are based on the package insert [25] and actual guidelines of the European association of Nuclear Medicine (EANM) and Society of Nuclear Medicine (SNM) in general. There is no dedicated EANM or SNM guideline for scintigraphy with ^{99m}Tc-TEKTROTYD®.

*No information is given on the hormonal effect of EDDA/HYNIC-Thr3-octreotide. However, the package insert states no significant pharmacologic side effects [25].

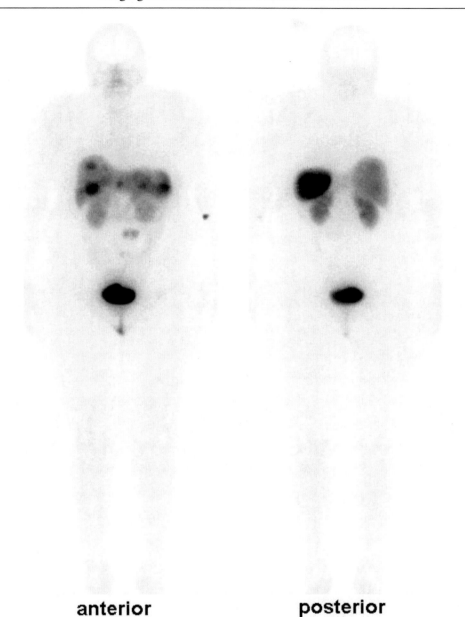

anterior   posterior

Figure 6.7. Planar images with 760 MBq of ^{99m}Tc-Tektotyd at 4,5 h p.i. in a 47 year-old female with suspected enteropancreatic NET. The images show the primary in the jejunum, an adjacent lymph node metastasis, and multiple liver metastases.

The pituitary or adrenal glands are more often visualized than with ^{111}In-pentetreotide. Other organs are imaged at different time points as a result of tracer excretion, including the urinary tract and bladder, gallbladder, and bowel.

The radiopharmaceutical is rapidly eliminated from the blood after intravenous administration. The activity accumulated in the blood cells is below 5% regardless of time after injection.

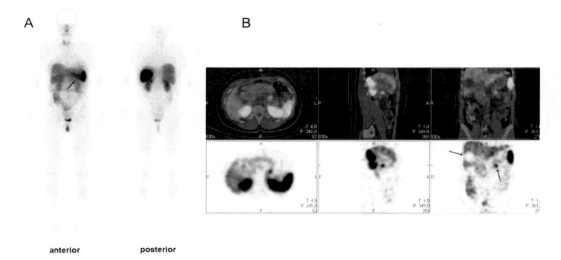

anterior   posterior

Figure 6.8. A: Planar images with 700 MBq of ^{99m}Tc-Tektotyd at 5 h p.i. in a 41-year-old female who had resection of a single liver metastasis of a NET of unknown origin 3 months before. The images show the resection defect in right liver lobe (arrow). B: The SPECT/CT reconstructions show a small focal tracer accumulation in the first jejunal loop that was retrospectively identified in the planar images as a small hot spot in front of the left kidney (A and B, arrows). Resection and histology confirmed it to be a NET of 4 mm, probably the primary tumor.

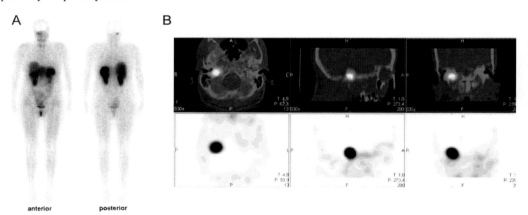

anterior   posterior

Figure 6.9. Scan with 690 MBq of ^{99m}Tc-Tektotyd at 5 h p.i. in a 46-year-old female. The images show a right-sided glomus jugulare paraganglioma. Planar images (A), low-dose SPECT/CT (B).

Binding to blood proteins is lower at earlier time points (e.g. 2–11% within 5 minutes after injection) in comparison to subsequent time points (33–51% after 20 hours). Excretion is predominantly renal, and hepatobiliary excretion is negligible. Cumulative urine excretion within 24 h falls in the range of 24–64% of the administered dose. Lesional uptake is usually fast and specific tracer accumulation can be seen after 10 minutes. Target-to-background is best at 4 hours after injection. Lesions are still visible after 24 hours. The tumor/liver and tumor/lungs ratios are about 1.4 and 1.2, respectively [25].

Imaging procedure and medications that may interfere with ^{99m}Tc-EDDA/HYNIC-TOC binding/internalization are listed in box 6-2.

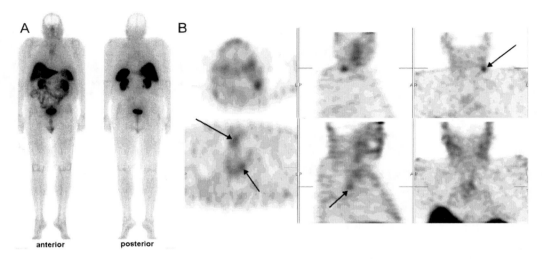

Figure 6.10. Scan with 750 MBq of ^{99m}Tc-Tektotyd at 4 h p.i. in a 71-year-old male with MEN 2 and metastasised medullary thyroid carcinoma. The images show weak to moderate tracer accumulation in cervical and mediastinal lymph node metastases (arrows). Planar images (A), SPECT reconstructions (B).

Reports on ^{99m}Tc-EDDA/HYNIC-TOC are still somewhat scarce but are steadily increasing. Early reports stated that ^{99m}Tc-EDDA/HYNIC-TOC was characterized by higher target-to-non-target ratios than ^{111}In-pentetreotide [26, 27]. ^{99m}Tc-EDDA/HYNIC-TOC also showed a higher sensitivity for NET detection in a direct comparison to ^{111}In-pentetreotide with the identification of more lesions, especially small liver and lymph node metastases (Figure 6-7 & 6-8) [27]. Overall, the sensitivity in abdominal NET is about 90% [3]. However, like ^{111}In-pentetreotide, the specificity tends to be rather moderate (40%) [27].

There are even fewer reports differentiating between the various types of NET:

^{99m}Tc-EDDA/HYNIC-TOC possesses a rather moderate sensitivity for adrenal pheochromocytoma (50%), but a high sensitivity for extra-adrenal pheochromocytoma (96%) (Figure 6-9) [28].

In contrast to ^{111}In-pentetreotide, a high sensitivity of 80% (specificity 83%) was reported in medullary thyroid cancer (Figure 6-10) [29].

Besides potential differences in sensitivity or accuracy one of the main advantages is the (usually) short examination duration compared to ^{111}In-pentetreotide, of less than half a day [30].

Other Radiolabelled Peptide Receptor Tracers

A second ^{99m}Tc-labelled sst radioligand, ^{99m}Tc-Depreotide (NeoSpect®), was approved for lung cancer studies but was withdrawn from the market for commercial reasons in 2010 as the substance was never extensively used for this clinical indication [6, 31]. Its applications for NET in the abdomen yielded inferior results in comparison to ^{111}In-pentetreotide [32]. However, ^{99m}Tc-Depreotide possesses a greater affinity for sst3 and sst5 than ^{111}In-pentetreotide or ^{99m}Tc-EDDA/HYNIC-TOC and may have some benefit in patients with a very high suspicion of NET and a negative ^{111}In-pentetreotide scan [33].

The simultaneous expression of multiple peptide receptors in NET provides the molecular basis for in-vivo multireceptor targeting (e.g., Glucagon-like peptide 1, cholecystokinin, bombesin/gastrin-releasing peptide, vasoactive intestinal peptide) [3]. However, all of these tracers remain experimental and none is available for routine clinical use.

Metabolic Imaging

Catecholamine Pathway - [123]I- and ^{131}I-Metaiodobenzylguanidine (MIBG) Imaging

Norepinephrine (NE), also called noradrenaline, is a catecholamine, i.e. a sympathomimetic biogenic amine that contains a catechol (1,2-dihydroxyphenyl) moiety and the aliphatic portion of amine. It acts as a neurotransmitter of most sympathetic postganglionic neurons and of certain tracts in the central nervous system. NE is also a neurohormone that is released from the chromaffin cells of the adrenal medulla in response to sympathetic stimulation. NE is synthesized from either tyrosine or phenylalanine as precursors. During synthesis or re-uptake NE is concentrated and stored in intracellular secretory (chromaffin) granules via vesicular monoamine transporters (VMAT), which are integrated into the membrane of the vesicles. NE acts systemically as a stress hormone underlying the fight-or-flight response. In the CNS NE exerts effects on large areas of the brain that are involved in alertness and arousal, and the reward system. The actions of NE are carried out by binding to and activating adrenergic α or β receptors, followed by signal termination, either by degradation, or (predominantly) by re-uptake. The re-uptake of NE into the cytosol is either accomplished via a high-affinity and low-capacity transport system (uptake 1 = the norepinephrine transporter) or by a low-affinity and high-capacity transport system (uptake 2) [18, 21].

MIBG is a meta isomer of the guanethidine (a neurosecretory vesicle depleting agent) derivative iodobenzylguanidine. As such it is a catecholamine analog structurally resembling NE. MIBG shares to some extent the biological behavior of NE in that it is taken up by the norepinephrine transporter of sympathomedullary tissues and is stored in secretory vesicles [17]. However, it is not significantly metabolized [17]. MIBG shows little binding to post-synaptic receptors but may evoke adrenergic side effects due to the release of catecholamines (see chapter 7).

MIBG can be labelled with either ^{131}I or [123]I. Due to favorable dosimetry and superior image quality the ^{123}I-labelled agent is to be considered the radiopharmaceutical of choice for diagnostic application [21]. ^{123}I-MIBG is registered for imaging tumors with an increased metabolic rate of catecholamines such as pheochromocytoma, neuroblastoma or carcinoids and their metastases, and for analysis of cardiac sympathetic innervation. ^{131}I-MIBG is registered for nuclear therapy of malignant neuroendocrine tumors and their metastases and for diagnostic use in conjunction with therapy planning (to proof sufficient ^{131}I-MIBG accumulation in tumor cells) (Figure 6-11).

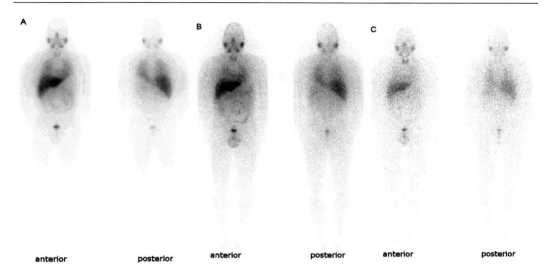

anterior   posterior   anterior   posterior   anterior   posterior

Figure 6.11. Planar images with 210 MBq of ^{123}I-MIBG in a 30-year-old male with MEN 2 showing a normal tracer distribution. Scans at 4 h (A), 24 h (B), 48 h (C) p.i.

Moreover, labelling with [124]I for PET imaging is possible, providing superior imaging quality compared to the gamma camera tracers. However, [124]I-MIBG is not registered for clinical use.

After intravenous injection approximately 50% of the administered radioactivity is recovered in the urine by 24 h, and 70–90% of the residual activity within 48 h. There is variable excretion into the gut (1 to 4%). The whole body half-life is about 24 hours, but the agent is retained in sympathetic nervous tissue for a prolonged period of time [21, 34].

Imaging procedure and medications that interfere with ^{131}I/^{123}I-MIBG uptake and/or vesicular storage are listed in table 6-3 [21, 34].

The uptake of MIBG in different organs is dependent on catecholamine excretion and/or adrenergic innervation, and in tumors is usually proportional to the number of neurosecretory granules. However, in neuroblastoma, MIBG is not stored within granules, but is retained within the cellular cytoplasm by rapid re-uptake of what has escaped the cell [21]. The normal scintigraphic pattern includes moderate accumulation in the liver, which is a major site of catecholamine degradation (Figure 6-11). This accumulation may show a physiologic accentuation of the left liver lobe [37, 38]. Uptake is inversely related to circulating catecholamine levels. Visualization of the normal adrenals differs between [131]I- and ^{123}I-MIBG. However, the intensity of uptake in the normal adrenal gland should be less than that in the liver. With ^{131}I-MIBG the adrenals are usually not seen, but may be faintly visualized in 10 to 20% on delayed images. Nevertheless, the larger the dose of tracer used, the more likely the normal adrenal gland will be seen. Due to the improved specific activity of MIBG used for imaging, a higher rate of visualization may now be possible compared to initial reports [39]. With ^{123}I-MIBG the normal adrenals are seen on planar images 24 h p.i. in 50–80% of patients. Although uptake is generally weak to moderate (less than or occasionally equal to liver intensity) and symmetric, it can be unilateral or asymmetric in up to 15% of patients [40]. Moreover, in patients with renal insufficiency elevated plasma levels of MIBG induce higher levels of accumulation of MIBG in the adrenals and thus may cause false-positive results [41, 42].

Box 6.3. MIBG scintigraphy: Protocol for ^{123}I-MIBG (e.g. AdreView®)

Patient Preparation:
- Patients should be well hydrated before and after injection.
- Thyroid blockade: Potassium iodine tablets/solution (Lugol's) containing an oral dose equivalent to 100 mg iodine starting 1 day (at least 30 min) before and continuing 3 days following MIBG administration (body weight adjusted in children). If iodine is contraindicated: Potassium perchlorate capsules/solution containing 300 mg b.i.d. starting 1 day (at least 30 min) before and continuing 3 days following MIBG administration (body weight adjusted in children).
- Caution: Many classes of drugs are known (or may be expected) to interfere with the uptake and/or vesicular storage of mIBG (v. EANM Guideline[34]).

Dosage and Route of Administration:
- 200 (200-400) MBq (slow intravenous injection, approx. 5-10 min).*
- Dosage in children according to the recommendations of the EANM Paediatric Task Group.
- Effective dose (ICRP 80) (mSv/MBq): Adults: 0,013, children (10 years): 0,026, children (1 year): 0,068.

Time of Imaging:
- 4 h p.i., 24 h p.i., up to 48 h in selected cases.
- SPECT/(CT) 4 h, 24 h p.i.

Acquisition protocol:
Collimator:
- Low energy, high resolution, parallel hole, or medium energy, parallel hole (to reduce septa penetration from small high energy photopeaks)
Energy window:
- [123]I photopeak (159 keV) with a 15 % window. When using a LEHR collimator, a scatter correction can improve image quality**.
Planar images:
- Both anterior and posterior of head, neck, chest, abdomen, pelvis and lower extremities
- 4 h p.i.: 7 min, 24 h p.i.: 15 min per view
- 128x128 or 256x265 matrix
Whole body:
- Max. scanning speed: 4 h p.i.: 10 cm/min, 24 & 48 h p.i.: 5 cm/min
- 256x1024 matrix
(Multidetector) SPECT:
- 360° of rotation
- 3° angular sampling
- 4 h p.i. 20 s per projection, 24 h p.i. 30 s per projection
- 128×128 acquisition matrix
- SPECT/CT imaging may help localise foci of abnormal tracer accumulation more accurately than planar imaging or SPECT alone and should be considered whenever indicated and available.

Image processing:
Due to the high variability of hardware and types of software of gamma camera systems recommendations are difficult. However, iterative reconstruction should be preferred (2D or 3D algorithms). Specific parameters and choice of collimators depend on vendor recommendations and local preferences. Attenuation correction based on CT or radioactive sources should be applied if available. However, caution must be taken in CT based attenuation correction in suspected adrenal pheochromocytoma as visualisation of the adrenals is heavily affected by attenuation correction (with regard to false positive or false negative results).

Recommendations are based on the actual guidelines of the European association of Nuclear Medicine (EANM) and Society of Nuclear Medicine (SNM) [21, 34].

*MIBG shows little binding to adrenergic receptors but may evoke adrenergic side effects due to release of catecholamines [21].

**Different methods have been published for scatter correction, which are mainly based on energy window subtraction. The efficiency of these techniques varies depending on the collimators used [35, 36].

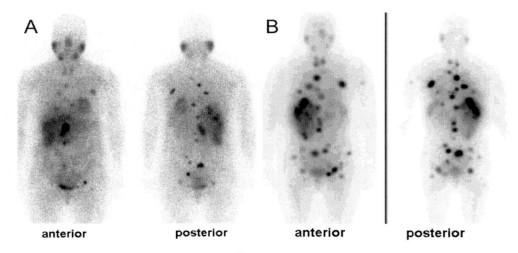

Figure 6.12. A: Planar images with 180 MBq of ^{123}I-MIBG in a 62-year-old female who had resection of an unspecified adrenal tumour 3 years ago. Actual referral was due to suspected metastasised malignant pheochromocytoma. The images show intense uptake in multiple metastases in the liver and skeleton. B: Post-therapeutic scan 3 days after therapy with 10 GBq of ^{131}I-MIBG.

Moderate uptake is present in the salivary glands and weak to moderate uptake in the spleen and heart (myocardial uptake is inversely related to circulating catecholamine levels). MIBG may accumulate to a variable degree in the nasal mucosa, lungs, gallbladder, and uterus. The thyroid may be visualized in a small number of patients, even if it was properly blocked (table 6-3). Due to the presence of brown fat, relatively symmetric uptake along the edge of the trapezius muscles may occur in children. Moreover, it may be seen over the top of each lung, and along either side of the spine to the level of the diaphragm (children and adults). Extremities show only slight muscular activity. No skeletal uptake should be seen. Other organs are imaged at different time points as a result of tracer excretion, primarily the urinary tract and also the bowel in 15–20% (or more) of patients.

Any sufficient non-physiological uptake indicates the presence of lesions with an increased density of norepinephrine transporters/neurosecretory granules, which is usually suspicious for a tumor manifestation.

Because of its characteristics as a "metabolic" tracer MIBG is mainly suitable for imaging of tumors with functional activity, but is highly specific in this setting. MIBG plays a more limited role in other NET when compared with its relevance in pheochromocytoma/paraganglioma or neuroblastoma. Overall sensitivity in NET ranges between 60 and 70% with a specificity of about 95% [6], but is again related to various factors such as tumor type, origin, grade of differentiation, and functionality [6, 19]. The best results are seen in GEP NET [6]. Only moderate results are obtained in bronchopulmonary NET and medullary thyroid cancer (sensitivity <50%) [18]. In general, radiolabelled somatostatin analogs are more sensitive in detecting NET, although less specific. However, MIBG may exert a complementary role to somatostatin receptor scintigraphy as there are reports of MIBG uptake in NET lesions that are not visualized with somatostatin receptor scintigraphy [17]. Additionally, it can be used for tumor characterization to evaluate MIBG uptake in known lesions preceding a potential ^{131}I-MIBG therapy.

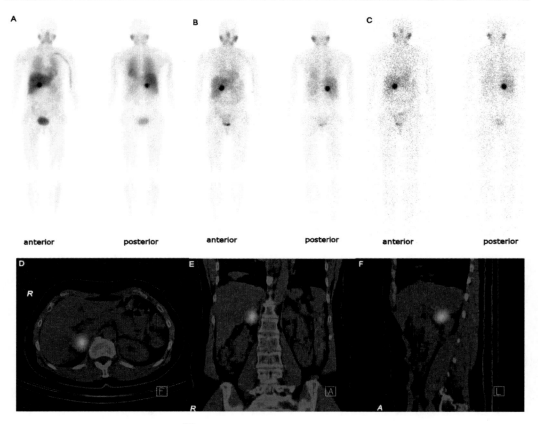

Figure 6.13. Scans with 200 MBq of ^{123}I-MIBG in a 58-year-old female with a history of hypertension and elevated plasma metanephrines showing a right-sided adrenal pheochromocytoma. Planar images at 4 h (A), 24 h (B), 48 h (C) p.i., SPECT/CT fusion of transversal (D), coronal (E), sagittal (F) sections at 24 h p.i.. R = right, V = ventral.

The main indication for MIBG scintigraphy is the imaging of pheochromocytomas, functioning paragangliomas, and neuroblastomas, which are visualized with high sensitivity and specificity. The sensitivity of MIBG imaging is lower in metastatic pheochromocytomas/paragangliomas, recurrences and some familial paraganglioma/pheochromocytoma syndromes [21]. In patients with MEN2, discriminating physiological uptake from mild adrenal medulla hyperplasia or small pheochromocytoma is challenging [21]. The overall sensitivity of ^{123}I-MIBG imaging is 80–90% (specificity 80–100%) [18, 21]. It is higher than that of diagnostic ^{131}I-MIBG scans due to its superior imaging characteristics. Both tracers also offer the option of performing SPECT imaging for improving contrast resolution to aid in lesion detection and localization (mainly in extra-adrenal lesions). This is particularly useful for detection of hepatic metastases, as physiologic uptake in the liver may obscure small intrahepatic lesions on planar imaging [21]. The sensitivity is higher for the identification of adrenal pheochromocytomas (about 90%) (Figure 6-13) than for extra-adrenal tumors (about 70%), which account for about 10% of lesions in adults [28, 43].

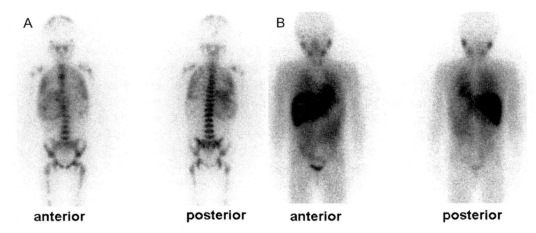

Figure 6.14. A: Planar images with 100 MBq of ^{123}I-MIBG at 24 h p.i. in a 7-year-old girl with neuroblastoma stage IV. The images show a large and mostly necrotic tumour in the right upper abdomen as well as disseminated bone marrow disease. B: Planar images with 110 MBq of ^{123}I-MIBG at 24 h p.i. after one year following chemotherapy, surgery, and bone marrow transplantation. The images show a complete remission.

However, the normal adrenal medulla is visualized in 50–80% of cases with ^{123}I-MIBG (see above) and this physiologic uptake may obscure tiny lesions with faint uptake [44]. Pheochromocytoma is bilateral in only 10% of patients, but this rate is much higher in MEN2 patients (up to 75%). Thus, physiologic uptake may be an issue in the initial staging of MEN patients or during follow-up after adrenal-sparing surgery. Moreover, although physiologic adrenal uptake is usually symmetric and only weak to moderate (less than or occasionally equal to liver intensity), it can be unilateral or asymmetric in up to 15% of patients [40]. This pattern may be difficult or impossible to differentiate from pheochromocytoma as unilateral uptake less than or equal to the liver can represent pheochromocytoma in about 10% of cases [40]. The absence of an anatomic lesion on the "abnormal" side can aid in excluding a tumor.

In addition to exclusively diagnostic scans, MIBG is used for tumor characterization in metastasized pheochromocytoma/paraganglioma to evaluate uptake in known lesions preceding a potential ^{131}I-MIBG therapy.

MIBG imaging is a standard procedure in the staging and re-staging of neuroblastoma, depicting primary and residual or recurrent disease, as well as metastatic lesions with an overall sensitivity of about 90% and specificity of approximately 95% [18]. The highest sensitivity (91–97%) is shown in the evaluation of the extent of metastatic bone and bone marrow disease (Figure 6-14). Additionally, MIBG is used for tumor characterization to evaluate uptake in known lesions preceding a potential ^{131}I-MIBG therapy. Imaging with somatostatin receptor scintigraphy possesses an inferior sensitivity (64%) and specificity in neuroblastoma in comparison to MIBG; however it may provide prognostic information in terms of longer survival in patients with neuroblastomas that express sst [18].

MIBG is a highly specific tracer and false positives due to accumulation in non-sympathomedullary/non-neuroendocrine tumors or other findings are rare (e.g. adrenocortical adenoma or carcinoma, retroperitoneal angiomyolipoma, hemangioma, focal pyelonephritis) [21]. MIBG may not differentiate between certain types of these NET but this rarely leads to a diagnostic dilemma in the clinical context in which a MIBG scan is usually performed [45].

Other Metabolic Pathways and Tracers

Overexpression of amino acid transporters constitutes the basis for another experimental type of metabolic imaging of NET: L-3-^{123}I-alpha-methyl-tyrosine (^{123}I-IMT) is an artificial amino acid derived from tyrosine that is accumulated in NET cells due to uptake via a large amino acid transporter (LAT1) [3]. However, a study in carcinoid patients showed an overall rate of lesion detection of only about 40% with lower lesion contrast and image quality than ^{111}In-pentetreotide [46]. Phosphate metabolism is another metabolic pathway for imaging of NET. Inorganic phosphate (Pi) molecules and Na^+ ions are taken up by cells via members of the Na^+/Pi co-transporter family [47]. Due to the overexpression of type III Na+/Pi transporters, a deficiency of type II Na+/Pi transporters, and a more acidic extra-cellular pH in tumor cells than normal tissue, tumor cells tend to have a higher uptake of phosphate than normal tissue [3]. [99m]Tc-(V)-dimercaptosuccinic acid ([99m]Tc-(V)-DMSA) resembles the phosphate molecule and is thus actively taken up in tumor cells [3]. [99m]Tc-(V)-DMSA was routinely used for imaging medullary thyroid cancer. However, the results were rather mediocre with an average sensitivity of about 50% [3].

Conclusion

Molecular imaging is an invaluable tool in the diagnostic work-up of NET. Several gamma-emitting radiopharmaceuticals that are capable of specifically imaging the different entities of NET are established in clinical routine. Their functional information complements that of morphology-based imaging techniques, such as sonography, CT and MRI. Thus, molecular imaging contributes in most clinical settings, including initial diagnosis, disease staging and re-staging, treatment planning and monitoring, and follow-up [31]. Moreover, functional information like receptor expression or metabolic properties may act as prognostic factors or may be used to predict treatment response [18]. Molecular imaging has been performed using planar imaging techniques and SPECT for about the last 30 years. But it is now the age of PET/CT and the dawn of PET/MR. Already, some have questioned the potential of SPECT to survive the challenges arising from PET/(CT). But there is life in the old dog yet.

In practice, gamma-emitting radiopharmaceuticals may not be replaceable by PET radiopharmaceuticals for various reasons, ranging from the lack of formal approval by regulatory authorities and general or commercial unavailability to important socio-economic considerations [10]. Moreover, SPECT imaging is still progressing: Integrated SPECT/CT has improved the localization and characterization of lesions and facilitated the detection of involvement of adjacent structures, issues that are particularly important in the management of NET. Moreover, the recent introduction of ^{99m}Tc-TEKTROTYD® to clinical routine has generally improved and simplified the scintigraphic imaging of NET. Thus, far from suggesting that SPECT in NET imaging is soon to be replaced by PET its future certainly lies in hybrid imaging and the development of new NET-specific gamma-emitting radiopharmaceuticals.

References

[1]   Gustafsson BI, Kidd M, Modlin IM. Neuroendocrine tumors of the diffuse neuroendocrine system. *Curr. Opin. Oncol.* 2008; 20: 1-12.

[2]   Modlin IM, Oberg K, Chung DC, Jensen RT, de Herder WW et al. Gastroenteropancreatic neuroendocrine tumours. *Lancet Oncol.* 2008; 9: 61-72.

[3]   Koopmans KP, Neels ON, Kema IP, Elsinga PH, Links TP et al. Molecular imaging in neuroendocrine tumors: molecular uptake mechanisms and clinical results. *Crit. Rev. Oncol. Hematol.* 2009; 71: 199-213.

[4]   Reubi JC, Waser B. Concomitant expression of several peptide receptors in neuroendocrine tumours: molecular basis for in vivo multireceptor tumour targeting. *Eur. J. Nucl. Med. Mol. Imaging* 2003; 30: 781-93.

[5]   Reubi JC, Waser B, Schaer JC, Laissue JA. Somatostatin receptor sst1-sst5 expression in normal and neoplastic human tissues using receptor autoradiography with subtype-selective ligands. *Eur. J. Nucl. Med.* 2001; 28: 836-46.

[6]   Bombardieri E, Coliva A, Maccauro M, Seregni E, Orunesu E et al. Imaging of neuroendocrine tumours with gamma-emitting radiopharmaceuticals. *Q. J. Nucl. Med. Mol. Imaging* 2010; 54: 3-15.

[7]   Modlin IM, Lye KD, Kidd M. A 5-decade analysis of 13,715 carcinoid tumors. *Cancer* 2003; 97: 934-59.

[8]   Zanzonico P. Principles of nuclear medicine imaging: planar, SPECT, PET, multi-modality, and autoradiography systems. *Radiat Res.* 2012; 177: 349-64.

[9]   Schillaci O. Somatostatin receptor imaging in patients with neuroendocrine tumors: not only SPECT? *J. Nucl. Med.* 2007; 48: 498-500.

[10]   Mariani G, Bruselli L, Kuwert T, Kim EE, Flotats A et al. A review on the clinical uses of SPECT/CT. *European journal of nuclear medicine and molecular imaging* 2010; 37: 1959-85.

[11]   Hoyer D, Bell GI, Berelowitz M, Epelbaum J, Feniuk W et al. Classification and nomenclature of somatostatin receptors. *Trends Pharmacol. Sci.* 1995; 16: 86-8.

[12]   Reubi JC, Schar JC, Waser B, Wenger S, Heppeler A et al. Affinity profiles for human somatostatin receptor subtypes SST1-SST5 of somatostatin radiotracers selected for scintigraphic and radiotherapeutic use. *Eur. J. Nucl. Med.* 2000; 27: 273-82.

[13]   Volante M, Bozzalla-Cassione F, Papotti M. Somatostatin receptors and their interest in diagnostic pathology. *Endocr Pathol* 2004; 15: 275-91.

[14]   Balon HR, Brown TL, Goldsmith SJ, Silberstein EB, Krenning EP et al. The SNM practice guideline for somatostatin receptor scintigraphy 2.0. *J. Nucl. Med. Technol.* 2011; 39: 317-24.

[15]   Bombardieri E, Ambrosini V, Aktolun C, Baum RP, Bishof-Delaloye A et al. 111In-pentetreotide scintigraphy: procedure guidelines for tumour imaging. *Eur. J. Nucl. Med. Mol. Imaging* 2010; 37: 1441-8.

[16]   Pepe G, Moncayo R, Bombardieri E, Chiti A. Somatostatin receptor SPECT. *Eur. J. Nucl. Med. Mol Imaging* 2012; 39 Suppl 1: S41-51.

[17]   Teunissen JJ, Kwekkeboom DJ, Valkema R, Krenning EP. Nuclear medicine techniques for the imaging and treatment of neuroendocrine tumours. *Endocr Relat Cancer* 2011; 18 Suppl 1: S27-51.

[18] Rufini V, Calcagni ML, Baum RP. Imaging of neuroendocrine tumors. *Semin. Nucl. Med.* 2006; 36: 228-47.

[19] Ezziddin S, Logvinski T, Yong-Hing C, Ahmadzadehfar H, Fischer HP et al. Factors predicting tracer uptake in somatostatin receptor and MIBG scintigraphy of metastatic gastroenteropancreatic neuroendocrine tumors. *J. Nucl. Med.* 2006; 47: 223-33.

[20] van der Harst E, de Herder WW, Bruining HA, Bonjer HJ, de Krijger RR et al. [(123)I]metaiodobenzylguanidine and [(111)In]octreotide uptake in begnign and malignant pheochromocytomas. *J. Clin. Endocrinol. Metab.* 2001; 86: 685-93.

[21] Taieb D, Timmers HJ, Hindie E, Guillet BA, Neumann HP et al. EANM 2012 guidelines for radionuclide imaging of phaeochromocytoma and paraganglioma. *Eur. J. Nucl. Med. Mol. Imaging* 2012; 39: 1977-95.

[22] Koopmans KP, Jager PL, Kema IP, Kerstens MN, Albers F et al. 111In-octreotide is superior to 123I-metaiodobenzylguanidine for scintigraphic detection of head and neck paragangliomas. *J. Nucl. Med.* 2008; 49: 1232-7.

[23] Behr TM, Gratz S, Markus PM, Dunn RM, Hufner M et al. Anti-carcinoembryonic antigen antibodies versus somatostatin analogs in the detection of metastatic medullary thyroid carcinoma: are carcinoembryonic antigen and somatostatin receptor expression prognostic factors? *Cancer* 1997; 80: 2436-57.

[24] Perri M, Erba P, Volterrani D, Lazzeri E, Boni G et al. Octreo-SPECT/CT imaging for accurate detection and localization of suspected neuroendocrine tumors. *Q J. Nucl. Med. Mol. Imaging* 2008; 52: 323-33.

[25] Energy IoA. 99mTc-Tektrotyd summary of product characteristics. 2007 [cited; Available from: http://www.polatom.pl/Tektrotyd/Collection_22.pdf

[26] Decristoforo C, Mather SJ, Cholewinski W, Donnemiller E, Riccabona G et al. 99mTc-EDDA/HYNIC-TOC: a new 99mTc-labelled radiopharmaceutical for imaging somatostatin receptor-positive tumours; first clinical results and intra-patient comparison with 111In-labelled octreotide derivatives. *Eur. J. Nucl. Med.* 2000; 27: 1318-25.

[27] Gabriel M, Decristoforo C, Donnemiller E, Ulmer H, Watfah Rychlinski C et al. An intrapatient comparison of 99mTc-EDDA/HYNIC-TOC with 111In-DTPA-octreotide for diagnosis of somatostatin receptor-expressing tumors. *J. Nucl. Med.* 2003; 44: 708-16.

[28] Chen L, Li F, Zhuang H, Jing H, Du Y et al. 99mTc-HYNIC-TOC scintigraphy is superior to 131I-MIBG imaging in the evaluation of extraadrenal pheochromocytoma. *J. Nucl. Med.* 2009; 50: 397-400.

[29] Czepczynski R, Parisella MG, Kosowicz J, Mikolajczak R, Ziemnicka K et al. Somatostatin receptor scintigraphy using 99mTc-EDDA/HYNIC-TOC in patients with medullary thyroid carcinoma. *Eur J. Nucl. Med. Mol. Imaging* 2007; 34: 1635-45.

[30] Hubalewska-Dydejczyk A, Sowa-Staszczak A, Tomaszuk M. Comment on Pepe et al.: somatostatin receptor SPECT. *Eur J. Nucl. Med. Mol. Imaging* 2012; 39: 1656-7.

[31] Brandon D, Alazraki A, Halkar RK, Alazraki NP. The role of single-photon emission computed tomography and SPECT/computed tomography in oncologic imaging. *Semin. Oncol.* 2011; 38: 87-108.

[32] Lebtahi R, Le Cloirec J, Houzard C, Daou D, Sobhani I et al. Detection of neuroendocrine tumors: 99mTc-P829 scintigraphy compared with 111In-pentetreotide scintigraphy. *J. Nucl. Med.* 2002; 43: 889-95.

[33] Shah T, Kulakiene I, Quigley AM, Warbey VS, Srirajaskanthan R et al. The role of 99mTc-depreotide in the management of neuroendocrine tumours. *Nucl. Med. Commun.* 2008; 29: 436-40.

[34] Bombardieri E, Giammarile F, Aktolun C, Baum RP, Bischof Delaloye A et al. 131I/123I-metaiodobenzylguanidine (mIBG) scintigraphy: procedure guidelines for tumour imaging. *Eur. J. Nucl. Med. Mol. Imaging* 2010; 37: 2436-46.

[35] Lagerburg V, de Nijs R, Holm S, Svarer C. A comparison of different energy window subtraction methods to correct for scatter and downscatter in I-123 SPECT imaging. *Nucl. Med. Commun.* 2012; 33: 708-18.

[36] Rault E, Vandenberghe S, Van Holen R, De Beenhouwer J, Staelens S et al. Comparison of image quality of different iodine isotopes (I-123, I-124, and I-131). *Cancer Biother Radiopharm.* 2007; 22: 423-30.

[37] Jacobsson H, Hellstrom PM, Kogner P, Larsson SA. Different concentrations of I-123 MIBG and In-111 pentetreotide in the two main liver lobes in children: persisting regional functional differences after birth? *Clin. Nucl. Med.* 2007; 32: 24-8.

[38] Jacobsson H, Jonas E, Hellstrom PM, Larsson SA. Different concentrations of various radiopharmaceuticals in the two main liver lobes: a preliminary study in clinical patients. *J. Gastroenterol.* 2005; 40: 733-8.

[39] Roelants V, Goulios C, Beckers C, Jamar F. Iodine-131-MIBG scintigraphy in adults: interpretation revisited? *J. Nucl. Med.* 1998; 39: 1007-12.

[40] Mozley PD, Kim CK, Mohsin J, Jatlow A, Gosfield E, 3rd et al. The efficacy of iodine-123-MIBG as a screening test for pheochromocytoma. *J. Nucl. Med.* 1994; 35: 1138-44.

[41] Gallar P, Oliet A, Hernandez E, Vigil A, Ortega O. Renal failure as a cause of false-positive on metaiodobenzilguanidine (MIBG) scan. *Nephrol. Dial Transplant* 1993; 8: 481.

[42] Tobes MC, Fig LM, Carey J, Geatti O, Sisson JC et al. Alterations of iodine-131 MIBG biodistribution in an anephric patient: comparison to normal and impaired renal function. *J. Nucl. Med.* 1989; 30: 1476-82.

[43] Wiseman GA, Pacak K, O'Dorisio MS, Neumann DR, Waxman AD et al. Usefulness of 123I-MIBG scintigraphy in the evaluation of patients with known or suspected primary or metastatic pheochromocytoma or paraganglioma: results from a prospective multicenter trial. *J. Nucl. Med.* 2009; 50: 1448-54.

[44] Taieb D, Neumann H, Rubello D, Al-Nahhas A, Guillet B et al. Modern nuclear imaging for paragangliomas: beyond SPECT. *J. Nucl. Med.* 2012; 53: 264-74.

[45] Leung A, Shapiro B, Hattner R, Kim E, de Kraker J et al. Specificity of radioiodinated MIBG for neural crest tumors in childhood. *J. Nucl. Med.* 1997; 38: 1352-7.

[46] Jager PL, Meijer WG, Kema IP, Willemse PH, Piers DA et al. L-3- [123I]Iodo-alpha-methyltyrosine scintigraphy in carcinoid tumors: correlation with biochemical activity and comparison with [111In-DTPA-D-Phe1]-octreotide imaging. *J. Nucl. Med.* 2000; 41: 1793-800.

[47] Werner A, Dehmelt L, Nalbant P. Na+-dependent phosphate cotransporters: the NaPi protein families. *J. Exp. Biol.* 1998; 201: 3135-42.

In: SPECT
Editors: Hojjat Ahmadzadehfar and Elham Habibi

ISBN: 978-1-62808-344-6
© 2013 Nova Science Publishers, Inc.

Chapter VII

Tumor Imaging with $^{123/131}$I-MIBG SPECT

Verena Hartung*, Marcus Ruhlmann, Andreas Bockisch and James Nagarajah

Department of Nuclear Medicine, University Hospital Essen, Essen, Germany

Introduction

MIBG (metaiodobenzylguanidine) scintigraphy is used to image tumors of neuroendocrine origin, particularly those of the neuro-ectodermal (sympatho-adrenal) system (pheochromocytomas, paragangliomas and neuroblastomas) [1]; however, other neuroendocrine tumors (NET) (e.g. carcinoids, medullary thyroid carcinoma) can also be visualized [2, 3]. In addition, MIBG can be employed to study disorders of sympathetic innervation, for example in ischemic and non-ischemic cardiomyopathy (see chapter 10) as well as in the differentiation between idiopathic Parkinson's syndrome and multisystem atrophy (see chapter 11).

MIBG or Iobenguane, a combination of an iodinated benzyl and a guanidine group, was developed in the early 1980s to visualize tumors of the adrenal medulla [4]. MIBG, which is structurally similar to norepinephrine, enters neuroendocrine cells by an active uptake mechanism via the (nor)epinephrine transporter and is stored in the neurosecretory granules, resulting in a specific concentration that differs from that in cells of other tissues. MIBG specifically concentrates in tissues expressing (nor)epinephrine transporter.

MIBG can be labeled with either ^{131}I or ^{123}I. ^{123}I is a gamma-emitting radionuclide with a physical half-life of 13.13 hours. The principal gamma photon is emitted at 159 keV (83% abundance). ^{131}I emits a principal gamma photon of 364 keV (81% abundance) with a

---

* Corresponding Author: Verena Hartung, MD - Department of Nuclear Medicine, University Hospital Essen, Hufelandstr. 55, D-45122 Essen. Phone: ++49-201-7232032, Fax: ++49-201-7235964. E-mail: verena.hartung@uk-essen.de.

physical half-life of 8.04 days and also beta particles with a maximum energy of 0.61 MeV (mean 0.192 MeV).

^{123}I-MIBG scintigraphy is preferable to ^{131}I-MIBG scintigraphy because (a) the 159 keV emission of ^{123}I can be detected better using conventional gamma cameras (especially when using SPECT) in contrast to the 360 keV photons of ^{131}I, which provide images of higher quality, (b) the lower radiation burden of ^{123}I permits a higher permissible administered activity, resulting in a higher count rate, which is more suitable for imaging and (c) with ^{123}I-MIBG scintigraphy the duration between injection and imaging is shorter (4-24 hours) than with ^{131}I-MIBG scintigraphy (48–72 hours), because with ^{131}I-MIBG delayed images may be required for optimal target-to-background ratios [5].

Theoretical considerations and clinical experience indicate that the ^{123}I-labelled agent is to be considered the radiopharmaceutical of choice as it has a more favorable dosimetry and provides better image quality, allowing accurate anatomical localization via the use of SPECT/CT. Nevertheless, ^{123}I-MIBG might not be available in every nuclear medicine facility. Although ^{131}I-MIBG is widely employed for most routine applications (mainly in adult patients) because of its ready availability and the possibility of obtaining delayed scans, it is not recommended because of low sensitivity and unfavorable dosimetry. Nonetheless, ^{131}I-MIBG may be preferred when estimation of tumor uptake and retention measurement is required for MIBG therapy planning.

Performing MIBG scintigraphy requires a gamma camera to acquire planar and/or tomographic (SPECT) images. Using SPECT/CT hybrid systems is highly recommended, because fusion images can improve diagnostic accuracy.

There exists a wide spectrum of oncological and non-oncological indications for MIBG imaging that are summarized in table 7-1.

Table 7-1. Indications for MIBG scintigraphy

Oncological indications	Other (non-oncological) indications
Detection, localization, staging (at initial presentation), restaging and follow-up of neuroendocrine tumors and their metastases, in particular: pheochromocytoma, neuroblastoma, ganglioneuroblastoma, ganglioneuroma, paraganglioma, carcinoid tumors, medullary thyroid carcinoma, Merkel cell tumors of skin and MEN2 syndromes.	Functional studies of the adrenal medulla (hyperplasia), sympathetic innervation of the myocardium (e.g. in ischemic and not ischemic cardiomyopathy as well as in the differentiation between idiopathic Parkinson's syndrome and multisystem atrophy), salivary glands and lungs [6].
Selection for targeted radiotherapy: study of tumor uptake and residence time in order to decide and plan a treatment with ^{131}I-MIBG. In this case the dosimetric evaluation should be individual and not based on the ICRP Tables, that have only an indicative value limited to diagnostic procedures [7-9].	
Evaluation of tumor response by measuring the intensity of MIBG uptake and the number of focal MIBG uptake sites [10, 11].	
Confirmation of suspected tumors derived from neuroendocrine tissue.	

Pathophysiology of the Diseases Relevant for MIBG Scintigraphy

MIBG accumulates in the normal adrenal gland, in adrenal hyperplasia, in tumors of neuroendocrine origin such as adrenal tumors, paragangliomas, pheochromocytomas, neuroblastomas, ganglioneuromas, ganglioneuroblastomas, carcinoid tumours, Merkel cell tumors of the skin and medullary thyroid carcinoma.

Paragangliomas are tumors that develop from neuroendocrine cells derived from neural crest stem cells. They may arise anywhere along the paraganglial system and can be associated with the sympathetic nervous system (derived from the adrenal medulla or other chromaffin cells that may persist beyond embryogenesis) or the parasympathetic nervous system (developing from neural crest cell derivates in the parasympathetic paraganglia, mainly located in the head and neck). Paragangliomas can be distributed from the skull base to the sacrum (with a predilection for the middle ear (glomus tympanicum), the dome of the internal jugular vein (glomus jugulare), at the bifurcation of the common carotid arteries (glomus caroticum), along the vagus nerve, in the mediastinum (from the aortopulmonary body or the thoracic sympathetic chain), in the adrenal medulla and in the abdominal and pelvic paraaortic regions. The term *pheochromocytoma* should be reserved solely for adrenal paraganglioma based on the classification published in 2004 by the World Health Organization.

Paragangliomas/pheochromocytomas are rare tumors (annual incidence of 0.1 to 0.6 per 100,000 population) that account for about 4% of adrenal incidentalomas. Pheochromocytomas and paragangliomas of the sympathetic nervous system usually cause symptoms of catecholamine over-secretion, such as hypertension, palpitations, headache, sweating, pallor, apprehension, anxiety and tremor. Accordingly there are also increased catecholamine levels in the plasma and urine. Pharmacological blockade of α - and β-adrenergic receptors can relieve the symptoms, but has no effect on tumor growth.

In contrast, head and neck and parasympathetic thoracic paragangliomas are almost always (up to 95%) non-secreting tumors that are revealed by symptoms of compression or infiltration of the adjacent structures (e.g. hearing loss, tinnitus, dysphagia, cranial nerve palsies), because of loco-regional extension, and/or are discovered on imaging studies.

Paragangliomas/pheochromocytomas are characterized by a high frequency of hereditary forms (35%) that may coexist with other tumor types in multiple neoplasia syndromes with a propensity for multifocal disease[12, 13], which, for instance, are associated with various familial syndromes such as multiple endocrine neoplasia (MEN IIA and IIB), von Hippel-Lindau syndrome and neurofibromatosis.

Paragangliomas/pheochromocytomas are usually benign and progress slowly and, in the absence of metastasis with complete resection, are curable. The rate of metastasization varies widely, ranging from less than 1% to more than 60%, depending on tumor location, size and genetic background.

Increased catecholamine levels in the plasma and urine and radiological features of anatomical imaging (CT/MRI) may also be suggestive of the diagnosis of paraganglioma/pheochromocytoma. However, in cases of a non-secreting adrenal mass, the high specificity of functional imaging such as MIBG scintigraphy may contribute to the diagnosis. Functional imaging is helpful in the preoperative work-up of patients < 40 years of age, positive family history and > 3.0 cm pheochromocytoma. Pretreatment imaging is important for providing accurate staging of the disease in extraadrenal pheochromocytoma, regardless of its size and/or hereditary syndromes, as well as in identifying metastatic paraganglioma.

MIBG scintigraphy may be used to restage and/or localize tumor sites in patients with positive biochemical results or suspicion of disease recurrence.

Neuroblastoma is the most common extracranial malignant tumor in children (8–10%) and occurs mainly in younger children: 50% up to the age to 2 years and 75% up to 4 years. The tumors are derived from the neural crest and arise in the adrenal gland (65%) or the sympathetic nervous system. Cancer stage IVS and I can regress spontaneously, while neuroblastoma stage IV is highly malignant (staging and assessment of treatment response according to the "International Neuroblastoma Staging System"). At stage IV more than half of children already have metastases at the time of diagnosis and a 5-year survival rate of only 30–40%.

Non-oncological indications are a functional test of the adrenal medulla in hyperplasia and analysis of the sympathetic innervation of the heart muscle, salivary glands and lungs. As in idiopathic Parkinson's disease the sympathetic innervation of the heart is reduced, while being normal in multiple system atrophy; ^{123}I-MIBG scintigraphy can be used to distinguish between these two conditions (see chapter 11) [14, 15].

^{123}I-MIBG-Scintigraphy with SPECT (/CT)

Conventional ^{123}I-MIBG scintigraphy with SPECT is a well-established nuclear imaging modality in the staging and restaging of pheochromocytoma and paraganglioma. Also, SPECT/CT has now become more widely available and has the advantage of the simultaneous acquisition of both morphological and functional data, thus increasing diagnostic confidence in image interpretation and enhancing sensitivity. However, these conventional examinations are associated with some practical constraints such as long imaging times, gastrointestinal tract artifacts requiring bowel cleansing in some patients, thyroid blockage and the need for withdrawal of certain medications that interfere with interpretation. The pre-examination procedures that are required prior to starting ^{123}I-MIBG scintigraphy are clearly represented in the current EANM (European Association of Nuclear Medicine) guidelines for radionuclide imaging of pheochromocytoma and paraganglioma (box 1) [16].

Prearrangements and Pre-Examination Procedure

Pharmaceutical. MIBG labeled with ^{123}I or ^{131}I is currently commercially available in a "ready to use" formulation and conforms to the criteria laid down in the European Pharmacopoeia.

The labeled product is available in a sterile solution for intravenous use. The activity of MIBG should be measured in a calibrated ionization chamber, and radiochemical purity can be determined using thin-layer chromatography.

Box 1. Protocol for MIBG-scintigraphy

Patient Preparation:
- slow intravenous injection (over about 2-3 min) to minimize rare adverse events (tachycardia, pallor, vomiting, abdominal pain)
- thyroid blockage (thyroid uptake of free iodide is prevented using stable iodine per os: 130 mg/day of potassium iodide; equivalent to 100 mg of iodine 1 day before tracer injection and continued for 2 days for ^{123}I-MIBG and 5 days for ^{131}I-MIBG or potassium perchlorate in iodine allergic patients 4 h before tracer injection and continued for 2 days (400–600 mg/day).
- need for withdrawal (for an adequate time prior imaging) of certain medications (like opioids, tricyclic antidepressants, sympathomimetics, antipsychotics, antihypertensive agents) that may interfere with MIBG uptake
- *Contraindications:* pregnancy, breast feeding should be discontinued for at least 2 days after scintigraphy using ^{123}I-MIBG and stopped completely if ^{131}I-MIBG is used.

Dosage and Route of Administration:
- 200–400 MBq for ^{123}I-MIBG and 40–80 MBq for ^{131}I-MIBG in adults
- the activity administered to children should be calculated on the basis of a reference dose for an adult, scaled to body weight according to the schedule proposed by the EANM Paediatric Task Group (^{123}I-MIBG 80–400 MBq) [11]
- effective doses: 0.013 mSv/MBq for ^{123}I-MIBG and 0.14 mSv/MBq for ^{131}I-MIBG in adults, 0.037 mSv/MBq for ^{123}I-MIBG and 0.43 mSv/MBq for ^{131}I-MIBG in children (5-year old).
- increased radiation dose from CT in SPECT/CT protocols (volume CT dose index: 3–5 mGy depending on acquisition parameters).

Time of Imaging:
- 4, 24, 48 h p.i. with ^{123}I-MIBG and 24, 48 up to 3 days (or later) with ^{131}I-MIBG
- SPECT(/CT) 24 (when indicated additionally 4 and/or 48 h) p.i.

Acquisition protocol:
- Collimator:
- high energy, parallel hole for ^{131}I-MIBG
- low/ medium energy, high resolution for ^{123}I-MIBG

Energy window:
- ^{123}I-MIBG: 159 keV with 20 % window
- ^{131}I-MIBG: 360 keV with 20 % window

Planar images:
- Whole body with additional limited-field images or spot images (both anterior and posterior limited-field or static spot views of head, neck, chest, abdomen, pelvis and upper/lower extremities
- *^{123}I-MIBG*: speed of 5 cm/min whole-body or static spot views with about 500 kcounts or 10-15 minutes acquisition per image using a 256x256 matrix or 128x128 matrix with zoom
- (optionally for whole-body (planar anterior and posterior) images 256x1,024 word matrix for a minimum of 30 min with a max. speed 6 cm/min. For spot views 75-100 kcounts to reduce acquisition time))
- *^{131}I-MIBG*: speed of 4 cm/sec for a total body scan with both anterior and posterior limited-field or static spot views (>150 kcounts) 128x128 or 256x256 matrix

(Multi-detector) SPECT(/CT):
- 360° of rotation (120 projections, in 3-degree steps (or 6° angle steps))
- continuous or step and shoot mode, 25-35 seconds per step (or 30–45 s per step).
- 128×128 acquisition matrix
- (to reduce acquisition time use 6 degree steps, or a 64x64 matrix with shorter time per frame)
- additionally SPECT/CT in adults and SPECT image alone in children may help localise foci of abnormal tracer accumulation more accurately than planar imaging and should be considered whenever indicated and available
- co-registered CT images from SPECT/CT enable attenuation and facilitate precise localisation of any focus of increased tracer (100–130 kV, low-dose CT (mAs modulation recommended))

Reconstructions:
- Due to the high variability of hardware and types of software of gamma camera systems recommendations are difficult. However, iterative reconstruction should be preferred (2D or 3D algorithms). Specific parameters depend on vendor recommendations and local preferences. Attenuation correction based on CT or radioactive sources should be applied if available.

Tracer Injection and Activity

Slow intravenous injection is recommended (over about 2-3 min) to minimize rare adverse events (tachycardia, pallor, vomiting and abdominal pain). No adverse allergic reactions are expected. The recommended activities in adults are 200–400 MBq for ^{123}I-MIBG and 40–80 MBq for ^{131}I-MIBG. The activity administered to children should be calculated on the basis of a reference dose for an adult, scaled to body weight according to the schedule proposed by the EANM Paediatric Task Group (^{123}I-MIBG 80–400 MBq) [17].

Radiation Exposure

Dosimetry can be obtained from the ICRP tables. The effective doses are 0.013 mSv/MBq for ^{123}I-MIBG and 0.14 mSv/MBq for ^{131}I-MIBG in adults, and 0.037 mSv/MBq for ^{123}I-MIBG and 0.43 mSv/MBq for ^{131}I-MIBG in children (5 years old) [8, 9]. There is an increased radiation dose from CT in SPECT/CT protocols (volume CT dose index: 3–5 mGy depending on acquisition parameters).

Contraindications

Clinical decisions should consider the benefits against the possible harm of carrying out any procedure in patients known or suspected to be pregnant. Breast feeding should be discontinued for at least 2 days after scintigraphy using ^{123}I-MIBG and stopped completely if ^{131}I-MIBG is used. Plasma clearance of ^{123}I-MIBG is reduced in patients with renal insufficiency. ^{123}I-MIBG is not cleared by dialysis [18].

Thyroid Blockade

Prior to intravenous tracer administration a thyroid blockade is obligatory. Thyroid uptake of free iodide is prevented using stable iodine per os. Thyroid blockade (130 mg/day of potassium iodide; equivalent to 100 mg of iodine) should be started 1 day before tracer injection and continued for 2 days for ^{123}I-MIBG and 5 days for ^{131}I-MIBG. Potassium perchlorate may be substituted for iodine in iodine-allergic patients and started 4 h before tracer injection and continued for 2 days (400–600 mg/day).

Drug Interactions

Drugs that are known (or expected) to modify the uptake and/or vesicular storage of MIBG and may interfere with MIBG imaging should be discontinued. For a review of drugs that may interact or interfere with MIBG uptake, the reader is referred to previous reviews and guidelines [16, 19-21]. Some of the most important substances that may affect the results of MIBG scintigraphy are medications such as opioids, tricyclic antidepressants, sympathomimetics, antipsychotics, antihypertensive agents (e.g. alpha- or beta-blocking treatment in metabolically active catecholamine secreting tumors) and/or some foods containing vanillin and catecholamine-like compounds (such as chocolate and blue-veined cheeses). Care must be taken to ensure that such drugs are discontinued (if possible) for sufficient time prior to imaging.

Image Acquisition

Instrumentation and Image Parameters

A single or multiple head gamma camera with a large field of view is necessary to acquire planar and/or tomographic (SPECT) images. For scintigraphy a large-field-of-view camera with a high-energy (parallel hole) collimator is used for ^{131}I-MIBG and a low-energy (high-resolution) collimator for ^{123}I-MIBG. Many nuclear medicine centers prefer medium-energy collimators because ^{123}I decay includes a small fraction (less than 3%) of high-energy photons (346,440,505,529,539 keV) that can scatter in the collimator or experience septal penetration, and medium-energy collimators may thus improve image quality by reducing scatter while preserving acceptable sensitivity (i.e. without increasing acquisition time).

Acquisition Modality

^{123}I-MIBG scans are usually obtained 20 to 24 h after tracer injection. Selected delayed images (never later than day 2) may be useful in the case of equivocal findings at day 1. Early static images at 4 to 6 h after injection can be performed optionally. Scanning with ^{131}I-MIBG is performed 1 and 2 days after injection and can be repeated at day 3 or later. Whole body imaging with additional limited-field images or spot images (recommended especially in pediatric patients) should be performed (patient in supine position). With ^{123}I-MIBG a total body scan with a speed of 5 cm/min or both anterior and posterior limited-field or static spot views of the head, neck, chest, abdomen, pelvis, upper and lower extremities with about 500 kcounts or 10–15 minutes acquisition per image using a 256x256 matrix or 128x128 matrix with zoom and a 20% window centered at the 159 keV photopeak is usually performed. For whole-body images, planar anterior and posterior images may be acquired into a 1024×512 word or 1024×256 word matrix for a minimum of 30 min (maximum speed 6 cm/min). In order to reduce acquisition time, spot views with 75–100 kcounts could be sufficient for upper and lower limbs. With ^{131}I-MIBG a total body scan with a speed of 4 cm/min or both anterior and posterior limited-field or static spot views (>150 kcounts) of the head, neck, chest, abdomen, pelvis, upper and lower extremities is requested. When performing multiple spot views of the body starting the exam with the abdomen/pelvis, spot views are recommended (cooperative patients should be encouraged to empty their bladder prior to imaging). In neuroblastoma patients requiring head imaging and both antero-posterior and lateral views are recommended. In young children spot views are often superior to whole body scans in terms of contrast and resolution, especially in low count regions (longer acquisition time in total, but with interruptions in between, improving their tolerance of the examination). Some authors consider that SPECT or SPECT/CT should be regarded as a mandatory part of MIBG scintigraphy.

SPECT

Single photon emission tomography can improve diagnostic accuracy and is useful mainly in cases where uncertainty exists regarding the localization and interpretation of tracer uptake. In the case of superimposed areas of high physiological (i.e. liver, bladder) or pathological (i.e. primary tumor) uptake, SPECT can improve the characterization of small lesions, which may not be evident on planar images. Fundamental in tumor grading is distinguishing between soft tissue and skeletal lesions (especially in the spine); in this case SPECT can help. SPECT can be fused or co-registered with CT or MRI images in order to interpret and identify the topographic location and nature of some doubtful lesions. Thus, whenever possible, SPECT should be performed, even if sedation is required in young children. SPECT should cover the region of interest (e.g. pelvis, abdomen and thorax), especially anatomical regions showing pathological tracer uptake on planar images. In SPECT one should take into account the different types of gamma camera and software available, as the acquisition parameters depend on the equipment available and the radioisotope used. Generally, SPECT images are obtained over a 360° orbit and the protocol consists of 120 projections, in 3-degree steps (or 6° angle steps), in continuous or step-and-shoot mode, 25–35 seconds per step (or 30–45 s per step). Data are acquired on a 128x128 word matrix. If acquisition time needs to be reduced (e.g. in non-cooperative patients), it is possible to use 6-degree steps, or a 64x64 matrix with a shorter time per frame [22, 23].

SPECT/CT

In children, in whom one normally abstains from performing SPECT/CT (to reduce radiation exposure), the SPECT image alone can be considered sufficient. In adults SPECT/CT can often be useful. Co-registered CT images from SPECT/CT cameras enable attenuation and facilitate the precise localization of any focus of increased tracer (100–130 kV, low-dose CT (mAs modulation recommended)). The CT image should be taken at high resolution in order to enable better characterization of the anatomical surroundings; this is also important for dosimetry calculations (uptake and size of the tumor).

Reconstructions

SPECT iterative reconstruction with a low pass post-filter often provides better images than filtered back projection, thus allowing accurate visualization of lesions. CT-based attenuation correction for SPECT/CT can be performed. Attenuation correction can also be performed on SPECT images alone based on the constant μ before or after processing (e.g. Chang, Sorenson), but this is not usually done. Scatter correction methods using spectral analysis can be used to improve the accuracy of quantification. Any reporting should clearly state the methodology adopted for image processing and quantification.

Image Interpretation

Physiological MIBG Uptake and Distribution

The uptake of radiolabelled MIBG in different organs depends on catecholamine excretion and/or adrenergic innervation. MIBG is normally taken up mainly by the liver; lower levels of uptake have been described in the spleen, lungs, salivary glands, skeletal muscles and myocardium. ^{123}I-MIBG uptake in the adrenal glands is considered normal if symmetrical or mild (less than or equal to liver uptake) and when the glands are not enlarged on the CT scan. Normal adrenals are usually faintly visible, but can be visualized in up to 75% of cases if using ^{123}I-MIBG, and 48–72 hours after injection in up to 15% of cases when using ^{131}I-MIBG. The majority of MIBG is excreted unaltered by the kidneys (60–90% of the injected dose is recovered in the urine within 4 days; 50% within 24 hours), and fecal elimination is weak (<2% up to day 4). In patients with pheochromocytoma and paraganglioma, uptake in the heart and liver is significantly lowered by about 40% [24]. No skeletal uptake should be seen. More common in children than in adults, brown fat uptake should be considered as a normal distribution of MIBG and this is usually quite symmetric, along the edge of the trapezius muscles [25], over the top of each lung, and along either side of the spine to the level of the diaphragm [4].

Pathological MIBG Uptake

Extra-adrenal sites of uptake that cannot be explained by normal physiological distribution are considered abnormal. Pathological MIBG uptake is observed in primary tumor (soft tissue) and in metastatic sites including lymph nodes, liver, bone and bone marrow (Figure 7-1–7-3).

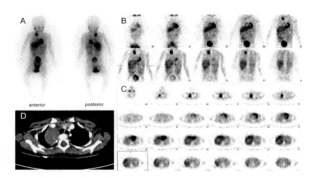

Figure 7-1. ^{123}I-MIBG scintigraphy of a 3-year old child with a neuroblastoma with a fokal pathological increased uptake in the right side of the chest. A: Planar whole body image after 1 day after tracer application. BandC: SPECT imaging coronal and transversal views. E: CT imaging (transversal) shows compression of the trachea, main bronchus and neighboring vessels.

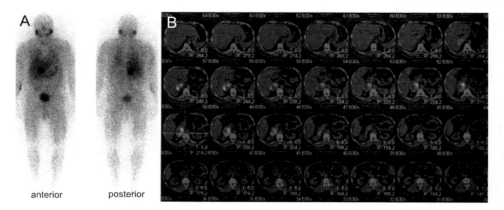

Figure 7-2. ¹²³I-MIBG scintigraphy (planar whole body image 1 day after tracer application) of a 61-year old man with a tumor of 7 cm diameter in the right adrenal and clinical suspected phaeochromoytoma with pathological increased marginal uptake in the right adrenal. A: Planar whole body image ,1 day after tracer application. B: SPECT/CT imaging (transversal).

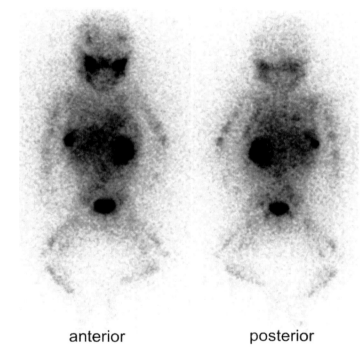

Figure 7-3. ¹²³I-MIBG scintigraphy of a 1-year old child with suspected Neuroblastoma. The scintigraphy shows a neuroblastoma Stadium IV (bone marrow involvement) with multiple pathological increased uptakes in an expanded retroperitoneal tumor on the left side paravertebral with liver metastasis and bone metastasis, especially in os sphenoidale.

High-intensity adrenal uptake (more intense than liver uptake) or inhomogeneous adrenal uptake with a concordant enlarged gland is abnormal. Note the compensatory increased diffuse MIBG uptake receiving the opposite side after adrenalectomy (hyperplastic adrenal gland after contralateral adrenalectomy). Increased uptake in the skeleton (focal or diffuse) is indicative of bone marrow involvement or skeletal metastases (Figure 7-3).

False-Positive Pitfalls

Increased diffuse physiological uptake in the urinary tract, bowel or urine contamination, uptake by the hyperplastic adrenal gland after contralateral adrenalectomy, and/or any other external contamination (salivary secretion) lead to false-positive results. CT-based attenuation correction often leads to enhanced physiological visualization of the adrenal medulla and may therefore lead to false-positive interpretation. In patients with MEN2, ^{123}I-MIBG scintigraphy is of limited value for discriminating physiological uptake from mild adrenal medulla hyperplasia or small pheochromocytoma. MIBG uptake has rarely been reported in adrenocortical adenoma or carcinoma, retroperitoneal angiomyolipoma and hemangioma. SPECT/CT may avoid misleading accumulations in the liver (inhomogeneous uptake, hepatic hemangioma, hepatocellular carcinoma), in the renal parenchyma (diffuse for renal artery stenosis, focal for acute pyelonephritis) or in the urinary tract (hydronephrosis, renal cysts).

False-Negative Pitfall

False-negative results may result from pharmaceutical interactions with MIBG uptake. Physiological uptake can mask cancer lesions. Tumor lesions close to areas of high physiological or pathological uptake can be overlooked (e.g. pelvic views cannot be correctly interpreted if the patient has not voided before the acquisition). Head and neck paraganglioma, retroperitoneal extra-adrenal paraganglioma, small lesions (below the resolution of scintigraphy) and tumor lesions that do not uptake MIBG (e.g. large pheochromocytoma/paraganglioma with substantial necrosis or hemorrhage, poorly differentiated tumors) can yield false-negative results [26-30].

Diagnostic Accuracy

^{123}I-MIBG scintigraphy has a sensitivity ranging from 83% to 100% and a high specificity (95–100%) for pheochromocytoma. Its specificity decreases in MEN2-related pheochromocytoma. Studies that have included high numbers of extra-adrenal, multiple or hereditary paragangliomas have shown reduced sensitivity of ^{123}I-MIBG scintigraphy (52–75%) [26-29]. In patients with metastatic disease, ^{123}I-MIBG scintigraphy may lead to a significant underestimation of the extent of disease with potentially inappropriate management. ^{131}I-MIBG has a high sensitivity (81–96%) and specificity (95–100%) in the diagnosis of pheochromocytoma and neuroblastoma, and a lower sensitivity in carcinoid (70%), medullary carcinoma (35%) and head and neck paragangliomas (18–50%).

Moreover, SPECT imaging is still progressing; integrated SPECT/CT has improved the localization and characterization of lesions and facilitated detection of the involvement of adjacent structures.

Recommendations for Clinical Practice

^{123}I-MIBG is as sensitive as PET imaging (^{18}F-FDOPA PET, ^{18}F-FDA PET, ^{18}F-FDG), and definitely superior to ^{111}In-pentetreotide SPECT(/CT) in localizing non metastatic apparently sporadic pheochromocytoma. ^{123}I-MIBG scintigraphy appears sufficient to confirm the diagnosis of pheochromocytoma even in rare cases of non-hypersecreting pheochromocytoma. With its ability for whole-body screening, it can rule out extra-adrenal disease and act as a guide for additional CT and MRI investigations. ^{123}I-MIBG scintigraphy is not sufficiently sensitive in head and neck paragangliomas or retroperitoneal extra-adrenal paragangliomas. ^{123}I-MIBG scintigraphy can be used in the detection of MEN2-related pheochromocytoma, but its sensitivity and specificity are suboptimal. Many of these patients do not need any specific functional imaging if a tumor is confined to the adrenal gland with concomitant and characteristic elevation of plasma or urine metanephrine levels.

Several studies have demonstrated the limitations of using ^{123}I-MIBG scintigraphy alone in the staging and restaging of hereditary and metastatic pheochromocytomas/paragangliomas.

The use of ^{123}I-MIBG may lead to significant underestimation of metastatic disease with potentially inappropriate management. The main purpose of ^{123}I-MIBG scintigraphy in a patient with metastases is to determine whether internal targeted radiotherapy is an appropriate treatment choice.

References

[1]   Rubello D, Bui C, Casara D, Gross MD, Fig LM et al. Functional scintigraphy of the adrenal gland. *European journal of endocrinology / European Federation of Endocrine Societies* 2002; 147: 13-28.

[2]   Leung A, Shapiro B, Hattner R, Kim E, de Kraker J et al. Specificity of radioiodinated MIBG for neural crest tumors in childhood. *Journal of nuclear medicine : official publication, Society of Nuclear Medicine* 1997; 38: 1352-7.

[3]   Sisson JC, Shulkin BL. Nuclear medicine imaging of pheochromocytoma and neuroblastoma. *The quarterly journal of nuclear medicine : official publication of the Italian Association of Nuclear Medicine* 1999; 43: 217-23.

[4]   Nakajo M, Shapiro B, Copp J, Kalff V, Gross MD et al. The normal and abnormal distribution of the adrenomedullary imaging agent m-[I-131]iodobenzylguanidine (I-131 MIBG) in man: evaluation by scintigraphy. *Journal of nuclear medicine : official publication, Society of Nuclear Medicine* 1983; 24: 672-82.

[5]   Shapiro B, Gross MD. Radiochemistry, biochemistry, and kinetics of 131I-metaiodobenzylguanidine (MIBG) and 123I-MIBG: clinical implications of the use of 123I-MIBG. *Medical and pediatric oncology* 1987; 15: 170-7.

[6]   Wafelman AR, Hoefnagel CA, Maes RA, Beijnen JH. Radioiodinated metaiodobenzylguanidine: a review of its biodistribution and pharmacokinetics, drug interactions, cytotoxicity and dosimetry. *European journal of nuclear medicine* 1994; 21: 545-59.

[7]   Stabin MG, Gelfand MJ. Dosimetry of pediatric nuclear medicine procedures. *The quarterly journal of nuclear medicine : official publication of the Italian Association of Nuclear Medicine* 1998; 42: 93-112.

[8]   Radiation dose to patients from radiopharmaceuticals. A report of a Task Group of Committee 2 of the International Commission on Radiological Protection. *Annals of the ICRP* 1987; 18: 1-377.

[9]   Radiation dose to patients from radiopharmaceuticals (addendum 2 to ICRP publication 53). *Annals of the ICRP* 1998; 28: 1-126.

[10]   Boubaker A, Bischof Delaloye A. Nuclear medicine procedures and neuroblastoma in childhood. Their value in the diagnosis, staging and assessment of response to therapy. *The quarterly journal of nuclear medicine: official publication of the Italian Association of Nuclear Medicine* 2003; 47: 31-40.

[11]   Perel Y, Conway J, Kletzel M, Goldman J, Weiss S et al. Clinical impact and prognostic value of metaiodobenzylguanidine imaging in children with metastatic neuroblastoma. *Journal of pediatric hematology/oncology* 1999; 21: 13-8.

[12]   Taieb D, Neumann H, Rubello D, Al-Nahhas A, Guillet B et al. Modern nuclear imaging for paragangliomas: beyond SPECT. *Journal of nuclear medicine : official publication, Society of Nuclear Medicine* 2012; 53: 264-74.

[13]   Karasek D, Shah U, Frysak Z, Stratakis C, Pacak K. An update on the genetics of pheochromocytoma. *Journal of human hypertension* 2013; 27: 141-7.

[14]   Braune S, Reinhardt M, Schnitzer R, Riedel A, Lucking CH. Cardiac uptake of [123I]MIBG separates Parkinson's disease from multiple system atrophy. *Neurology* 1999; 53: 1020-5.

[15]   Lipp A, Sandroni P, Ahlskog JE, Fealey RD, Kimpinski K et al. Prospective differentiation of multiple system atrophy from Parkinson disease, with and without autonomic failure. *Archives of neurology* 2009; 66: 742-50.

[16]   Taieb D, Timmers HJ, Hindie E, Guillet BA, Neumann HP et al. EANM 2012 guidelines for radionuclide imaging of phaeochromocytoma and paraganglioma. *European journal of nuclear medicine and molecular imaging* 2012; 39: 1977-95.

[17]   Lassmann M, Biassoni L, Monsieurs M, Franzius C. The new EANM paediatric dosage card: additional notes with respect to F-18. *Eur J Nucl Med Mol Imaging* 2008; 35: 1666-8.

[18]   Tobes MC, Fig LM, Carey J, Geatti O, Sisson JC et al. Alterations of iodine-131 MIBG biodistribution in an anephric patient: comparison to normal and impaired renal function. *Journal of nuclear medicine : official publication, Society of Nuclear Medicine* 1989; 30: 1476-82.

[19]   Solanki KK, Bomanji J, Moyes J, Mather SJ, Trainer PJ et al. A pharmacological guide to medicines which interfere with the biodistribution of radiolabelled meta-iodobenzylguanidine (MIBG). *Nuclear medicine communications* 1992; 13: 513-21.

[20]   Bombardieri E, Aktolun C, Baum RP, Bishof-Delaloye A, Buscombe J et al. 131I/123I-metaiodobenzylguanidine (MIBG) scintigraphy: procedure guidelines for tumour imaging. *European journal of nuclear medicine and molecular imaging* 2003; 30: BP132-9.

[21]   Bombardieri E, Giammarile F, Aktolun C, Baum RP, Bischof Delaloye A et al. 131I/123I-metaiodobenzylguanidine (MIBG) scintigraphy: procedure guidelines for

tumour imaging. *European journal of nuclear medicine and molecular imaging* 2010; 37: 2436-46.

[22]   Rufini V, Fisher GA, Shulkin BL, Sisson JC, Shapiro B. Iodine-123-MIBG imaging of neuroblastoma: utility of SPECT and delayed imaging. *Journal of nuclear medicine : official publication, Society of Nuclear Medicine* 1996; 37: 1464-8.

[23]   Rufini V, Giordano A, Di Giuda D, Petrone A, Deb G et al. [123I]MIBG scintigraphy in neuroblastoma: a comparison between planar and SPECT imaging. *The quarterly journal of nuclear medicine : official publication of the Italian Association of Nuclear Medicine* 1995; 39: 25-8.

[24]   Sinclair AJ, Bomanji J, Harris P, Ross G, Besser GM et al. Pre- and post-treatment distribution pattern of 123I-MIBG in patients with phaeochromocytomas and paragangliomas. *Nuclear medicine communications* 1989; 10: 567-76.

[25]   Okuyama C, Sakane N, Yoshida T, Shima K, Kurosawa H et al. (123)I- or (125)I-metaiodobenzylguanidine visualization of brown adipose tissue. *Journal of nuclear medicine : official publication, Society of Nuclear Medicine* 2002; 43: 1234-40.

[26]   Ilias I, Chen CC, Carrasquillo JA, Whatley M, Ling A et al. Comparison of 6-18F-fluorodopamine PET with 123I-metaiodobenzylguanidine and 111in-pentetreotide scintigraphy in localization of nonmetastatic and metastatic pheochromocytoma. *Journal of nuclear medicine : official publication, Society of Nuclear Medicine* 2008; 49: 1613-9.

[27]   Timmers HJ, Eisenhofer G, Carrasquillo JA, Chen CC, Whatley M et al. Use of 6-[18F]-fluorodopamine positron emission tomography (PET) as first-line investigation for the diagnosis and localization of non-metastatic and metastatic phaeochromocytoma (PHEO). *Clinical endocrinology* 2009; 71: 11-7.

[28]   Timmers HJ, Chen CC, Carrasquillo JA, Whatley M, Ling A et al. Comparison of 18F-fluoro-L-DOPA, 18F-fluoro-deoxyglucose, and 18F-fluorodopamine PET and 123I-MIBG scintigraphy in the localization of pheochromocytoma and paraganglioma. *The Journal of clinical endocrinology and metabolism* 2009; 94: 4757-67.

[29]   Fiebrich HB, Brouwers AH, Kerstens MN, Pijl ME, Kema IP et al. 6-[F-18]Fluoro-L-dihydroxyphenylalanine positron emission tomography is superior to conventional imaging with (123)I-metaiodobenzylguanidine scintigraphy, computer tomography, and magnetic resonance imaging in localizing tumors causing catecholamine excess. *The Journal of clinical endocrinology and metabolism* 2009; 94: 3922-30.

[30]   Fonte JS, Robles JF, Chen CC, Reynolds J, Whatley M et al. False-negative (1)(2)(3)I-MIBG SPECT is most commonly found in SDHB-related pheochromocytoma or paraganglioma with high frequency to develop metastatic disease. *Endocrine-related cancer* 2012; 19: 83-93.

In: SPECT
Editors: Hojjat Ahmadzadehfar and Elham Habibi

ISBN: 978-1-62808-344-6
© 2013 Nova Science Publishers, Inc.

Chapter VIII

Cardiac SPECT

Tomoaki Nakata[1,2,*] *and Akiyoshi Hashimoto*[2]

[1]Cardiology Department, Hakodate Goryoukaku Hospital, Hakodate-city,
Hokkaido, Japan
[2]Second (Cardiology) Department of Internal Medicine,
Sapporo Medical University School of Medicine, Sapporo, Hokkaido, Japan

Introduction

Single photon emission computed tomography (SPECT) techniques have been widely applied for diagnosis, disease severity assessment, risk-stratification for selecting treatment strategies, evaluation of therapeutic efficacies and prognosis prediction in cardiology practice. Among recent advances in cardiac imaging modalities, SPECT imaging has a unique position as a molecular imaging. This imaging procedure can provide various types of specific functional information, such as information on myocardial perfusion, viability, fatty acid metabolism and sympathetic nerve innervation, rather than anatomical information, in patients with coronary artery disease, heart failure or cardiomyopathies. There are several international guidelines [1-5] and textbooks providing a wide range of information on nuclear cardiology techniques [6]. This chapter outlines recent applications and advances in SPECT procedures and future perspectives, but does not introduce an overall guide of SPECT technology or delve into details of procedural aspects.

Tracers

Cardiac SPECT imaging is widely used in routine clinical practice. There are several radiopharmaceutical agents available for the assessment of myocardial perfusion, fatty acid

---

* Address for correspondence: Tomoaki Nakata, MD-PhD, Clinical Associate Professor. S-1, W-16, Chuo-ku, Sapporo 060-0061, Japan. Phone: +81-138-51-2295. Fax: +81-138-56-2695, E-mail: tnakata@sapmed.ac.jp.

metabolism and autonomic function. ^{99m}Technetium (^{99m}Tc)-labeled myocardial perfusion traces (sestamibi and tetrofosmin) are most commonly used for myocardial perfusion imaging in patients with suspected or known coronary artery disease; these tracers have several advantages over ^{201}Thallium (^{201}Tl), such as a greater photo-peak (140 KeV), a shorter half-life (6 hours) and easy preparation for urgent use [6]. These features contribute to an improvement in image quality and diagnostic accuracy, lowering of radiation exposure, the application of an electrocardiogram (ECG)-gating approach and ultimately better cost-effectiveness. ^{123}I-labeled tracers, metaiodobenzylguanidine (^{123}I-MIBG) and beta-methyl-p-iodophenylpentadecanoic acid (^{123}I -BMIPP), enable the delineation of cardiac sympathetic innervation and fatty acid metabolism in clinical practice, respectively.

Myocardial Perfusion SPECT Imaging

Myocardial perfusion SPECT imaging is the most well-established diagnostic technique for the detection of coronary artery disease in nuclear cardiology practice. This technique is widely used for the diagnosis of reversible ischemia and myocardial infarction, the assessment of disease severity, the assessment of myocardial viability, risk-stratification and prediction of prognosis, the determination of indication for a revascularization procedure, and the evaluation of therapeutic effects.

A stress approach using exercise or pharmacological agents enables noninvasive assessment of the area, severity and location of reversible myocardial ischemia and limited coronary flow reserve, contributing to risk-stratification and prognosis assessment; these are indispensable for selecting therapeutic strategy in patients with suspected or known coronary artery disease and in patients with multiple coronary risk factors. Exercise-stress testing is performed using a treadmill or ergometer with a standard step-wise protocol. Pharmacological stress testing is performed using coronary dilator agents such as dipyridamole, adenosine and selective A2a receptor agonists (regadenoson) or by using dobutamine as a cardiac inotrope and chronotrope, with established protocols. Because of the very short half-life (less than ten seconds) and safety, adenosine and its analogues are widely used. Regadenoson, which has recently become available in North-America and Europe, contributes to a very simple and short protocol (a bolus injection of a fixed dose without an infusion pump or specialized tubing) and to an improvement in safety due to highly selective A2a stimulation; therefore, it is promising for use in patients with COPD and/or bronchial asthma. Resting perfusion SPECT imaging can provide information on myocardial viability in post-myocardial infarction patients with heart failure and in patients with cardiomyopathy, by quantifying tracer activity (relative percent tracer uptake); this information is useful for the selection of medical and surgical treatments.

For visual SPECT analysis, myocardial uptake is semi-quantitatively scored in 17 segments with a 5-point model from normal (score 0) to absent (score 4) as recommended by the ACC/AHA/ASNC guidelines [2, 6]. Global tracer uptake in the left ventricle is calculated as summed scores, such as summed rest score (SRS), summed stress score (SSS) and summed difference score (SDS), the latter being derived from SSS minus SRS, using the 17-segment, 5-point model. These scores are useful for risk-stratification (low-, intermediate- and high-risk categories) and have been established as predictors of both low-risk and high-risk categories for major cardiac events in patients with coronary artery disease. As a more quantitative analysis, percent tracer activity can be regionally measured on SPECT images. Myocardium with a regional percent tracer uptake of 50% or more has residual viability, and if the regional wall is impaired at a corresponding area, the recovery of regional dysfunction is expected as stunned or hibernating myocardium. The former has no ischemia and the latter has residual ischemia, both of which can be evaluated by stress myocardial perfusion SPECT imaging. Ischemic but viable myocardium with wall motion abnormalities can be salvaged by revascularization therapy. On the other hand, myocardium with asynergic wall motion and regional percent tracer activity of less than 40% has far less or no viability, and regional wall abnormality is unlikely to be recovered, even by coronary revascularization. Thus, semi-quantitative and quantitative analyses of myocardial perfusion SPECT imaging have high clinical efficacies for the management of patients with suspected or known coronary artery disease.

ECG-Gating Approach in Myocardial Perfusion SPECT

In the past decade, instead of conventional first-pass or equilibrium-gated radionuclide angiography using ^{99m}Tc-labeled red blood cells or albumin, an ECG-gating approach in myocardial perfusion SPECT has been widely used for the measurement of left ventricular function [1, 2]. There are several reasons for this: first, ^{99m}Tc-labled perfusion tracers (sestamibi and tetrofosmin) currently used for myocardial perfusion SPECT imaging improve image quality with a high count rate and allow flexible acquisition protocols; second, advances in multi-detector gamma cameras and computer systems have significantly shortened the acquisition and processing time; third, reliable software programs have been developed for the analysis of global and regional left ventricular functions using SPECT images, which are routinely available; and finally, this approach enables the simultaneous evaluation of myocardial perfusion and left ventricular function within a single study. Software programs for gated SPECT have automated data processing systems and provide 2- and 3-dimensional images with a cine-mode, making this technique a routine application for nuclear cardiology practice. Several established software programs that are highly reproducible, practical and easily operated are available for clinical use: *Cedars-Sinai QGS (Quantitative Gated SPECT), Sapporo pFAST (Perfusion and Function Assessment for gated SPECT) program, Emory Cardiac Toolbox* and *Michigan 4D-MSPECT*. An ECG-gating approach provides functional information, such as information on left ventricular volume, ejection fraction and regional wall motion, which is useful for better differentiation from the appearance of artifacts, with better cost-effectiveness (less necessity of conventional radionuclide ventriculography).

It is of great importance to note that gated perfusion SPECT imaging enables the simultaneous assessment of myocardial perfusion and wall motion. The mild-to-moderate reduction of tracer uptake with normal or near-normal wall motion can be identified as artifacts or less pathological, resulting in an improvement in specificity (low-risk assessment) of perfusion SPECT imaging. On the other hand, reduced regional wall motion with normal, near-normal or reversibly reduced tracer uptake can be identified as stunned or hibernating myocardium; the former has no residual ischemia and the latter has persistent ischemia. Quantification of the degree and extent of left ventricular dysfunction enables a systematic assessment of the disease process of myocardial injury, provides objective prognostic information for risk stratification and therapeutic strategy, and allows functional outcomes after optimal medical therapy or a revascularization procedure to be traced. More importantly, gated SPECT information provides incremental information over the perfusion data and conventional clinical risks, particularly using end-systolic volume and left ventricular ejection fraction in patients with suspected or known coronary artery disease [7, 8]. Thus, the gated SPECT technique contributes to improvements in diagnostic accuracy, pathophysiological understanding of myocardial ischemia and viability assessment in patients with coronary artery disease or heart failure. The addition to functional data, myocardial perfusion information by the gated SPECT approach improves risk-stratification of low- or high-risk patients for heart failure, myocardial infarction or cardiac death, contributing to the selection of the optimal therapeutic strategy based on cardiac risk factors. Future improvement in spatial and temporal resolutions of gated SPECT images, however, is necessary for the accurate detection of epicardial and endocardial surfaces, particularly in a small heart, as well as for a more precise diastolic function analysis.

Myocardial Sympathetic Nerve Imaging Using ^{123}I-MIBG

^{123}I-MIBG enables the assessment of cardiac sympathetic innervation and function in clinical settings. This tracer is a norepinephrine analogue but is inactive, and was originally developed as an imaging agent for adrenal medulla [9]. This molecule is specifically taken up and retained at pre-synaptic sympathetic nerve terminals without being metabolized, reflecting the distribution and function of sympathetic nerve terminals in the myocardium. Because of the elimination of contaminated (i.e., non-neuronal) activity, cardiac ^{123}I-MIBG uptake is assessed as myocardial sympathetic innervation several hours after tracer injection. Cardiac ^{123}I-MIBG activity on a planar image is quantified as heart-to-mediastinal ratio (HMR) by manually setting the region of interest on the upper mediastinum and the whole cardiac region on a planar image [9]. Clearance rate of ^{123}I-MIBG from the heart reflects sympathetic nerve activity. For the calculation of washout kinetics of ^{123}I-MIBG from the heart, cardiac MIBG imaging is performed twice, 15-30 minutes (early image) and 4-6 hours (late image) after tracer injection.

Myocardial ^{123}I-MIBG activity (HMR) and clearance rate (washout rate) from the myocardium are well known to be closely related to lethal cardiac events in patients with heart failure [11-15]. Cardiac ^{123}I-MIBG activity has incremental prognostic efficacies in combination with known cardiac risks such as left ventricular ejection fraction, New York Heart Association functional class, brain natriuretic peptide level, diabetes mellitus and chronic kidney disease in heart failure [16-18]. Global innervation (HMR) of the myocardium assessed by planar imaging is closely related to heart failure outcomes, but washout kinetics is related to sudden cardiac death [19, 20]. ^{123}I-MIBG SPECT imaging is useful for the detection of local denervation in patients with coronary artery disease [21-23]. By comparing with myocardial perfusion SPECT images, ^{123}I-MIBG SPECT imaging enables the detection of ischemia-related denervation in the viable myocardium in patients with acute coronary syndrome and stable coronary artery disease. This is because nerve terminals are more sensitive to ischemia than cardiomyocytes. However, it is not clear whether regional MIBG abnormality has prognostic value in patients with heart failure when compared to global cardiac MIBG parameters. It is also known that there are several clinical conditions that reduce myocardial MIBG uptake, even in the absence of cardiac disease, such as aging, a diabetic state, central nervous system disorders such as Parkinsonism and Shy-Drager syndrome, the use of some drugs such as reserpine and tricyclic antidepressants, and markedly increased liver uptake. Myocardial MIBG activity is useful not only for assessment of disease severity and prognosis but also for monitoring pharmacological [24-27] and non-pharmacological (i.e., implantable cardioverter defibrillator and cardiac re-synchronization therapy) [28, 29] treatment effects in patients with heart failure.

Myocardial Fatty Acid Metabolism Imaging Using ^{123}I-BMIPP

^{123}I-BMIPP is a side-branched long-chain fatty acid and is taken up via a specific sarcolemmal transporter (CD36) of long-chain fatty acids, such as palmitate. This molecule is retained at the triglyceride pool of the cytoplasm without being metabolized by beta-oxidation at mitochondria because of the presence of a methyl branch [30]. Long retention of the tracer enables the assessment of cardiac myocardial fatty acid metabolism in clinical settings. In fasting and resting conditions, myocardial BMIPP imaging is performed using ^{123}I-BMIPP of 111 MBq for adults 30 minutes after intravenous injection. Like semi-quantitative analysis of myocardial perfusion SPECT, myocardial uptake is scored visually from normal (score 0) to absent (score 4) in 17 segments on SPECT images with a 5-point model based on ACC/AHA/ASNC guidelines.

This technique is useful for the diagnosis of coronary artery disease, particularly for the detection of ischemia-related metabolic injury in patients with atypical, suspected, or definitive acute coronary syndrome even after coronary reperfusion [31-33]. It is also useful for the detection of ischemic injury in patients who have difficulty in undergoing stress tests and for diagnosis of coronary vasospastic angina [34-37]. This is because myocardial fatty acid metabolism is very sensitive to ischemia and is rapidly impaired by a transient or persistent ischemic event. Beta-oxidation of fatty acids is a major energy-producing system in the myocardium but requires a lot of oxygen for the function. Myocardial ischemia, therefore, rapidly impairs beta-oxidation and uptake of fatty acids, resulting in cessation of the energy-producing system and fatty acid uptake in the myocardium. This feature explains the mechanism by which myocardial BMIPP imaging is useful for detecting myocardial metabolic injury in the ischemic myocardium at rest [38]. Impaired fatty acid metabolism in the viable myocardium is identified as perfusion-metabolism mismatch (i.e., greater BMIPP defect relative to perfusion defect on SPECT images) in coronary artery disease [31, 39-40]. This phenomenon is known as metabolic stunning or ischemic memory in viable myocardium in coronary artery disease. BMIPP-perfusion mismatch is closely related to regional wall motion abnormality and global left ventricular dysfunction and is known to recover several weeks to months following the success of acute coronary reperfusion or elective coronary revascularization. Discordance of impaired BMIPP uptake and preserved perfusion indicates stunned myocardium that is often observed at a recovery process from acute myocardial ischemia or hibernating myocardium that has persistent ischemia [42-44]. Myocardial fatty acid metabolism imaging with ^{123}I-BMIPP has prognostic value in patients with coronary artery disease [45-49]. A large BMIPP defect and a persistent large BMIPP-perfusion mismatch are closely related to future major cardiac events. The prognostic efficacies increase in combination with known cardiac risks such as a history of myocardial infarction, left ventricular ejection fraction, diabetes mellitus, myocardial perfusion SPECT defect size and advanced chronic kidney disease. Thus, this metabolic imaging technique is useful not only for the diagnosis and risk-stratification of coronary patients but also for understanding the pathophysiology of intracellular metabolic alterations in the ischemic myocardium.

Advances in Quantitative Analysis of SPECT Images

Besides conventional semi-quantitative visual analysis using a 5-point, 17-segment model, there are software tools available for more quantitative analysis of SPECT images. Some software programs for myocardial SPECT imaging offer an automated scoring system in which percent tracer uptake (% activity) is converted into a conventional regional visual score (5-point, 17-segment model) and global score is also calculated as SSS, SRS, SDS or percent myocardial ischemia. The automated quantitative analysis of myocardial SPECT imaging is highly objective, reproducible, cost-effective and widely available at any medical facility, even without an experienced nuclear expert. *Cedars-Sinai QPS (Quantitative Perfusion SPECT)*, *Heart-Score-View*, *Heart-Risk-View* and *cardio Bull* programs can automatically provide quantitative scores of regional and global tracer uptakes (SSS, SRS, SDS). The quantitative SPECT score scan contribute to the assessment of cardiac event risks by combining clinical information and by comparing with a normal or specific patient database, such as *Heart-Risk-View* using the J-ACCESS (Japanese Assessment of Cardiac Events and Survival Study by Quantitative Gated SPECT) database and *cardio Bull* using a normal database [50-52]. Although these software programs were originally developed for myocardial perfusion SPECT analysis, recent studies have demonstrated possible applications to myocardial BMIPP SPECT imaging in comparison with expert visual analysis [52, 53]. There is another type of PC-operated tool named *Cardio GRAF* that can quantify dys-synchrony by modifying a gated SPECT software program (*pFAST* program). The quantitative index of dys-synchrony is calculated from end-systolic phase distribution of SPECT segments and is useful for determining the indication for and therapeutic effects of cardiac resynchronization therapy [54].

High-Resolution, High-Speed SPECT Imaging

Rapid and easy access to a diagnostic procedure is essential in daily practice. Particularly in clinically high-risk patients with known or suspected coronary artery disease, this is crucial for precise diagnosis and early risk-stratification. High-speed SPECT imaging can improve patient throughput (cost-effectiveness and amenity) at a SPECT laboratory and enables the rapid reporting of results for physicians. Recently, because of advances in "high-resolution" collimators and SPECT camera systems, high-speed SPECT imaging has become possible [55, 56]. Compared with conventional collimators such as general-purpose or all-purpose collimators, "high-resolution" collimators have a longer hole-length, smaller hole-diameter and thinner septa. Instead of parallel-hole geometry, which is commonly used in SPECT cameras, fan-beam geometry is recently noted and a hybrid system combining fan-beam properties in the center of the field of view and a gradual approach to parallel-hole design toward the edge of the field of view has been applied for a dual detector Anger-based SPECT system. A right-angle SPECT camera with highly sensitive detectors, such as cadmium zinc telluride (CZT) crystal arrays, at a sitting position can reduce radiotracer doses (radiation exposure) and shorten imaging time by 50-70%. This system can also increase temporal and spatial resolutions with fewer artifacts and ultimately contribute to the better identification of ischemia and scars and to the more accurate analysis, including analysis of cardiac function and myocardial blood flow.

In patients with coronary artery disease, quantitative assessment of coronary flow reserve with high-speed SPECT could be useful for functional evaluation of coronary artery narrowing. Although these approaches are still suboptimal and have issues to be resolved, it is expected that future technical advances will result in the realization of high-resolution, high-speed, high-quality quantitative SPECT imaging.

Hybrid Imaging System: SPECT/ CT Scanner

Because of recent advances in multi-slice CT scanners, coronary CT angiography is now widely used in patients with suspected or known coronary artery disease. Coronary CT angiography, however, has limitations in the precise assessment of functional implications of coronary artery narrowing, particularly at a highly calcified segment and in cases of the appearance of non-negligible artifacts, which result in a low positive predictive value in detection of ischemia-related coronary artery narrowing. An important clinical issue to be resolved is the fact that morphological information provided by coronary angiography shows discrepancies with clinical symptoms or inducible ischemia assessed by stress tests with ECG and/or perfusion SPECT imaging. Despite advances in computer-assisted fusion techniques using separate imaging data sources, there are still difficulties in the precise registration of anatomical CT angiographic and SPECT functional data. The use of a cardiac hybrid SPECT/CT system is a new approach using one machine and blending two essential imaging techniques; this has certain advantages compared to traditional SPECT imaging [6]. CT-based attenuation correction of SPECT data contributes to better diagnostic accuracy, particularly because of improvements in the specificity of myocardial perfusion SPECT imaging without attenuation correction.

This system enables the anatomically accurate positioning of CT angiographic and SPECT images and contributes to the combination of physiological assessment of perfusion, function, sympathetic innervation or fatty acid metabolism with an anatomic assessment of atherosclerotic or structural heart disease. Calcium scoring (i.e., an Agatston calcium score) of coronary arteries adds incremental diagnostic and prognostic values to perfusion SPECT data. Multi-functional images derived from one SPECT/CT study allow rapid and reasonable decision-making by physicians for diagnosis and treatment. For more widespread clinical use of this system, studies must be carried out to more clearly define the roles of a SPECT/CT scanner in the management of patients with cardiovascular disorders and to establish a more cost-effective and lower radiation-exposure approach [57].

Perspectives

SPECT imaging has limited spatial resolution and attenuation correction is still suboptimal. Moreover, SPECT tracer activity is quantified as a "relative", but not absolute, value. In contrast, positron emission tomography (PET) can provide high-quality images with fewer artifacts and high spatial resolution and real quantitative information on myocardial blood flow, coronary flow reserve and metabolic state. Compared to SPECT imaging, however, PET has more difficult access and is less cost-effective, limiting its routine clinical application. As mentioned above, advances in SPECT technologies will enhance the advantages of cardiac molecular/functional imaging and overcome the disadvantages in a cost-effective manner.

References

[1]   JCS Joint Working Group. Guidelines for clinical use of cardiac nuclear medicine (JCS 2010) – digest version –*Circ. J.* 2012;76:761-7.
[2]   Klocke FJ, Baird MG, Lorell BH, et al. ACC/AHA/ASNC guidelines for the clinical use of cardiac radionuclide imaging--executive summary: a report of the American College of Cardiology/American Heart Association Task Force on Practice Guidelines (ACC/AHA/ASNC Committee to Revise the 1995 Guidelines for the Clinical Use of Cardiac Radionuclide Imaging). Circulation. 2003 Sep 16;108: 1404-18., *J. Am. Coll. Cardiol.* 2003 Oct 1;42:1318-33.
[3]   Hendel RC, Berman DS, Di Carli MF, et al. ACCF/ASNC/ACR/AHA/ASE/SCCT/ SCMR/SNM 2009 Appropriate Use Criteria for Cardiac Radionuclide Imaging: A Report of the American College of Cardiology Foundation Appropriate Use Criteria Task Force. Circulation 2009 Jun 9;119:e561-87. *J. Am. Coll. Cardiol.* 2009 Jun 9;53: 2201-29.
[4]   Henzlova MJ, Cerqueira MD, Hansen CL, et al. ASNC Imaging Guidelines for Nuclear Cardiology Procedures: Stress protocols and tracers. *J. Nucl. Cardiol.* 2009. http://www.asnc.org/imageuploads/ImagingGuidelinesStressProtocols021109.pdf.
[5]   Hendel RC, Berman DS, Di Carli MF, et al. ACCF/ASNC/ACR/AHA/ASE/SCCT/ SCMR/SNM 2009 Appropriate Use Criteria for Cardiac Radionuclide Imaging: A Report of the American College of Cardiology Foundation Appropriate Use Criteria Task Force. Circulation 2009 Jun 9;119:e561-87. *J. Am. Coll. Cardiol.* 2009 Jun 9;53: 2201-29.

[6]   Heller GV, Hendel RC. *Nuclear Cardiology Practical Applications*, 2011, The McGraw-Hill Medical, Inc.

[7]   Sharir T, Germano G, Kavanagh PB, et al. Incremental prognostic value of post-stress left ventricular ejection fraction and volume by gated myocardial perfusion single photon emission computed tomography. *Circulation*. 1999;100:1035-42.

[8]   Nakata T, Hashimoto A, Wakabayashi T, Kusuoka H, Nishimura T. Prediction of new-onset refractory congestive heart failure using stress/rest gated perfusion SPECT imaging in patients with known or suspected coronary artery disease: Sub-analysis of the J-ACCESS. *J. Am. Coll. Cardiol. Cardiovsc. Imag.* 2009;2:1393-1400.

[9]   Wieland DM, Wu JI, Brown LE, Mangner TJ, Swanson DP, Beierwaltes WH. Radiolabeled adrenergic neuron-blocking agents: adrenomedullary imaging with 123 I-metaiodobenzylguanidine. *J. Nucl. Med.* 1980;21:349-353.

[10] Merlet P, Dubois-Rande JL, Adnot S, et al. Myocardial beta-adrenergic desensitization and neuronal norepinephrine uptake function in idiopathic dilated cardiomyopathy. *J. Cardiovasc. Pharmacol.* 1992;19:10-16.

[11] Nakata T, Miyamoto K, Doi A, et al. Cardiac death prediction and impaired cardiac sympathetic innervations assessed by metaiodobenzylguanidine in patients with failing and non-failing heart. *J. Nucl. Cardiol.* 1998;5:579-590.

[12] Momose M, Kobayashi H, Iguchi N, et al. Comparison of parameters of 123I-mIBG scintigraphy for predicting prognosis in patients with dilated cardiomyopathy. *Nucl. Med. Commun.* 1999;20:529-535.

[13] Agostini D, Verberne HJ, Burchert W, et al.I-123-mIBG myocardial imaging for assessment of risk for a major cardiac event in heart failure patients: insights from a retrospective European multicenter study. *Eur. J. Nucl. Med. Mol. Imaging.* 2008; 35: 535-46.

[14] Jacobson AF, Senior R, Cerqueira MD, et al. Myocardial iodine-123 meta-iodobenzylguanidine imaging and cardiac events in chronic heart failure. Results of the prospective ADMIRE-HF (AdreView myocardial imaging for risk evaluation in heart failure) study. *J. Am. Coll. Cardiol.* 2010;55:2212-21.

[15] Kuwahara Y, Tamaki N, Nakata T, Yamashina S, Yamazaki J. Determination of the survival rate in patients with congestive heart failure stratified by 123I-MIBG imaging: a meta-analysis from the studied performed in Japan. *Ann. Nucl. Med.* 2011; 25: 101-107.

[16] Wakabayashi T, Nakata T, Hashimoto A, et al. Assessment of underlying etiology and cardiac sympathetic innervation to identify patients at high risk of cardiac death. *J. Nucl. Med.* 2001;42:1757-1767.

[17] Kyuma M, Nakata T, Hashimoto A, et al. Incremental prognostic implications of brain natriuretic peptide, cardiac sympathetic nerve innervation, and noncardiac disorders in patients with heart failure. *J. Nucl. Med.* 2004;45:155-163.

[18] Doi T, Nakata T, Hashimoto A, et al. Cardiac mortality assessment improved by evaluation of cardiac sympathetic nerve activity in combination with hemoglobin and kidney function in chronic heart failure patients. *J. Nucl. Med.* 2012;53:731- 740.

[19] Arora A, Ferrick KJ, Nakata T, et al. I-123 MIBG imaging and heart rate variability analysis to predict the need for an implantable cardioverter defibrillator. *J. Nucl. Cardiol.* 2003;10:121-31.

[20] Yamada T, Shimonagata T, Fukunami M, et al. Comparison of the prognostic value of cardiac iodine-123 metaiodobenzylguanidine imaging and heart rate variability in patients with chronic heart failure: a prospective study. *J. Am. Coll. Cardiol.* 2003; 41: 231-8.

[21] Parthenakis FI, Prassopoulos VK, Koukouraki SI, et al. Segmental pattern of myocardial sympathetic denervation in idiopathic dilated cardiomyopathy: relationship to regional wall motion and myocardial perfusion abnormalities. *J. Nucl. Cardiol.* 2002; 9:15-22.

[22] Nakata T, Nagao K, Tsuchihashi K, Hashimoto A, Tanaka S, Iimura O. Regional cardiac sympathetic nerve dysfunction and the diagnostic efficacy of metaiodobenzylguanidine tomography in stable coronary artery disease. *Am. J. Cardiol.* 1996;78:292-7.

[23] Sakata K, Shirotani M, Yoshida H, Kurata C. Iodide-123 metaiodobenzylguanidine cardiac imaging to identify and localize vasospastic angina without significant coronary artery narrowing. *J. Am. Coll. Cardiol.* 1997;30:370-376.

[24] Yamazaki J, Muto H, Kabano T, Yamashina S, Nanjo S, Inoue A. Evaluation of beta-blocker therapy in patients with dilated cardiomyopathy- Clinical meaning of iodine 123-metaiodobenzylguanidine myocardial single-photon emission computed tomography. *Am. Heart J.* 2001;141:645-652.

[25] Kasama S, Toyama T, Kumakura H, et al. Spironolactone improves cardiac sympathetic nerve activity and symptoms in patients with congestive heart failure. *J. Nucl. Med.* 2002; 43:1279-1285.

[26] Agostini D, Belin A, Amar MH, et al. Improvement of cardiac neuronal function after carvedilol treatment in dilated cardiomyopathy: a 123I-MIBG scintigraphic study. *J. Nucl. Med.* 2000;41:845-51.

[27] Nakata T, Wakabayashi T, Kyuma M, et al. Cardiac metaiodobenzylguanidine activity can predict the long-term efficacy of angiotensin- converting enzyme inhibitors and/or beta-adrenoceptor blockers in patients with heart failure. *Eur. J. Nucl. Med. Mol. Imaging* 2005;32:186-194.

[28] Nagahara D, Nakata T, Hashimoto A, et al. Predicting the need for an implantable cardioverter defibrillator using cardiac metaiodobenzylguanidine activity together with plasma natriuretic peptide concentration or left ventricular function. *J. Nucl. Med.* 2008; 49:225-233.

[29] Nishisato K, Hashimoto A, Nakata T,et al. Impaired Cardiac Sympathetic Innervation and Myocardial Perfusion Are Related to Lethal Arrhythmia: Quantification of Cardiac Tracers in Patients with ICDs. *J. Nucl. Med.* 2010;51:1241–1249.

[30] Knapp FF, Jr., Ambrose KR, Goodman MM. New radioiodinated methyl-branched fatty acids for cardiac studies. *Eur. J. Nucl. Med.* 1986;12 Suppl:S39-44.

[31] Hashimoto A, Nakata T, Tsuchihashi K, Tanaka S, Fujimori K, Iimura O. Postischemic functional recovery and BMIPP uptake after primary percutaneous transluminal coronary angioplasty in acute myocardial infarction. *Am. J. Cardiol.* 1996;77:25-30.

[32] Nakata T, Hashimoto A, Eguchi M. Cardiac BMIPP imaging in acute myocardial infarction. *Int. J. Card. Imaging.* 1999;15:21-6.

[33] Franken PR, De Geeter F, Dendale P, Demoor D, Block P, Bossuyt A. Abnormal free fatty acid uptake in subacute myocardial infarction after coronary thrombolysis: correlation with wall motion and inotropic reserve. *J. Nucl. Med.* 1994;35:1758-65.

[34] Kawai Y, Tsukamoto E, Nozaki Y, Morita K, Sakurai M, Tamaki N. Significance of reduced uptake of iodinated fatty acid analogue for the evaluation of patients with acute chest pain. *J. Am. Coll. Cardiol.* 2001;38:1888-94.

[35] Morimoto K, Tomoda H, Yoshitake M, Aoki N, Handa S, Suzuki Y. Prediction of coronary artery lesions in unstable angina by iodine 123 beta-methyl iodophenyl pentadecanoic acid (BMIPP), a fatty acid analogue, single photon emission computed tomography at rest. *Angiology.* 1999;50:639-48.

[36] Takeishi Y, Fujiwara S, Atsumi H, Takahashi K, Sukekawa H, Tomoike H. Iodine-123-BMIPP imaging in unstable angina: a guide for interventional strategy. *J. Nucl. Med.* 1997; 38:1407-11.

[37] Nakajima K, Shimizu K, Taki J, Uetani Y, Konishi S, Tonami N, et al. Utility of iodine-123-BMIPP in the diagnosis and follow-up of vasospastic angina. *J. Nucl. Med.* 1995; 36: 1934-40.

[38] Dilsizian V, Bateman TM, Bergmann SR, Des Prez R, Magram MY, Goodbody AE, et al. Metabolic imaging with beta-methyl-p-[(123)I]-iodophenyl-pentadecanoic acid identifies ischemic memory after demand ischemia. *Circulation.* 2005;112:2169-74.

[39] Tamaki N, Kawamoto M, Yonekura Y, Fujibayashi Y, Takahashi N, Konishi J, et al. Regional metabolic abnormality in relation to perfusion and wall motion in patients with myocardial infarction: assessment with emission tomography using an iodinated branched fatty acid analog. *J. Nucl. Med.* 1992;33:659-67.

[40] Nakata T, Hashimoto A, Kobayashi H, Miyamoto K, Tsuchihashi K, Miura T, et al. Outcome significance of thallium-201 and iodine-123-BMIPP perfusion-metabolism mismatch in preinfarction angina. *J. Nucl. Med.* 1998;39:1492-9.

[41] Kawai Y, Tsukamoto E, Nozaki Y, Kishino K, Kohya T, Tamaki N. Use of 123I-BMIPP single-photon emission tomography to estimate areas at risk following successful revascularization in patients with acute myocardial infarction. *Eur. J. Nucl. Med.* 1998;25(10):1390-5.

[42] Sato H, Iwasaki T, Toyama T, Kaneko Y, Inoue T, Endo K, et al. Prediction of functional recovery after revascularization in coronary artery disease using (18)F-FDG and (123)I-BMIPP SPECT. *Chest.* 2000;117:65-72.

[43] Shimonagata T, Nanto S, Kusuoka H, Ohara T, Inoue K, Yamada S, et al. Metabolic changes in hibernating myocardium after percutaneous transluminal coronary angioplasty and the relation between recovery in left ventricular function and free fatty acid metabolism. *Am. J. Cardiol.* 1998;82:559-63.

[44] Taki J, Nakajima K, Matsunari I, Bunko H, Takata S, Kawasuji M, et al. Assessment of improvement of myocardial fatty acid uptake and function after revascularization using iodine-123-BMIPP. *J. Nucl. Med.* 1997;38:1503-10.

[45] Nakata T, Kobayashi T, Tamaki N, Kobayashi H, Wakabayashi T, Shimoshige S, et al. Prognostic value of impaired myocardial fatty acid uptake in patients with acute myocardial infarction. *Nucl. Med. Commun.* 2000;21:897-906.

[46] Hashimoto A, Nakata T, Tamaki N, Kobayashi T, Matsuki T, Shogase T, et al. Serial alterations and prognostic implications of myocardial perfusion and fatty acid metabolism in patients with acute myocardial infarction. *Circ. J.* 2006;70:1466-74.

[47] Chikamori T, Fujita H, Nanasato M, Toba M, Nishimura T. Prognostic value of I-123 15-(p-iodophenyl)-3-(R,S) methylpentadecanoic acid myocardial imaging in patients with known or suspected coronary artery disease. *J. Nucl. Cardiol.* 2005;12:172-8.

[48] Matsuki T, Tamaki N, Nakata T, Doi A, Takahashi H, Iwata M, et al. Prognostic value of fatty acid imaging in patients with angina pectoris without prior myocardial infarction: comparison with stress thallium imaging. *Eur. J. Nucl. Med. Mol. Imaging.* 2004; 31:1585-91.

[49] Sasaki R, Mitani I, Usui T, Kitamura Y, Yoshii Y, Ishikawa T, et al. Clinical value of iodine-123 beta-methyliodophenyl pentadecanoic acid (BMIPP) myocardial single photon emission computed tomography for predicting cardiac death among patients with chronic heart failure. *Circ. J.* 2003;67:918-24.

[50] Nakajima K, Nishimura T. Prognostic table for predicting major cardiac events based on J-ACESS investigation. *Ann. Nucl. Med.* 2008;22:891-897.

[51] Yamamoto A, Hosoya T, Takahashi N, et al. Quantification of myocardial perfusion SPECT using freeware package (cardioBull). *Ann. Nucl. Med.* 2011;25:571-579.

[52] Yoshinaga K, Matsuki T, Hashimoto A, et al. Validation of automated quantification of myocardial perfusion and fatty acid metabolism abnormalities on SPECT images. *Circ. J.* 2011; 75: 2187-95.

[53] Nakata T, Hashimoto A, Matsuki T, et al. Prognostic value of automated SPECT scoring system for coronary artery disease in stress myocardial perfusion and fatty acid metabolism imaging. *Int. J. Cardiovasc. Imaging.* 2013;29:253-62.

[54] Okuda K, Nakajima K, Hosoya T, et al. Quantification of left ventricular regional functions using ECG-gated myocardial perfusion SPECT – validation of left ventricular systolic functions. *Ann. Nucl. Med.* 2006;20:449-456.

[55] Funk T, Kirch DL, Koss JE, Botvinick E, Hasegawa BH. A novel approach to multipinhole SPECT for myocardial perfusion imaging *J. Nucl. Med.* 2006;47:595-602.

[56] Sharir T, Ben-Haim S, Merzon K, et al. High-speed myocardial perfusion imaging: initial clinical comparison with conventional dual detector Anger camera imaging *J. Am. Coll. Cardiol. Img.* 2008;1:156-63.

[57] Singh B, Bateman TM, Case JA, Heller G. Attenuation artifact, attenuation correction, and the future of myocardial perfusion SPECT. *J. Nucl. Cardiol.* 2007; 14:153-64.

In: SPECT
Editors: Hojjat Ahmadzadehfar and Elham Habibi

ISBN: 978-1-62808-344-6
© 2013 Nova Science Publishers, Inc.

Chapter IX

The Story of Myocardial Infarction - Before, When it Strikes, and Afterwards: A Tale in Images

Elly L. van der Veen[1,2], Hans J. de Haas[2,3], Artiom D. Petrov[2], Chris P. M. Reutelingsperger[4], Jos G. W. Kosterink[1], Clark J. Zeebregts[5], René A. Tio[6], Riemer H. J. A. Slart[3] and Hendrikus H. Boersma[1,3]*

[1]Department of Clinical and Hospital Pharmacy, University Medical Center Groningen, University of Groningen, Groningen, the Netherlands.
[2]Zena and Michael A. Wiener Cardiovascular Institute, Mount Sinai School of Medicine, New York, New York, US
[3]Department of Nuclear Medicine and Molecular Imaging, Cardiovascular Imaging Group Groningen, University Medical Center Groningen, University of Groningen,the Netherlands
[4]Department of Biochemistry, Maastricht University Medical Center, Maastricht, the Netherlands
[5]Division of Vascular Surgery, Department of Surgery, Cardiovascular Imaging Group Groningen, University Medical Center Groningen, University of Groningen, the Netherlands
[6]Department of Cardiology, Cardiovascular Imaging Group Groningen, University Medical Center Groningen, University of Groningen, the Netherlands

* Hendrikus H. Boersma, PharmD, PhD. Dept of Hospital and Clinical Pharmacy EB 70, University Medical Center Groningen, P.O. Box 30.001, NL-9700 RB Groningen. Email: h.h.boersma@umcg.nl.

Introduction

Cardiovascular diseases are a major cause of death worldwide. Many people die due to an acute cardiovascular event such as myocardial infarction (MI) or ischemic stroke [1]. The process towards the development of myocardial infarction evolves from atherosclerosis. Loss of thrombus particles by an atherosclerotic plaque may lead to the formation of obstructive thrombi within the heart. This process reduces coronary blood flow, and is followed by ischemia; subsequently, MI may occur. After MI, many complications can occur. First, scar tissue will be formed, leading to fibrosis and cardiac hypertrophy; the latter ultimately results in heart failure. Molecular imaging techniques focusing on cardiovascular diseases are important for developing new therapeutic options. In this chapter the different molecular imaging techniques are outlined first, together with their most important imaging tracers. Second, the process towards myocardial infarction and its damage afterwards is discussed. Pathology, therapy and recent imaging developments will be elucidated.

Imaging Techniques

Currently, molecular imaging techniques are increasingly important within cardiovascular research. These techniques can be divided in three types: conventional imaging (duplex ultrasound, computed tomography (CT) and magnetic resonance imaging (MRI)), nuclear imaging positron emission tomography (PET) and single photon emission tomography (SPECT) and bio-optical imaging. These are techniques that are used worldwide to image and detect many disorders [2, 3]. In the next section the advantages and disadvantages of these different types of imaging techniques are outlined.

Conventional Imaging Techniques

The three types of conventional imaging techniques are duplex ultrasound, CT and MRI.

Duplex ultrasound imaging has the advantage that it offers a high spatial resolution (<1mm); it also provides good anatomical information for co-registration with molecular information. Imaging agents for ultrasound imaging are designed using microbubbles, liposomes or perfluorocarbon emulsions as scaffolds. The limitation of ultrasound imaging, however, is the relatively large size of imaging agent particles. These can restrict tissue penetration and thereby limit applications to vascular targets [3-5].

CT imaging has the advantage of high resolution, which makes it possible to image differences in tissues with different physical densities. Therefore, it gives good anatomical information.

An important advantage of MRI is its ability to provide soft tissue and functional information by exploiting proton density, perfusion, diffusion and biochemical contrasts. In a single imaging mode the molecular information is combined with anatomical information. MRI provides high resolution (<1mm) and good depth penetration (>10cm). A disadvantage of MRI is the lower sensitivity for detection of targeted agents; however, this problem is solved by signal amplification strategies, generating a higher contrast between target and background. Examples of imaging agents for MRI are gadolinium and iron oxide [3, 6-9].

Nuclear Imaging Techniques

The nuclear imaging techniques SPECT and PET have the advantage of high intrinsic sensitivity, unlimited depth penetration and a broad range of clinically available molecular imaging agents in order to depict the functionality of organs as well as other disease related targets within the human body. PET is fully quantitative and provides a higher resolution than SPECT. A disadvantage of PET is that a cyclotron is required for the generation of most imaging agents. Another limitation of both PET and SPECT is that patients are exposed to radiation and the anatomical resolution in clinical imaging is lower than for other molecular imaging modalities (5-10mm).

Nowadays, fusion systems of PET and SPECT with CT are used to overcome this last limitation. These fusion systems integrate the lower resolution molecular information from PET or SPECT with the higher resolution anatomical detail achieved by CT [3].

Another novel strategy for molecular imaging is the combination of PET and MRI. PET can image a radionuclide with high detection sensitivity, while simultaneous non-invasive MRI provides high-resolution anatomical images with a large variety of tissue contrasts. With the combination of PET and MRI the registration errors will be minimized and the total imaging time will be reduced [10, 11].

Bio-optical Imaging Techniques

Optical imaging techniques are based on the detection of photons after their interaction with tissue. When photons within the visible or near infrared wavelengths travel through tissue, they are subsequently absorbed and scattered along the way. This effect can be quantified. It is a good method for imaging the blood vessel wall, because there is a relatively low background signal from autofluorescence and also because fluorescence energy transfer or bioluminescence can be used to target relevant metabolic processes. Advantages of optical imaging over other imaging techniques include the fact that they use non-ionizing radiation and provide high spatial resolution. Limitations are the inability to penetrate deeper tissues and the need to use invasive detection for imaging of underlying tissues.

Optical imaging techniques are used for example to visualize biological processes in an atherosclerotic plaque, such as inflammation, endothelial dysfunction, thrombus formation, microcalcifications, apoptosis and angiogenesis [12].

Two important optical imaging methods are near-infrared fluorescence (NIRF) imaging and fluorescence-mediated tomographic imaging. The first uses photons emitted in the near-infrared range. In this wavelength band (650-950 nm), hemoglobin has a lower light absorption, which enables practical photon detection through several centimeters in tissue (up to 10 cm). Another advantage is the reduced autofluorescence in the near infrared range [13]. Fluorescence-mediated tomographic imaging is a preclinical non-invasive fluorescence imaging method, reconstructing light similarly to ultrasound [3].

Advantages of the fluorescence imaging methods are improved relative sensitivity, high resolution and the availability of imaging reports and signal amplification strategies. Besides, surface anatomical information is combined with molecular information [3, 14-17].

Imaging Agents

In molecular imaging, the use of suitable tracers makes it possible to visualize different cardiac disorders. These agents consist of a signal detection compound and an affinity ligand that recognizes the intended molecular or cellular target [18]. In this section, the most important radiotracers for the nuclear imaging techniques SPECT and PET will be discussed.

Perfusion Tracers

PET Myocardial Perfusion Tracers

PET uses radionuclides that decay with positron emission. The masses of positrons and electrons are comparable, but positrons have a positive charge. The positron travels a short distance of a few millimeters and interacts with an electron. The two undergo annihilation, which results in the production of two 511-keV gamma photons, in opposite directions. These photons are detected in a ring detector system, which leads to imaging with high-quality images. The three most commonly used clinical tracers for PET cardiac perfusion imaging are ^{13}N-ammonia, ^{15}O-water (both cyclotron dependent) and Rb-82 chloride (Sr/Rb generator produced) [19]. The advantage of PET myocardial perfusion versus SPECT is the possibility of absolute quantification (mL/min/g) by using specific compartment modeling.

^{13}N-ammonia

In blood, ^{13}N-ammonia consists of neutral ammonia (NH_3) and its charged ammonium (NH_4^+) ion, between which there is equilibrium. Because of its lipid solubility, the neutral NH_3-molecule can diffuse across the plasma and cell membrane and form a new equilibrium with its ammonium form inside the cell [20]. This ammonium form is trapped in glutamine via the enzyme glutamine synthase. There is back-diffusion, but the first-pass trapping of ^{13}N-ammonia at rest is high; however, this decreases with higher blood flow. ^{13}N-ammonia is used for absolute quantification of perfusion at rest and after the application of vasodilating agents to assess myocardial perfusion reserve (Figure 9-1). It has a short half life of 10 minutes [19, 21-23]. LV-function can also be assessed with gated ^{13}N-ammonia.

^{15}O- water

^{15}O-water is a good tracer to determine myocardial blood flow, because it diffuses freely across plasma membranes. However, ^{15}O-water also circulates in the blood, so a poor contrast between the myocardium and cardiac blood pool is achieved. As a consequence, subtraction of blood pool activity is required [21,22]. The proportion of the total tissue that is capable of rapidly exchanging water can be used as a marker for tissue viability [21, 24-25].

^{82}Rb

Rubidium-82 (^{82}Rb) is produced in a generator by decay of ^{82}Sr attached to an elution column. ^{82}Rb decays by positron emission and has a short half-life of 75s. Because of this short half-life it can be used for the rapid completion of a series of resting and stress myocardial perfusion studies. ^{82}Rb is a cation and an analogue of potassium. Extraction from plasma by myocardial cells occurs via the Na$^+$/K$^+$ ATPase pump and is altered during severe acidosis, hypoxia and ischemia. Uptake is thus a function of blood flow and myocardial cell integrity. PET imaging with ^{82}Rb is accurate for the detection and functional assessment of coronary artery stenosis. One Disadvantaged of ^{82}Rb include the high energy of the positron, the long range of the positron and a relative low extraction fraction (65%) [21]. LV-function can also be assessed with gated ^{82}Rb.

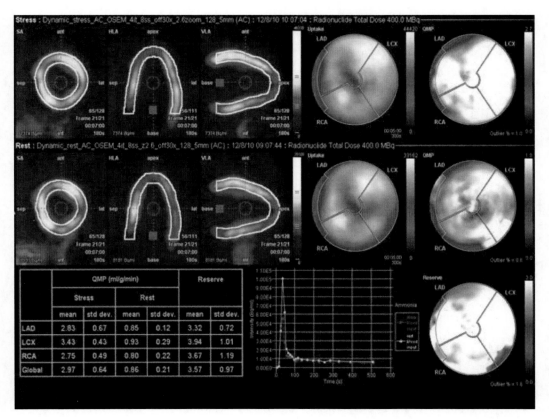

	QMP (ml/g/min)				Reserve	
	Stress		Rest			
	mean	std dev.	mean	std dev.	mean	std dev.
LAD	2.83	0.67	0.85	0.12	3.32	0.72
LCX	3.43	0.43	0.93	0.29	3.94	1.01
RCA	2.75	0.49	0.80	0.22	3.67	1.19
Global	2.97	0.64	0.86	0.21	3.57	0.97

Figure 9-1. Dynamic ^{13}N-ammonia PET: absolute quantification. First row shows adenosine stress ^{13}N-ammonia, second row shows rest ^{13}N-ammonia. Absolute flow numbers are presented in the table and flow reserve is automatically calculated for the different territories and also for the whole left ventricle (global) (previously unpublished, courtesy of Dr. R.H.J.A. Slart).

SPECT Myocardial Perfusion Tracers

The three most important radiotracers for SPECT myocardial perfusion imaging are ^{201}Thallium, ^{99m}Tc-sestamibi (^{99m}Tc-MIBI) and ^{99m}Tc-tetrofosmin [26, 27].

^{201}Thallium

Thallium is a metallic element in group III-A of the periodic table of elements. The uptake of ^{201}Tl by myocardial cells depends on myocardial blood flow and active transport [21]. Overall, 60% of uptake occurs via active transport by a Na^+-K^+-adenosine triphosphate mechanism and requires an intact cell membrane. After intravenous injection, the uptake reaches its peak within several minutes. ^{201}Tl is rapidly cleared from the blood.

Unlike ^{99m}Tc-MIBI and ^{99m}Tc-tetrofosmin, ^{201}Tl has redistribution properties. This means that after the initial phase of extraction, ^{201}Tl is constantly exchanged with new ^{201}Tl from the circulation, instead of being fixed in myocardial cells [22].

Major limitations of ^{201}Tl are the long half-life (physical half-life 73 hours, biological half-life 10 days, effective half-life 56 hours) and the low energy of gamma photons, resulting in poor quality of images [28].

^{99m}Tc-MIBI

Technetium-99m labeled sestamibi (^{99m}Tc-methoxy-isobutyl-isonitrile or ^{99m}Tc-MIBI) is also a tracer which is used as a SPECT perfusion tracer. It is a lipophilic cationic complex and it is an alternative to ^{201}Tl. Uptake of ^{99m}Tc-MIBI is related to the large negative transmembrane potential [29]. It is passively transported across both plasma and mitochondrial membranes. When myocytes are injured, the mitochondrial membranes are depolarized and the uptake of ^{99m}Tc-MIBI is impaired. After initial myocardial uptake, the clearance of ^{99m}Tc-MIBI is slow [22].

^{99m}Tc-Tetrofosmin

Tetrofosmin is a compound of the diphosphine group, with the chemical name 1,2-bis[bis(2-ethoxyethyl)phosphinol]ethane. ^{99m}Tc-tetrofosmin is a lipophilic cationic complex and is rapidly cleared form the blood but has, like ^{99m}Tc-MIBI, a slow myocardial clearance. The uptake by myocardial tissue is in proportion to blood flow and myocardial cellular viability. Like ^{99m}Tc-MIBI, it accumulates in the mitochondria [22]. Advantages of ^{99m}Tc-tetrofosmin in comparison to ^{99m}Tc-MIBI are faster excretion in the gastrointestinal tract, the possibility of creating an image earlier after injection and an easier preparation.

Viability Tracers

The term myocardial viability is used when the myocardium is dysfunctional, but is not entirely necrotic or fibrotic; this indicates that the myocardium is potentially recoverable. A state of dysfunctional but viable myocardium follows mostly after a short period of reversible ischemia, in non-transmural infarction, myocardial stunning or hibernation. There are different methods to estimate myocardial viability; for example SPECT imaging with ^{201}Tl, ^{99m}Tc-based SPECT imaging and ^{18}F-fluorodeoxy-glucose (^{18}F-FDG) PET imaging [31].

^{18}F-FDG

The assessment of oxidative metabolism plays an important role in myocardial viability studies; for this purpose, the PET-tracer ^{18}F-FDG is used. Under normal conditions, the preferential energy substrate of the heart is fatty acids; however, under ischemic conditions, utilization of this free fatty acid is impaired. On the other hand, glucose utilization is increased. FDG competes with glucose in metabolically active cells, such as activated macrophages, for facilitated transport sites and phosphorylation by hexokinase to yield FDG-6-phosphate. FDG-6-phosphate has low membrane permeability and is not a substrate for the glycolytic or glycogen synthetic pathways. Therefore, it accumulates in cells and can be imaged and quantified with PET [2, 30]. Also, a combination of perfusion imaging with ^{201}Tl and imaging of FDG uptake can be used to identify the viable myocardium [31].

Other Tracers

There are many other tracers developed for imaging of the (diseased) cardiovascular system. Different processes are used as a target, for example inflammation, proteolysis, apoptosis/necrosis and angiogenesis. Some examples are outlined below.

Inflammation

Folate

Folate can be used to identify activated macrophages in atherosclerotic plaques. Activated macrophages are an important diagnostic and therapeutic target for atherosclerosis, since they accumulate in inflammation at sites of plaque rupture. The activated macrophages express folate receptor β (FR-β), while this receptor is not present on quiescent macrophages or immune cells. Folate bound to an optical fluorescent contrast agent is used to visualize the FR-β on activated macrophages by optical imaging. An example is fluorescine-isothiocynate (FITC) conjugated with folate, which may be used to identify vulnerable sites within an atherosclerotic plaque [32-35]. Furthermore, it was also demonstrated that folate can be labeled using ^{99m}Tc pertechnetate. Although this tracer was used up until now only as a tumor tracer, it also bears promise to be used as a cardiovascular tracer [36].

^{99m}Tc-Fucoidan

Fucoidan is a sulfated polysaccharide derived from brown seaweed and is a naturally occurring mimic of Sialil Lewis X (SLe^x), a ligand of P-selectin. P-selectin is an important target in acute and chronic cardiovascular diseases. It is an adhesion molecule expressed at the surface of endothelial cells and platelets on activation, which interacts with the counter-receptor P-selectin glycoprotein ligand 1, and in inflammation this results in tethering of leukocytes, followed by rolling over the endothelium and migration into the tissue. On platelets it mediates the formation of platelet-leukocyte complexes, which enhances migration. During vascular thrombus formation, platelet-leukocyte complexes are also formed, causing growth and stabilization of the thrombus.

Because of its important role in cardiovascular diseases, imaging agents targeting P-selectin have been developed. These agents were either P-selectin antibodies or synthetic mimics of SLe^x. However, these agents were quite expensive and the antibodies presented a risk of immunogenicity. Fucoidan overcomes these limitations and is therefore a good target for P-selectin imaging. It can detect platelet-rich arterial thrombus and endothelial activation after an acute ischemic event [37, 38].

Proteolysis

Metalloproteinase Inhibitors

[99m]Tc-labeled matrix metalloproteinase inhibitors (MPIs) are used in imaging of matrix metalloproteinase (MMP) activity in atherosclerotic plaques. MMPs are cytokines secreted from macrophages and SMCs in atherosclerotic plaques. Secretion of MMP leads to collagen and elastin degradation, resulting in rupture of the fibrous cap. A reduction of MMP activity, e.g. with statin treatment, would therefore stabilize the plaque. To evaluate the efficacy of such treatments, SPECT imaging with MPIs can be performed. One common MPI is ^{99m}Tc-RP805. This MPI binds specifically to a broad range of active MMPs and not to other proteases. After intravenous administration, the MPI uptake in plaques can be determined by SPECT/CT (Figure 9-2) [39].

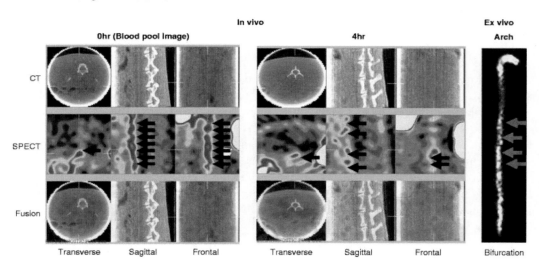

Figure 9-2. MicroCT, microSPECT and fusion images (rows) showing uptake of RP805 (a broad-spectrum MMP ligand) demonstrating MMP expression in an atherosclerotic rabbit on an uninterrupted diet. The three columns display transverse, sagittal, and frontal projections. Left set of three columns: images immediately (0 h) after radiotracer administration (representing blood pool images). Right set of three columns: images obtained at 4 h (representing tracer uptake in target tissue). "With kind permission from Springer Science+Business Media: Eur J Nucl Med, Small-animal SPECT and SPECT/CT: application in cardiovascular research, 37(9), 2010, p. 1766-1777, Golestani R et al., Fig 3.

Apoptosis/necrosis

Glucarate

[99m]Tc-Glucarate is a SPECT tracer used to visualize necrotic tissue and helps to detect MI in an early stage. It is also used to detect the anti-necrotic effect of drugs in models of ischemic heart diseases.

Glucarate is a six-carbon dicarbocylic acid sugar, a small molecular weight compound, and has an affinity for histone proteins. In necrotic cells, ^{99m}Tc-Glucarate can bind to histone proteins because of lesions in the cellular and nuclear membranes. ^{99m}Tc-Glucarate is excreted principally via the urinary system and localizes rapidly into the infarcted myocardium after intravenous administration [41-43].

Annexin A5

Annexin A5 is a human protein that is used to measure apoptosis, which is the major form of programmed cell death (PCD). Traditionally, it has been thought that the heart muscle cells are lost by necrosis during ischemia, but from the nineties onwards, it was recognized that apoptosis also has an important role.

Annexin A5 binds to the negatively charged phospholipid phospatidylserine (PS), which is normally located in the inner leaflet of the membrane. However, this is expressed on the outer cell membrane in apoptotic cells. Annexin was first discovered as a result of its ability to inhibit blood coagulation. [99m]Tc is the most used radionuclide for Annexin A5 (Figure 9-3) [44].

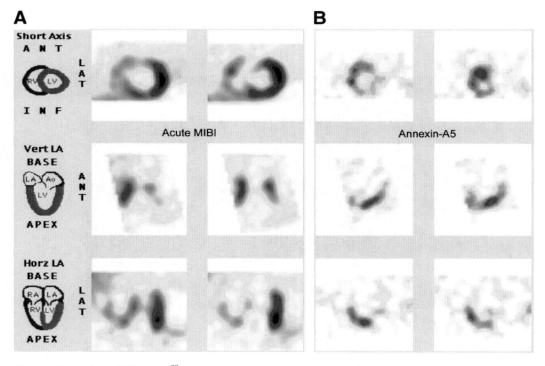

Figure 9-3. Imaging of MI, using ^{99m}Tc-annexin A5. (A) Methoxyisobutylisonitrile (MIBI) scintigraphy depicting area of perfusion, indicating area at risk. (B) Binding of ^{99m}Tc-anxA5 to reperfused myocardium, indicative of presence of programmed cell death (PCD). ANT = anterior; LAT = lateral; INF = inferior; Vert LA = vertical long axis; Horz LA = horizontal long axis; RV = right ventricle; LV = left ventricle; LA = left atrium; Ao = aorta; RA = right atrium. This research was originally published in JNM. Boersma HH, Kietselaer BL, Stolk LM, et al. Past, present, and future of annexin A5: from protein discovery to clinical applications. J Nucl Med 2005;46(12):2035-2050 © by the Society of Nuclear Medicine and Molecular Imaging, Inc (Ref. 44).

Other Apoptosis Tracers

There are also other tracers to detect apoptosis, including a new PS-binding peptide, synaptotagmin C2A. This is a possible alternative for Annexin A5. It is a 128-amino acid residue peptide that also binds to PS in a calcium-dependent, specific way. It has been conjugated to magnetic nanoparticles for MRI and also to ^{99m}Tc for apoptosis SPECT imaging. However, more research has to be done on this peptide to ensure safety and efficacy in humans [45]. To detect apoptosis, caspase activity can also be imaged with radiolabeled imaging agents. One example is an ^{18}F-isatin sulfonamide analogue, which targets activated macrophages [45, 46].

Angiogenesis

Angiogenesis, the formation of new blood vessels, plays an important role following myocardial infarction. It is necessary to provide the infarcted myocardium with nutrients and oxygen. Therefore, many pro-angiogenic drugs are being developed. To evaluate the efficacy of these treatments, non-invasive imaging methods are needed.

During angiogenesis, cell-cell and cell-matrix interactions are performed by endothelial cells. These interactions are mediated by integrins. In angiogenesis, $\alpha_v\beta_3$ integrin plays an important role, since it is overexpressed on the surface of newly-formed endothelium. It is thought to play a role in migration, adhesion and signal transduction.

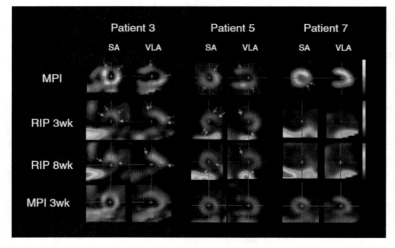

Figure 9-4. Example of stress MPI at discharge and ^{99m}Tc-RIP imaging at 3 and 8 weeks post-MI in 3 patients. The upper rows show myocardial perfusion imaging (MPI), the middle rows (2 and 3) show ^{99m}Tc-RIP images at 3 and 8 weeks post-MI and the last row shows fusion images of 3-week ^{99m}Tc-RIP and baseline MPL. MPI images of patient #3 demonstrate short axis (SA) and vertical long axis (VLA) views of perfusion defects in the anterolateral region (red arrows). ^{99m}Tc-RIP images at 3 and 8 weeks post-MI show uptake (blue arrows) corresponding to the infarct and border zone defined by MIPI (red arrows). Images of patient #5 show a LAD region perfusion defect in MPL. ^{99m}Tc-RIP uptake in SA view extends beyond the infarct border zone at 3 and 8 weeks (red vs. blue arrows). Images of patient #7 show a small RCA infarct (red arrows) and little or no uptake of ^{99m}Tc-RIP at 3 and 8 weeks. "With kind permission from Springer Science+Business Media: J Nucl Cardiol, Early molecular imaging of interstitial changes in patients after myocardial infarction: comparison with delayed contrast-enhanced magnetic resonance imaging, 17(6), 2010, p. 1065-1072, Verjans J et al., fig 2." (Ref. 50).

^{18}F-Galacto-RGD or ^{18}F-RGD-K5 bind to $\alpha_v\beta_3$ integrins and can be used as PET tracers to target $\alpha_v\beta_3$ expression. In an earlier stage, an RGD-Imaging Peptide (RIP, NC100692) was developed and labeled with ^{99m}Tc (Figure 9-4). Both compounds contain the tripeptide sequence arginine-glycine-aspartic acid (RGD) in a constant conformation, have a high affinity for $\alpha_v\beta_3$ integrin and are rapidly cleared from the blood. This makes both promising tracers for non-invasive PET and SPECT imaging [47-49].

Pathology, Therapy and Imaging Studies

In the next section the pathophysiology of the different stages before and after myocardial infarction are discussed, together with therapeutic strategies and examples of different imaging studies, using the radiotracers discussed in the previous section.

Pathology

Myocardial infarction results from myocardial ischemia, mostly caused by partial or complete epicardial coronary artery occlusion from a vulnerable atherosclerotic plaque [51]. A vulnerable atherosclerotic plaque is characterized by the presence of a large lipid-rich core, containing inflammatory cells and a thin fibrous cap.

The process of atherosclerosis starts with a change in the arterial endothelial cells. This change is caused by atherogenic stimuli like dyslipidemia, hypertension or pro-inflammatory mediators and leads to dysfunctioning of these cells. Dysfunction of the endothelial cells causes smooth muscle cells (SMCs) to proliferate, leading to intimal thickening. Due to the change in endothelial permeability, cholesterol-containing low-density lipoprotein (LDL) particles enter the artery wall and accumulate in the arterial intima. LDL is oxidatively modified and causes an inflammatory response.

At the same time, endothelial cells express adhesion molecules to which leukocytes bind (e.g. (VCAM)-1, E-selectin, P-selectin). The activated SMCs secrete chemokines such as CCL2, CCL5, CXCL10 and CX3CL1. These adhesion molecules and chemokines together attract monocytes and lymphocytes into the intima, followed by maturation of monocytes into macrophages stimulated by monocyte chemoattractant protein-1 (MCP-1). Macrophages become foam cells after endocytosis of the lipoprotein particles, which is regulated by scavenger receptors (SR-A, CD 36, LOX-1). T-cells are recruited by cytokines and chemokines, producing factors favoring atherogenesis. Proliferation of smooth muscle cells (SMCs) and production of extracellular matrix molecules, like interstitial collagen and elastin, leads to the formation of a fibrous cap covering the plaque. Apoptosis and necrosis of foam cells leads to lipid accumulation in the plaque [52, 53].

Foam cells interact with T-lymphocytes through coupling of CD40 and its ligand expressed on both cell types. This process leads to a greater immune response. Cytokines, adhesion molecules and matrix degrading proteases are produced. One cytokine that is produced is interferon-gamma (IFN-γ), which stimulates the proliferation of SMCs and inhibits the formation of collagen by SMCs. This disruption of collagen interferes with the maintenance and repair of the collagen framework on the fibrous cap [54]. Activation of macrophages leads to the secretion of matrix metalloproteinases (MMPs), supporting the breakdown of collagen and elastin. Disruption of the fibrous cap leads to thrombosis and formed thrombi can interrupt the blood flow. Plaques that are likely to rupture have thin, collagen-poor fibrous caps, few SMCs and a large amount of macrophages [52].

An important risk factor for developing atherosclerosis is hypertension. Other risk factors are smoking, diabetes mellitus, obesity and genetic predisposition [52, 55, 56].

Therapy

Acute coronary events are mainly caused by the disruption of an atherosclerotic plaque. Lowering the risk of plaque disruption is therefore an important therapeutic target. There are a number of different therapeutic strategies aimed at achieving this goal.

The first therapeutic target is lipids, because high levels of LDL increase the cardiovascular risk. Lowering LDL would therefore be a good target to prevent atherosclerotic events. Therapy with inhibitors of hydroxymethyl glutaryl coenzyme A reductase (statins) is a well-known therapy for the reduction of LDL levels, but there are also other biological targets that may reduce the LDL levels to a greater degree than achieved by statin-therapy [52].

Another approach for lowering plaque disruption is to increase the level of HDL, which correlates inversely with cardiovascular risk. There are different ways to increase HDL levels. One way is by inhibiting the plasma protein cholesteryl ester transfer protein (CETP). This protein facilitates the exchange of cholesteryl esters in HDL for triglycerides from apolipoprotein-B-containing lipoproteins. Another therapeutic target is apolipoprotein A-1 (Apo-A1), the major component of HDL. Stimulation of the peroxisome proliferator-activated receptor-α (PPAR-α) increases the Apo-A1 level and would therefore be a promising therapeutic target. A third way to increase HDL levels is by stimulating nicotinic acid [52].

Cardiovascular risk is also reduced by lowering triglycerides. The most important way to reduce the levels of triglycerides is by lifestyle changes, including weight loss, improving physical activity and low-carbohydrate diets. Triglyceride levels are also lowered by fibrates and omega-3-fatty acids, but their clinical benefit has not yet been proven [52].

The prevention of apoptosis of inflammatory cells is also a target for plaque stabilization. Apoptosis can be prevented by statin therapy or dietary modification [57].

Imaging Studies of Atherosclerosis

There are many imaging studies that have focused on atherosclerosis and especially vulnerable plaque formation. Some examples are outlined below.

Effect of Antimicrobial Agents

In a limited number of studies, the effect of antimicrobial agents on atherosclerotic plaque formation has been evaluated. Oshima et al. used ^{99m}Tc-MPI SPECT imaging for the noninvasive assessment of matrix metalloproteinase (MMP) activity in atherosclerotic plaques after minocycline intervention. MMP activity contributes to plaque instability and minocycline might reduce this activity. The study was performed in rabbits, and it was concluded that minocycline reduces plaque MMP activity and thus contributes to plaque stabilization [39].

Identification of Vulnerable Plaques with ^{18}F-FDG

Macrophages play an important role in inflammation in coronary plaques. Therefore, imaging of macrophages seems a good approach to detect the extent of inflammation in plaques. An approach for imaging macrophages is by using ^{18}F-FDG (Figure 9-5). Many studies with ^{18}F-FDG are done. For example, in a study by Masteling et al., whether enhanced FDG uptake on high-resolution micro PET correlates with macrophage infiltration and therefore with plaque instability and with neurological symptom status was evaluated. Plaques of patients with planned carotid endarterectomy were used. The plaques were incubated in FDG and imaged with micro-PET. The amount of macrophages was evaluated by immunohistochemistry. Plaque calcification was examined with CT and correlated to FDG uptake. FDG uptake and macrophage infiltration were compared with patient symptomatology. It was concluded that a micro-PET system can be used to visualize the carotid atherosclerotic plaque *ex vivo*. The FDG uptake correlated well with macrophage infiltration [58].

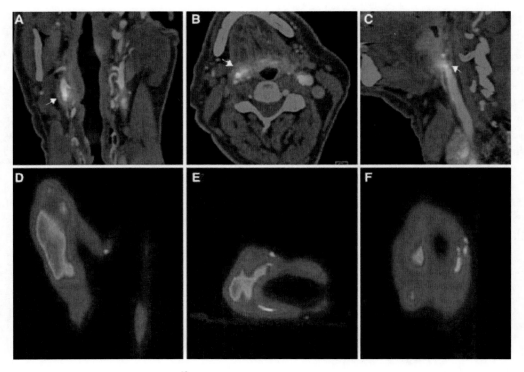

Figure 9-5. Example of imaging with ^{18}F-FDG, using PET. Coronal (A), transverse (B), and sagittal (C) plane slices of a patient showing FDG uptake in the affected right carotid artery (arrows). Coronal (D), transverse (E), and sagittal plane (F) of corresponding μPET images of the same patient showing also patchy FDG uptake and calcified areas. "With kind permission from Springer Science+Business Media: J Nucl Cardiol, High-resolution imaging of human atherosclerotic carotid plaques with micro 18F-FDG PET scanning exploring plaque vulnerability, 18(6), 2011, p. 1066-1075, Masterling MG et al., fig 1." (Ref. 58).

Figueroa et al. evaluated the relationship between inflammation in human atherosclerotic plaques and the number of high-risk morphological features of plaques, using FDG-PET. They concluded that inflammation, as assessed by both FDG uptake and histology, is increased in plaques containing high-risk morphological features, and FDG increases with an increasing number of high-risk morphological features. Thus, inflammation accumulates relative to the burden of morphological abnormalities [59].

Myers et al. performed a prospective, multicenter, ^{18}F-FDG PET/CT imaging study to estimate the correlations between arterial FDG uptake and macrophage content of excised plaque tissue. They found no significant correlation between the macrophage content and FDG uptake in the peripheral arteries. This result was unexpected, because previous studies showed a strong correlation. The result is probably due to differences in extraction technique, lesion size, degree of inflammation and imaging co-registration techniques [60].

Other Methods for Imaging Macrophages

Another way to image macrophages is with nanoparticle-enhanced MRI, which is a method where clinical dextran-coated magnetic nanoparticles (MNPs) are used. These nanoparticles consist of a 3-nm superparamagnetic iron oxide core that induces strong MRI contrast. This method is used in the detection of cancer metastases, but has now also been applied for detection of macrophage accumulation in carotid atheromata [18].

Another approach for imaging macrophages is based on the folate receptor β (FR-β). This receptor is present on activated macrophages, but not on quiescent macrophages or other immune cells. Jager et al. performed a folate imaging study on carotid specimens from 20 patients. The ligand folate was conjugated with a fluorescent contrast agent, fluoresceine-isothiocyanate (FITC), and activated macrophages could be visualized by optical fluorescence imaging to distinguish vulnerable sites from more stable regions. They concluded that in areas of high folate-FITC uptake within the atherosclerotic plaque, an increased number of activated macrophages and higher areas of hypoxia were present, compared to areas with low folate-FITC uptake. It seems that molecular imaging of folate receptor β could be a good indicator for plaque vulnerability [35].

Imaging Foam Cell Formation

Foam cell formation plays a role in the process of atherosclerosis. Ogawa et al. evaluated the effects of foam cell formation on ^{18}F-FDG uptake using cultured mouse peritoneal macrophages. They found that ^{18}F-FDG can detect the early stage of foam cell formation. The uptake of ^{18}F-FDG was decreased to control levels after complete differentiation to foam cells [61].

Myocardial Infarction

Pathology

MI is mainly caused by the loss of particles from a vulnerable atherosclerotic plaque. Most commonly, disruption of the atherosclerotic plaque is caused by a rupture of the fibrous cap. Blood coagulation components are able to come into contact with tissue factors in the plaques' interior. This leads to formation of thrombi in the vessel lumen. These thrombi reduce the coronary artery flow, leading to cardiac ischemia and subsequent infarction [51, 62].

Due to oxygen deficiency, the process of mitochondrial phosphorylation stops. The amount of adenosine triphosphate (ATP) will be decreased, since mitochondrial phosphorylation is the major source of ATP production for energy metabolism. To compensate for this loss of ATP, anaerobic glycolysis increases. Hydrogen ions and lactate accumulate, resulting in intracellular acidosis and an inhibition of glycolysis [63-66].

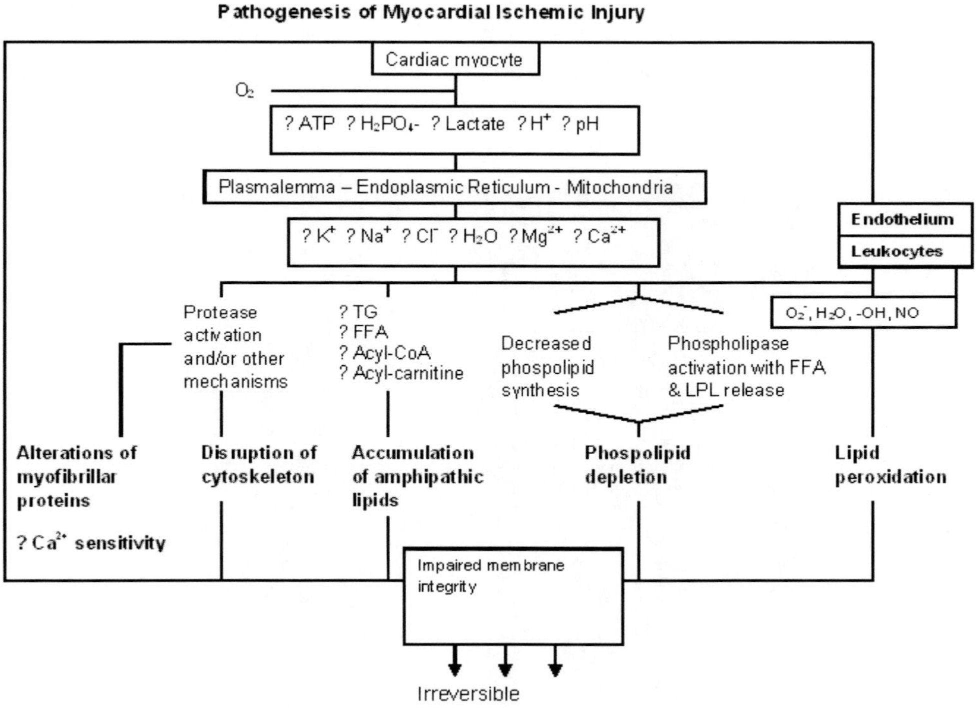

Pathogenesis of Myocardial Ischemic Injury

Figure 9-6. Pathogenesis of myocardial ischemic injury. Adapted from "Myocardial ischemia and reperfusion injury, 14(4), Buja LM, p. 170-175, 2005, with permission from Elsevier." (Ref. 63).

Contraction is impaired, but electrical activity continues. This leads to the development of ventricular arrhythmias. There are also alterations in ion transport systems. Accumulation of metabolites and inorganic phosphate result in an increased osmotic gradient. K^+-efflux is increased and the free Mg^{2+}-levels increase. This results in a decrease in total Mg^{2+}. Due to the loss of ATP, the Na^+-K^+-ATPase is inhibited and thereby K^+ further decreases and Na^+ increases. Influx of Na^+, Cl^- and water leads to cell swelling. The increased Ca^{2+}-level leads to the activation of proteases and phospholipases. The activation of phospholipases results in phospholipid degradation with the release of free fatty acids (FFA) and lysophospholipids. Phospholipid synthesis decreases and inhibition of the mitochondrial fatty acid metabolism results in an accumulation of amphiphilic molecules, which impair the function of the membranes. Due to an attack of free radicals, lipid peroxidation occurs. Because of the phospholipid loss, lipid peroxidation and cytoskeletal damage, an irreversible phase of injury is mediated. Followed by these triggers, the tissue cell may die by apoptosis or necrosis (Figure 9-6) [63, 66-68].

The acute MI can be divided into two major types: transmural and subendocardial. In transmural myocardial infarction, the necrosis involves full thickness of the ventricular wall. In the subendocardial type, necrosis remains confined to the inner layers [69, 70].

Another approach to categorize MI is determining whether there is an elevation in the ST interval in the ECG. There are two types: STEMI (ST-elevation myocardial infarction) and non-STEMI (non-ST-elevation myocardial infarction). It is estimated that each year over 3 million people have a STEMI and over 4 million people a non-STEMI [51].

MI leads to a number of changes in the heart, in a process known as cardiac remodeling. The workload of the remaining cardiomyocytes increases, leading to hypertrophy, dilatation and collagen formation. The infarction is followed by inflammation. The necrotic tissue is replaced by granulation tissue, which eventually matures into a scar [62].

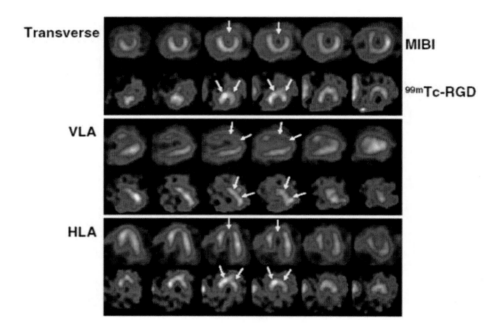

Figure 9.7. Example of ^{99m}Tc-RGD imaging. Figure shows scar formation 3 weeks after MI. Previously unpublished. Courtesy of Dr. J. Narula.

Therapy

The treatment of MI is based on improving the oxygen supply/demand ratio for the heart. There are two ways to achieve this, including the restoration of normal coronary blood flow and the lowering of myocardial oxygen consumption.

Restoring the normal coronary blood flow can be achieved with the administration of a thrombolytic drug to induce clot lysis, which is often combined with percutaneous coronary intervention (PCI), and/or the placement of an intracoronary stent to inhibit new clot formation, anticoagulant drugs need to be administered. Treatment with anti-platelet drugs is also required, in order to prevent recurrent thrombosis. Vasodilators such as nitroglycerin are often given to prevent or reverse vasospasm, which can also play a role via the reduction of perfusion [51].

The principal treatment for improving survival for patients with STEMI (not for non-STEMI) is pharmacological reperfusion with fibrinolysis. Fibrinolysis has to start as soon as possible, as a timely initiation improves the benefit of preservation of left-ventricular function and reduction in mortality [51].

Myocardial oxygen consumption can be decreased by decreasing the heart rate, contractility, and ventricular pre- and afterload. To reduce ventricular preload, vasodilators such as nitroglycerin are given. This reduces the oxygen demand of the heart. Beta-blockers inhibit sympathetic activity and are mostly given because the heart is stimulated by sympathetic activity. To reduce systemic vascular resistance, systemic vasodilators are given, but this can also lead to hypotension, so care must be taken. Other drugs that are given are: antiarrhythmic drugs, analgesic drugs and diuretics. Long-term treatment includes anti-platelet therapy, statins, beta-blockers and ACE-inhibitors [51].

Imaging Studies to Assess Myocardial Infarction

There are many imaging studies focusing on myocardial infarction, especially on the processes towards and after MI.

Perfusion Imaging

After MI, deterioration of left ventricular (LV) function is a major cause of heart failure. To this context, myocardial perfusion performance plays an important role. Slart et al. performed an imaging study to evaluate the myocardial perfusion reserve (MPR) and stress perfusion in deteriorating and non-deteriorating LV segments in patients after MI by PET and MRI, respectively. They concluded that there is an additional value of myocardial perfusion assessment in relation to the functional integrity of the injured myocardium. Dysfunctional segments had a lower myocardial perfusion PET value than improved segments [71]. Myocardial perfusion imaging has been shown to be a strong predictor for survival in patients with ischemic heart disease [72]. Also, a combination of perfusion imaging with PET imaging with ^{18}F-FDG can be used to assess myocardial function (see 1.3.2).

Imaging Inflammation after MI

Lee et al. used ^{18}FDG PET/MRI imaging to measure the inflammatory response after myocardial infarction. The activity of monocytes/macrophages was measured with ^{18}FDG. They concluded that the inflammatory response can be measured with this tracer, but that it has its limitations. Viable myocytes metabolize glucose, showing therefore high ^{18}FDG uptake, which may contribute to the signal. Suppressing myocardial uptake is therefore needed [11].

Imaging of Apoptosis

Kenis et al. performed a study with ^{99m}Tc-Annexin A5 in rabbits to evaluate whether apoptosis was initiated in brief episodes of myocardial ischemia and whether Annexin A5 was useful for the detection of ischemia. They concluded that after a single episode of ischemia, cardiomyocytes express phosphatidylserine, which can be targeted by Annexin A5 for at least 6 hours. It was also found that cardiomyocytes recover after restoration of the blood flow. Binding of Annexin A5 to phosphatidylserine leads to internalization of Annexin A5 into vesicles [73].

Radiolabeled Annexin A5 can thus be used to image apoptosis. Golestani et al. used Annexin A5 to evaluate whether minocycline, when administered upon reperfusion, reduced myocardial ischemia and reperfusion (IR) injury. The study was performed in both mice and rabbits. It was found that treatment with minocycline at reperfusion reduces the amount of apoptotic cells and thus can be a good therapeutic treatment for patients receiving primary interventions for acute coronary events [74].

Scar Formation

Pathology

After MI, the healing processes starts, beginning with the release of chemokines and cytokines that attract circulating leukocytes (neutrophils, monocytes) to the infarcted area. Monocytes differentiate into macrophages, which clear away dead cells and other necrotic debris. They also release factors that are important for formation of granulation tissue and also initiate endothelial cell proliferation and angiogenesis. This provides the blood flow needed to support the process of wound healing. Proliferation of fibroblasts, which generate extracellular matrix proteins (collagen), leads to strengthening of the infarcted area. However, over time the initial region of injury is replaced by a collageneous scar [75].

Therapy

Cardiac remodeling is stimulated by the up-regulation of the renin-angiotensin-aldosterone system (RAAS). Therefore, it has been proven that anti-angiotensin and anti-aldosterone therapy controls the process of remodeling and can delay or prevent the development of heart failure [50, 76]. Therapy leads to a reduction of the amount of interstitial collagen deposition [76].

Imaging Studies Scar Formation

RGD-Imaging

Verjans et al. performed a molecular imaging study with ^{99m}Tc-Cy5.5-RGD-imaging peptide (^{99m}Tc-CRIP). Arg-Gly-Asp (RGD) peptide binds to myofibroblasts in the infarcted area and correlates to the extent of new collagen deposition after MI. RIP imaging was compared to initial MPI and to the extent of scar formation defined by late gadolinium-enhanced (LGE) cardiac magnetic resonance (CMR) imaging 1 year after MI. The study demonstrated that RGD-based imaging early after MI may predict the eventual extent of scar formation, which often exceeds initial MPI but co-localizes with LGE in CMR imaging performed subsequently (Figure 9-7). [50]

Fibrosis

Pathology

After myocardial infarction, the necrotic tissue forms scar tissue, in a process known as myocardial fibrosis. In fibrosis, the heart muscle cells, the myocytes, are replaced by tissue that is unable to contract. Fibrosis leads therefore to myocardial stiffness and impairment of cardiac function [77]. In cases of fibrosis, an excessive amount of matrix proteins such as collagen is produced [78].

The fibrotic process starts with the secretion of pro-collagen molecules into the extracellular space [77]. Pro-collagen molecules are synthesized and secreted by myofibroblasts. These cells are differentiated from fibroblasts in response to factors like angtiotensin II, transforming growth factor-β (TGF-β) and hormones like aldosterone [79, 80]. They are also responsive to pro- inflammatory cytokines secreted by inflammatory cells like macrophages, T-cells and mast cells. Examples are tumor necrosis factor (TNF) and interleukin (IL)-1 [79].

Pro-collagen molecules are composed of a triple helix of three α-chains, containing amino acid residues. The collagen proteins found in the heart are types I, II and V, with type I being the most predominant [79, 81]. In the extracellular space, their end-terminal pro-peptides are cleaved by procollagen N- and C-proteinases to enable collagen fiber formation. Crosslinks are formed between lysine and hydroxylysine residues within and between the collagen molecules, after deamination of the residues by lysyl oxidase [77].

Collagen turnover is mediated by matrix metalloproteinases (MMP) and tissue inhibitors of metalloproteinases (TIMP). In myocardial fibrosis there is an increased deposition of type I collagen fibers [77].

Therapy

Therapy based on the reduction of fibrosis is an increasingly important strategy to reduce the development of heart failure (discussed in section 3.6). There are several drugs which have a direct effect on the turnover of the extracellular matrix. Examples are drugs affecting the RAAS, like aldosterone antagonists, TII receptor blockers and ACE inhibitors [78].

Imaging Studies in Fibrosis

RGD-imaging

Van den Borne et al. performed an RGD-imaging study on mice to evaluate the myofibroblastic proliferation, which could provide an indirect evidence of the extent of fibrosis. They used radiolabeled Cy5.5-RGD imaging peptide (CRIP) and concluded that this can be used for noninvasive visualization of interstitial alterations during cardiac remodeling [76].

Cardiac Hypertrophy

Pathology

Cardiac hypertrophy describes enlargement of the heart in response to altered contractility or an increase in wall stress [62, 82]. It is a response of the heart muscle to compensate for the decrease of cardiac output.

In cardiac hypertrophy there is an increased cardiomyocyte size, increased fibrosis, increased protein synthesis and up-regulation of fetal genes, normally activated in the developing heart, for example a-actin, b-myosin heavy chain (b-MHC), atrial natriuretic factor (ANF) and brain natriuretic peptide (BNP). Transcription factors which drive this process are NF-κB (nuclear factor-κB), GATA4 (GATA binding protein 4), NFAT (nuclear factor of activated T cells), SRF (serum response factor) and MEF2 (myocyte enhancer factor-2). The process is stimulated by different signaling pathways, with stimuli like angiotensin II (ANGII), endothelin-1 (ET-1) and phenylephrine (PE) [62, 83-88].

Hypertrophy is divided into two types: the concentric form and the eccentric form. The first is caused by pressure overload and leads to an increase in wall thickness by the addition of sarcomeres in parallel. Also, the left ventricular lumen is reduced. The eccentric form is caused by volume overload and leads to ventricle dilation and thinning of the ventricle wall by the addition of sarcomeres in series [62, 82].

Cardiac hypertrophy starts with an initial compensatory phase, but in the long-term it can result in decompensation, contractile dysfunction and heart failure. Another form of hypertrophy is physiological hypertrophy, which is caused by intensive exercise or pregnancy. It is activated by growth factors like insulin-like growth factor (IGF) and growth hormone (GF). This form is beneficial for the heart and does not lead to heart failure [62, 82].

Therapy

A possible new therapeutic approach for hypertrophy is calpain inhibitors. Proteases of the calpain family are thought to play a role in the development of cardiac hypertrophy. Calpain is involved in the degradation of proteins in cardiomyocytes. Inhibition of this process can reduce hypertrophy. Some studies have proven the effectiveness of calpain inhibition, but the safety and long-term effects remain to be determined [83, 89-91].

On the other hand, calpains also play a role in cell death, especially after myocardial ischemia-reperfusion, by causing sarcolemmal injury and promoting myofibrillar degradation. To protect for this, myocardial cell death ischemic pre-conditioning or post-conditioning can be done [92-94].

Imaging Studies Cardiac Hypertrophy

Breitenbach et al. performed an MRI study under patients after aortic valve replacement (AVR) to determine the decrease in left ventricular mass index. They compared this with the most common approach to determine this mass, which is transthoracic echocardiography (TTE). They concluded that MRI should be preferred, because of higher accuracy and reproducibility. In TTE there is an overestimation of the decrease in left ventricular mass index [95].

Goldstein et al. performed a PET study to evaluate whether the myocardial perfusion reserve (MPR) is influenced by left ventricular hypertrophy (LVH). They found that there is in abnormality in MPR in patients with LVH [96].

Heart Failure

Pathology

Heart failure (HF) is a complex clinical syndrome, which can result from any cardiac disorder that impairs the ability of the ventricle to fill or eject blood. Therefore, the oxygen supply is deficient for meeting the demands of the body. Many cardiac disorders can lead to heart failure. It can be a result of an ischemic heart disease due to coronary heart disease (CAD), but it can also be caused by other etiologies, for example hypertension, fibrosis, myocarditis and hypertrophy [97]. Cardinal manifestations of HF are dyspnea and fatigue. Patients are limited in (daily) exercise and pulmonary congestion and peripheral edema are caused by fluid retention. There are many different forms of HF and symptoms are diverse in patients.

Heart failure is present in many different forms and rates of progression, but HF ultimately leads to death or the need for cardiac transplantation or mechanical ventricular assistance [98-100].

Heart failure is classified by The American College of Cardiology/American Heart Association (AC/AHA) in 4 stages, which are based on risk factors, underlying heart diseases and symptoms [100].

For pharmacological treatment, HF is also classified into systolic versus diastolic left ventricular dysfunction. In left ventricular systolic dysfunction (LVSD) there is a decrease in contractility of the left ventricle to provide adequate blood supply to the rest of the body. In diastolic left ventricular dysfunction there is an impaired relaxation of the left ventricle, which is usually related to chronic hypertension or ischemic heart disease [99].

Another classification is made by the New York Heart Association (NYHA) [99, 100].

Therapy

Most patients with (chronic) HF are treated with a combination of drugs including diuretics, ACE-inhibitors and beta-blockers. The combination of these three types of drugs has been shown to be effective in many clinical trials. Digoxin can be added to the therapy to reduce symptoms, prevent hospitalization, control rhythm and enhance exercise tolerance.

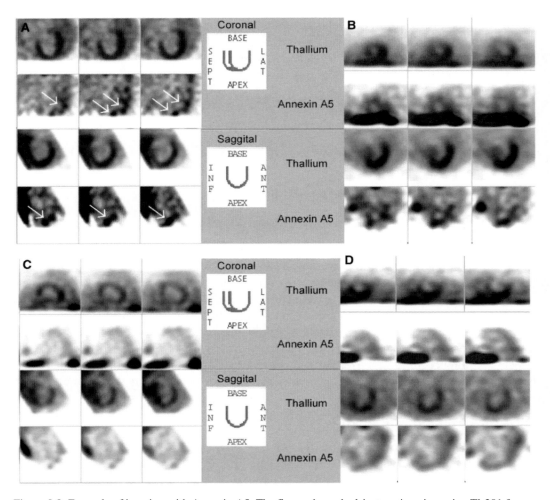

Figure 9.8. Example of imaging with Annexin A5. The figure showsdual-isotope imaging using Tl-201 for left ventricular contour detection and, simultaneously, radiolabeled annexin A5 in patients with dilated cardiomyopathy. (A) Dilated cardiomyopathy patient with rapid deterioration of left ventricular function. Note focal uptake in apex and lateral wall, and slight septal uptake. (B) Dilated cardiomyopathy patient in acute heart failure. Note global uptake of radiolabeled annexin A5. (C) Dilated cardiomyopathy patient in stable clinical condition. Uptake is absent even when image is enhanced to the extent that background radioactivity can be observed. (D) Family member of patient in panel B. No clinical evidence is seen of dilated cardiomyopathy. Note absence of uptake of radiolabeled annexin A5. ANT = anterior; INF = inferior; LAT = lateral; SEPT = septal. This research was originally published in JNM. Kietselaer BL, Reutelingsperger CP, Boersma HH, et al. Noninvasive detection of programmed cell loss with ^{99m}Tc-labeled annexin A5 in heart failure. JNM 2007;48(4):562-567. © by the Society of Nuclear Medicine and Molecular Imaging, Inc. (Ref. 102).

Since apoptosis of cardiomyocytes plays an important role in the progression towards heart failure, methods based on reversing apoptosis are developed. It is believed that cells can be in a state of 'apoptosis interruptus'. In this state, the apoptosis pathway is activated but there is a lack of terminal morphological features of apoptosis. The interruption is caused by a simultaneous activation of a protective mechanism that limits the damage due to activated caspases. These cardiomyocytes can avoid cell death or dysfunction if they are supported until rescue. For example, this rescue is achieved by LVAD (left ventricular assist device), which restores the cytoplasm of the cardiomyocytes [101].

Imaging Studies Heart Failure

Imaging of Apoptosis

Kietselaer et al. performed a study to evaluate the role of Annexin A5 imaging for the detection of apoptosis in heart failure patients. They concluded that Annexin A5 imaging may identify accelerated myocardial cell loss in non-ischemic dilated cardiomyopathy patients with a recent worsening of heart failure. This imaging method can be used for studying interventions to minimize the progression of heart failure (Figure 9-8) [102].

Conclusion

The process towards myocardial infarction is complex and compromises a lot of different stages. Also, the aftermath of a myocardial infarction is very complicated and scar formation, remodeling, hypertrophy and fibrosis can ultimately lead to heart failure. By the means of molecular imaging techniques, pathophysiology of the different stages can be evaluated and new therapeutic strategies can be developed. Therefore, the development of new molecular imaging agents is important, leading to new insights and strategies.

References

[1] Task Force for Diagnosis and Treatment of Non-ST-Segment Elevation Acute Coronary Syndromes of European Society of Cardiology, Bassand JP, Hamm CW, *et al.* Guidelines for the diagnosis and treatment of non-ST-segment elevation acute coronary syndromes. *Eur Heart J* 2007;28(13):1598-1660.

[2] Vancraeynest D, Pasquet A, Roelants V, Gerber BL, Vanoverschelde JL. Imaging the vulnerable plaque. *J Am Coll Cardiol* 2011;57(20):1961-1979.

[3] Jaffer FA, Weissleder R. Molecular imaging in the clinical arena. *JAMA* 2005;293(7):855-862.

[4] Lindner JR. Microbubbles in medical imaging: current applications and future directions. *Nat Rev Drug Discov* 2004;3(6):527-532.

[5] Lanza GM, Wickline SA. Targeted ultrasonic contrast agents for molecular imaging and therapy. *Curr Probl Cardiol* 2003;28(12):625-653.

[6] Jaffer FA, Weissleder R. Seeing within: molecular imaging of the cardiovascular system. *Circ Res* 2004;94(4):433-445.

[7] Weissleder R, Elizondo G, Wittenberg J, Rabito CA, Bengele HH, Josephson L. Ultrasmall superparamagnetic iron oxide: characterization of a new class of contrast agents for MR imaging. *Radiology* 1990;175(2):489-493.

[8]   Harisinghani MG, Barentsz J, Hahn PF, *et al.* Noninvasive detection of clinically occult lymph-node metastases in prostate cancer. *N Engl J Med* 2003;348(25):2491-2499.

[9]   Kooi ME, Cappendijk VC, Cleutjens KB, *et al.* Accumulation of ultrasmall superparamagnetic particles of iron oxide in human atherosclerotic plaques can be detected by in vivo magnetic resonance imaging. *Circulation* 2003;107(19):2453-2458.

[10]   Yamamoto S, Watabe T, Watabe H, *et al.* Simultaneous imaging using Si-PM-based PET and MRI for development of an integrated PET/MRI system. *Phys Med Biol* 2012;57(2):N1-N13.

[11]   Lee WW, Marinelli B, van der Laan AM, *et al.* PET/MRI of Inflammation in Myocardial Infarction. *J Am Coll Cardiol* 2012;59(2):153-163.

[12]   Subramanian S, Jaffer FA, Tawakol A. Optical molecular imaging in atherosclerosis. *J Nucl Cardiol* 2010;17(1):135-144.

[13]   Calfon MA, Vinegoni C, Ntziachristos V, Jaffer FA. Intravascular near-infrared fluorescence molecular imaging of atherosclerosis: toward coronary arterial visualization of biologically high-risk plaques. *J Biomed Opt* 2010;15(1):011107.

[14]   Ntziachristos V, Tung CH, Bremer C, Weissleder R. Fluorescence molecular tomography resolves protease activity in vivo. *Nat Med* 2002;8(7):757-760.

[15]   Ntziachristos V, Ripoll J, Weissleder R. Would near-infrared fluorescence signals propagate through large human organs for clinical studies? *Opt Lett* 2002;27(5):333-335.

[16]   Funovics MA, Weissleder R, Mahmood U. Catheter-based in vivo imaging of enzyme activity and gene expression: feasibility study in mice. *Radiology* 2004;231(3):659-666.

[17]   Weissleder R, Ntziachristos V. Shedding light onto live molecular targets. *Nat Med* 2003;9(1):123-128.

[18]   Jaffer FA, Libby P, Weissleder R. Molecular imaging of cardiovascular disease. *Circulation* 2007;116(9):1052-1061.

[19]   Machac J. Cardiac positron emission tomography imaging. *Semin Nucl Med* 2005;35(1):17-36.

[20]   Schelbert HR, Phelps ME, Huang SC, *et al.* N-13 ammonia as an indicator of myocardial blood flow. *Circulation* 1981;63(6):1259-1272.

[21]   Slart RH, Bax JJ, van Veldhuisen DJ, van der Wall EE, Dierckx RA, Jager PL. Imaging techniques in nuclear cardiology for the assessment of myocardial viability. *Int J Cardiovasc Imaging* 2006;22(1):63-80.

[22]   Beller GA, Bergmann SR. Myocardial perfusion imaging agents: SPECT and PET. *J Nucl Cardiol* 2004;11(1):71-86.

[23]   Schelbert HR, Phelps ME, Hoffman EJ, Huang SC, Selin CE, Kuhl DE. Regional myocardial perfusion assessed with N-13 labeled ammonia and positron emission computerized axial tomography. *Am J Cardiol* 1979;43(2):209-218.

[24]   de Silva R, Yamamoto Y, Rhodes CG, *et al.* Preoperative prediction of the outcome of coronary revascularization using positron emission tomography. *Circulation* 1992;86(6):1738-1742.

[25]   Yamamoto Y, de Silva R, Rhodes CG, *et al.* A new strategy for the assessment of viable myocardium and regional myocardial blood flow using 15O-water and dynamic positron emission tomography. *Circulation* 1992;86(1):167-178.

[26]   Russell RR,3rd, Zaret BL. Nuclear cardiology: present and future. *Curr Probl Cardiol* 2006;31(9):557-629.

[27] Rischpler C, Park MJ, Fung GS, Javadi M, Tsui BM, Higuchi T. Advances in PET myocardial perfusion imaging: F-18 labeled tracers. *Ann Nucl Med* 2012;26(1):1-6.

[28] Strauss HW, Bailey D. Resurrection of thallium-201 for myocardial perfusion imaging. *JACC Cardiovasc Imaging* 2009;2(3):283-285.

[29] Omur O, Ozcan Z, Argon M, Acar ET. A comparative evaluation of Tl-201 and Tc-99m sestamibi myocardial perfusion spect imaging in diabetic patients. *Int J Cardiovasc Imaging* 2008;24(2):173-181.

[30] Pierard LA, Lancellotti P, Benoit T. Myocardial viability. Stress echocardiography vs nuclear medicine. *Eur Heart J* 1997;18 Suppl D:D117-23.

[31] Mylonas I, Beanlands RS. Radionuclide Imaging of Viable Myocardium: Is it Underutilized? *Curr Cardiovasc Imaging Rep* 2011;4(3):251-261.

[32] Tiwari RL, Singh V, Barthwal MK. Macrophages: an elusive yet emerging therapeutic target of atherosclerosis. *Med Res Rev* 2008;28(4):483-544.

[33] Fuster V. Lewis A. Conner Memorial Lecture. Mechanisms leading to myocardial infarction: insights from studies of vascular biology. *Circulation* 1994;90(4):2126-2146.

[34] Antohe F, Radulescu L, Puchianu E, Kennedy MD, Low PS, Simionescu M. Increased uptake of folate conjugates by activated macrophages in experimental hyperlipemia. *Cell Tissue Res* 2005;320(2):277-285.

[35] Jager NA, Westra J, van Dam GM, *et al.* Targeted folate receptor beta fluorescence imaging as a measure of inflammation to estimate vulnerability within human atherosclerotic carotid plaque. *J Nucl Med* 2012;53(8):1222-1229.

[36] Muller C, Forrer F, Schibli R, Krenning EP, de Jong M. SPECT study of folate receptor-positive malignant and normal tissues in mice using a novel 99mTc-radiofolate. *J Nucl Med* 2008;49(2):310-317.

[37] Boersma HH, de Haas HJ, Reutelingsperger CP, Slart RH. P-selectin imaging in cardiovascular disease: what you see is what you get? *J Nucl Med* 2011;52(9):1337-1338.

[38] Rouzet F, Bachelet-Violette L, Alsac JM, *et al.* Radiolabeled fucoidan as a p-selectin targeting agent for in vivo imaging of platelet-rich thrombus and endothelial activation. *J Nucl Med* 2011;52(9):1433-1440.

[39] Ohshima S, Fujimoto S, Petrov A, *et al.* Effect of an antimicrobial agent on atherosclerotic plaques: assessment of metalloproteinase activity by molecular imaging. *J Am Coll Cardiol* 2010;55(12):1240-1249.

[40] Hofstra L, Liem IH, Dumont EA, *et al.* Visualisation of cell death in vivo in patients with acute myocardial infarction. *Lancet* 2000;356(9225):209-212.

[41] Golestani R, Wu C, Tio RA, *et al.* Small-animal SPECT and SPECT/CT: application in cardiovascular research. *Eur J Nucl Med Mol Imaging* 2010;37(9):1766-1777.

[42] Okada DR, Johnson G, Liu Z, Hocherman SD, Khaw BA, Okada RD. Early detection of infarct in reperfused canine myocardium using 99mTc-glucarate. *J Nucl Med* 2004;45(4):655-664.

[43] Khaw BA, Nakazawa A, O'Donnell SM, Pak KY, Narula J. Avidity of technetium 99m glucarate for the necrotic myocardium: in vivo and in vitro assessment. *J Nucl Cardiol* 1997;4(4):283-290.

[44] Boersma HH, Kietselaer BL, Stolk LM, *et al.* Past, present, and future of annexin A5: from protein discovery to clinical applications. *J Nucl Med* 2005;46(12):2035-2050.

[45] Korngold EC, Jaffer FA, Weissleder R, Sosnovik DE. Noninvasive imaging of apoptosis in cardiovascular disease. *Heart Fail Rev* 2008;13(2):163-173.

[46] Zhou D, Chu W, Rothfuss J, *et al.* Synthesis, radiolabeling, and in vivo evaluation of an 18F-labeled isatin analog for imaging caspase-3 activation in apoptosis. *Bioorg Med Chem Lett* 2006;16(19):5041-5046.

[47] Dimastromatteo J, Riou LM, Ahmadi M, *et al.* In vivo molecular imaging of myocardial angiogenesis using the alpha(v)beta3 integrin-targeted tracer 99mTc-RAFT-RGD. *J Nucl Cardiol* 2010;17(3):435-443.

[48] Higuchi T, Bengel FM, Seidl S, *et al.* Assessment of alphavbeta3 integrin expression after myocardial infarction by positron emission tomography. *Cardiovasc Res* 2008;78(2):395-403.

[49] Doss M, Kolb HC, Zhang JJ, *et al.* Biodistribution and radiation dosimetry of the integrin marker 18F-RGD-K5 determined from whole-body PET/CT in monkeys and humans. *J Nucl Med* 2012;53(5):787-795.

[50] Verjans J, Wolters S, Laufer W, *et al.* Early molecular imaging of interstitial changes in patients after myocardial infarction: comparison with delayed contrast-enhanced magnetic resonance imaging. *J Nucl Cardiol* 2010;17(6):1065-1072.

[51] White HD, Chew DP. Acute myocardial infarction. *Lancet* 2008;372(9638):570-584.

[52] Libby P, Ridker PM, Hansson GK. Progress and challenges in translating the biology of atherosclerosis. *Nature* 2011;473(7347):317-325.

[53] Falk E. Pathogenesis of atherosclerosis. *J Am Coll Cardiol* 2006;47(8 Suppl):C7-12.

[54] Finn AV, Nakano M, Narula J, Kolodgie FD, Virmani R. Concept of vulnerable/unstable plaque. Arterioscler *Thromb Vasc Biol* 2010;30(7):1282-1292.

[55] Libby P, DiCarli M, Weissleder R. The vascular biology of atherosclerosis and imaging targets. *J Nucl Med* 2010;51 Suppl 1:33S-37S.

[56] Alsheikh-Ali AA, Kitsios GD, Balk EM, Lau J, Ip S. The vulnerable atherosclerotic plaque: scope of the literature. *Ann Intern Med* 2010;153(6):387-395.

[57] Hartung D, Sarai M, Petrov A, *et al.* Resolution of apoptosis in atherosclerotic plaque by dietary modification and statin therapy. *J Nucl Med* 2005;46(12):2051-2056.

[58] Masteling MG, Zeebregts CJ, Tio RA, *et al.* High-resolution imaging of human atherosclerotic carotid plaques with micro 18F-FDG PET scanning exploring plaque vulnerability. *J Nucl Cardiol* 2011;18(6):1066-1075.

[59] Figueroa AL, Subramanian SS, Cury RC, *et al.* Distribution of inflammation within carotid atherosclerotic plaques with high-risk morphological features: a comparison between positron emission tomography activity, plaque morphology, and histopathology. *Circ Cardiovasc Imaging* 2012;5(1):69-77.

[60] Myers KS, Rudd JH, Hailman EP, *et al.* Correlation Between Arterial FDG Uptake and Biomarkers in Peripheral Artery Disease. *JACC Cardiovasc Imaging* 2012;5(1):38-45.

[61] Ogawa M, Nakamura S, Saito Y, Kosugi M, Magata Y. What Can Be Seen by 18F-FDG PET in Atherosclerosis Imaging? The Effect of Foam Cell Formation on 18F-FDG Uptake to Macrophages In Vitro. *J Nucl Med* 2012;53(1):55-58.

[62] Ter Horst P, Smits JF, Blankesteijn WM. The Wnt/Frizzled pathway as a therapeutic target for cardiac hypertrophy: where do we stand? *Acta Physiol* (Oxf) 2012;204(1):110-117.

[63] Buja LM. Myocardial ischemia and reperfusion injury. *Cardiovasc Pathol* 2005;14(4):170-175.

[64] Buja LM, Hagler HK, Willerson JT. Altered calcium homeostasis in the pathogenesis of myocardial ischemic and hypoxic injury. *Cell Calcium* 1988;9(5-6):205-217.

[65] Buja LM. Lipid abnormalities in myocardial cell injury. *Trends Cardiovasc Med* 1991;1(1):40-45.

[66] Thandroyen FT, Bellotto D, Katayama A, Hagler HK, Willerson JT, Buja LM. Subcellular electrolyte alterations during progressive hypoxia and following reoxygenation in isolated neonatal rat ventricular myocytes. *Circ Res* 1992;71(1):106-119.

[67] Yellon DM, Hausenloy DJ. Myocardial reperfusion injury. *N Engl J Med* 2007;357(11):1121-1135.

[68] Zweier JL. Measurement of superoxide-derived free radicals in the reperfused heart. Evidence for a free radical mechanism of reperfusion injury. *J Biol Chem* 1988;263(3):1353-1357.

[69] Basso C, Rizzo S, Thiene G. The metamorphosis of myocardial infarction following coronary recanalization. *Cardiovasc Pathol* 2010;19(1):22-28.

[70] Roberts WC, Buja LM. The frequency and significance of coronary arterial thrombi and other observations in fatal acute myocardial infarction: a study of 107 necropsy patients. *Am J Med* 1972;52(4):425-443.

[71] Slart RHJA, Glauche J, Golestani R, *et al.* PET and MRI for the evaluation of regional myocardial perfusion and wall thickening after myocardial infarction. *Eur J Nucl Med Mol Imaging* 2012; 39(6):1065-1069.

[72] Tio RA, Dabeshlim A, Siebelink HM, *et al.* Comparison between the prognostic value of left ventricular function and myocardial perfusion reserve in patients with ischemic heart disease. *J Nucl Med* 2009;50(2):214-219.

[73] Kenis H, Zandbergen HR, Hofstra L, *et al.* Annexin A5 uptake in ischemic myocardium: demonstration of reversible phosphatidylserine externalization and feasibility of radionuclide imaging. *J Nucl Med* 2010;51(2):259-267.

[74] Golestani R, de Haas H, Petrov AD, *et al.* Minocyclin inhibits myocardial cell death in animal models of myocardial ischemia and reperfusion. *European Journal of Nuclear Medicine and Molecular Imaging* 2010;37(2):S240-S240.

[75] Naresh NK, Ben-Mordechai T, Leor J, Epstein FH. Molecular Imaging of Healing After Myocardial Infarction. *Curr Cardiovasc Imaging Rep* 2011;4(1):63-76.

[76] van den Borne SW, Isobe S, Zandbergen HR, *et al.* Molecular imaging for efficacy of pharmacologic intervention in myocardial remodeling. *JACC Cardiovasc Imaging* 2009;2(2):187-198.

[77] Jellis C, Martin J, Narula J, Marwick TH. Assessment of nonischemic myocardial fibrosis. *J Am Coll Cardiol* 2010;56(2):89-97.

[78] de Jong S, van Veen TA, de Bakker JM, Vos MA, van Rijen HV. Biomarkers of myocardial fibrosis. *J Cardiovasc Pharmacol* 2011;57(5):522-535.

[79] van den Borne SW, Diez J, Blankesteijn WM, Verjans J, Hofstra L, Narula J. Myocardial remodeling after infarction: the role of myofibroblasts. *Nat Rev Cardiol* 2010;7(1):30-37.

[80] de Haas HJ, van den Borne SW, Boersma HH, Slart RH, Fuster V, Narula J. Evolving role of molecular imaging for new understanding: targeting myofibroblasts to predict remodeling. *Ann N Y Acad Sci* 2012;1254:33-41.

[81]   Sun Y. Myocardial repair/remodelling following infarction: roles of local factors. *Cardiovasc Res* 2009;81(3):482-490.

[82]   Harvey PA, Leinwand LA. The cell biology of disease: cellular mechanisms of cardiomyopathy. *J Cell Biol* 2011;194(3):355-365.

[83]   Patterson C, Portbury AL, Schisler JC, Willis MS. Tear me down: role of calpain in the development of cardiac ventricular hypertrophy. *Circ Res* 2011;109(4):453-462.

[84]   Frey N, Olson EN. Cardiac hypertrophy: the good, the bad, and the ugly. *Annu Rev Physiol* 2003;65:45-79.

[85]   Molkentin JD, Robbins J. With great power comes great responsibility: using mouse genetics to study cardiac hypertrophy and failure. *J Mol Cell Cardiol* 2009;46(2):130-136.

[86]   Sugden PH, Fuller SJ, Weiss SC, Clerk A. Glycogen synthase kinase 3 (GSK3) in the heart: a point of integration in hypertrophic signalling and a therapeutic target? A critical analysis. *Br J Pharmacol* 2008;153 Suppl 1:S137-53.

[87]   Van der Heiden K, Cuhlmann S, Luong le A, Zakkar M, Evans PC. Role of nuclear factor kappaB in cardiovascular health and disease. *Clin Sci (Lond)* 2010;118(10):593-605.

[88]   Wilkins BJ, Dai YS, Bueno OF, *et al.* Calcineurin/NFAT coupling participates in pathological, but not physiological, cardiac hypertrophy. *Circ Res* 2004;94(1):110-118.

[89]   Mani SK, Shiraishi H, Balasubramanian S, *et al.* In vivo administration of calpeptin attenuates calpain activation and cardiomyocyte loss in pressure-overloaded feline myocardium. *Am J Physiol Heart Circ Physiol* 2008;295(1):H314-26.

[90]   Greyson CR, Schwartz GG, Lu L, *et al.* Calpain inhibition attenuates right ventricular contractile dysfunction after acute pressure overload. *J Mol Cell Cardiol* 2008;44(1):59-68.

[91]   Arthur GD, Belcastro AN. A calcium stimulated cysteine protease involved in isoproterenol induced cardiac hypertrophy. *Mol Cell Biochem* 1997;176(1-2):241-248.

[92]   Letavernier E, Zafrani L, Perez J, Letavernier B, Haymann JP, Baud L. The role of calpains in myocardial remodelling and heart failure. *Cardiovasc Res* 2012.

[93]   Garcia-Dorado D, Rodriguez-Sinovas A, Ruiz-Meana M, Inserte J, Agullo L, Cabestrero A. The end-effectors of preconditioning protection against myocardial cell death secondary to ischemia-reperfusion. *Cardiovasc Res* 2006;70(2):274-285.

[94]   Portbury AL, Willis MS, Patterson C. Tearin' up my heart: proteolysis in the cardiac sarcomere. *J Biol Chem* 2011;286(12):9929-9934.

[95]   Breitenbach I, Harringer W, Tsui S, *et al.* Magnetic resonance imaging versus echocardiography to ascertain the regression of left ventricular hypertrophy after bioprosthetic aortic valve replacement: Results of the REST study. *J Thorac Cardiovasc Surg* 2011.

[96]   Goldstein RA, Haynie M. Limited myocardial perfusion reserve in patients with left ventricular hypertrophy. *J Nucl Med* 1990;31(3):255-258.

[97]   Lin D, Hollander Z, Meredith A, *et al.* Molecular signatures of end-stage heart failure. *J Card Fail* 2011;17(10):867-874.

[98]   Cheng JW, Nayar M. A review of heart failure management in the elderly population. *Am J Geriatr Pharmacother* 2009;7(5):233-249.

[99] De Boer RA, Pinto YM, Van Veldhuisen DJ. The imbalance between oxygen demand and supply as a potential mechanism in the pathophysiology of heart failure: the role of microvascular growth and abnormalities. *Microcirculation* 2003;10(2):113-126.

[100] Hunt SA, Abraham WT, Chin MH, *et al.* 2009 Focused update incorporated into the ACC/AHA 2005 Guidelines for the Diagnosis and Management of Heart Failure in Adults A Report of the American College of Cardiology Foundation/American Heart Association Task Force on Practice Guidelines Developed in Collaboration With the International Society for Heart and Lung Transplantation. *J Am Coll Cardiol* 2009;53(15):e1-e90.

[101] Masri C, Chandrashekhar Y. Apoptosis: a potentially reversible, meta-stable state of the heart. *Heart Fail Rev* 2008;13(2):175-179.

[102] Kietselaer BL, Reutelingsperger CP, Boersma HH, *et al.* Noninvasive detection of programmed cell loss with 99mTc-labeled annexin A5 in heart failure. *J Nucl Med* 2007;48(4):562-567.

In: SPECT   ISBN: 978-1-62808-344-6
Editors: Hojjat Ahmadzadehfar and Elham Habibi   © 2013 Nova Science Publishers, Inc.

Chapter X

Cardiac ^{123}I-MIBG SPECT

Ji Chen and *Weihua Zhou*
Emory University, Atlanta, US

Introduction

Heart failure (HF) is a prevalent, costly, and potentially deadly disease [1]. In the United States, more than 6 million people have HF and more than 0.5 million people are newly diagnosed with HF every year [2]. In developed countries, around 2% of adults suffer from HF [1-3].

HF is a major cause of mortality and morbidity, and sudden arrhythmic death is the cause of death in 30-50% of fatalities. Therapies with anti-arrhythmic drugs (AAD) and an implantable cardioverter defibrillator (ICD) have been developed to prevent arrhythmias. A number of clinical trials have demonstrated the superiority of ICD over AAD in the prevention of death from ventricular arrhythmias. The Sudden Cardiac Death in Heart Failure Trial (SCD-HeFT)[4] showed that HF patients with ICD therapy had an all-cause death risk with 23% lower than placebo and an absolute decrease in mortality of 7.2% after 5-year follow-up in the overall population.

Left ventricular ejection fraction (LVEF) is the main criterion for selecting HF patients for ICD therapy. An LVEF of less than 40% may confirm a diagnosis of HF. An LVEF of less than 35% increases the risk of life-threatening arrhythmia. The ACC/AHA/HRS guidelines [5] suggest that ICD therapy is recommended for the primary prevention of sudden cardiac death to reduce total mortality in patients with non-ischemic dilated cardiomyopathy or ischemic heart disease at least 40 days post-MI, an LVEF less than or equal to 35%, and New York Heart Association (NYHA) functional class II or III symptoms while receiving chronic optimal medical therapy, and who have reasonable expectation of survival with a good functional status for more than 1 year (Class I, Level of Evidence: A).

---

* Contact Information: Ji Chen, PhD, FACC, FASNC. Associate Professor, Department of Radiology and Imaging Sciences, Emory University, 1364 Clifton Road NE, Atlanta, GA 30322, USA. Phone: +1 (404) 712-4024; Fax: +1 (404) 727-3488; Email: jchen22@emory.edu.

Although the recommendations based on LVEF provide an important guide for ICD patient selection, pivot trials and post-hoc studies have demonstrated that this predictor has a number of limitations. On the one hand, ICD never discharges in a considerable number of patients who receive ICD therapy. In the SCD-HeFT trial [4], the average annual rate of appropriate ICD shocks was only about 5%. On the other hand, a lot of arrhythmic deaths occur in a population who have an LVEF higher than 35% and are not qualified for ICD therapy according to the guidelines [6].

Therefore, a better parameter than LVEF is needed to improve patient selection for ICD therapy. Abnormalities of the autonomic nervous system are thought to play an important role in the development of ventricular tachyarrhythmia [7, 8]. Moreover, it was recently found that the inducibility of ventricular tachyarrhythmia is related to regional cardiac sympathetic denervation, as assessed by ^{123}I-MIBG SPECT imaging [9]. Thus, cardiac ^{123}I-MIBG SPECT imaging may be a useful tool for detecting abnormalities of the myocardial adrenergic nervous system and predicting ventricular arrhythmia in HF patients. This chapter reviews the technical background of ^{123}I-MIBG SPECT imaging and introduces its clinical application in predicting ventricular arrhythmia and selecting HF patients for ICD therapy.

The Physical Characteristics of ^{123}I

[123]I emits 159-keV photopeak photons as well as multiple low-abundance, high-energy photons (Table 10-1).

Table 10-1. ^{123}I photons

Energy (keV)	Photons per decay
159	0.8280
248	0.0007
281	0.0008
346	0.0013
440	0.0043
505	0.0031
529	0.0138
539	0.0038
625	0.0008
688	0.0003
736	0.0006
784	0.0006

The high-energy photons can penetrate the septa of low-energy high-resolution (LEHR) collimators, which are widely used for ^{99m}Tc and ^{201}Tl myocardial perfusion imaging. Since the LEHR collimator blocks many 159-keV photopeak photons while it is almost transparent to the high-energy photons, a prominent plateau is observed in the ^{123}I spectrum, which is measured extrinsically with a low-energy collimator compared to that measured intrinsically (Figure 10-1).

Septal penetration can degrade image quality and quantitative accuracy of ^{123}I-MIBG imaging [10-15]. Since medium-energy all-purpose (MEAP) collimators have thicker septa and lower transparency to the high-energy photons than LEHR collimators, they have been shown to reduce the influence of septal penetration and improve accuracy in the quantification of ^{123}I-MIBG cardiac uptake [16, 17]. However, the sensitivity of MEAP collimators (approximately 8.0 counts/kBq/min) is much lower than LEHR collimators (approximately 14.3 counts/kBq/min) [18]; therefore, they require a longer acquisition to achieve a comparable count density to that of LEHR collimators. In addition, MEAP collimators are not available with many small field-of-view, dedicated cardiac SPECT systems. Therefore, its applicability in nuclear cardiology is limited.

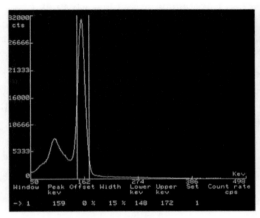
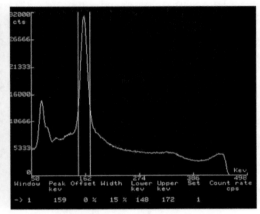

A. Intrinsic I-123 spectrum.   B. Extrinsic I-123 spectrum.

Figure 10.1. ^{123}I energy spectrum measured by a gamma camera without (A) and with a collimator (B). The high-energy component is much more prominent when measured with a collimator, because the collimator blocks a lot of the photopeak photons, but is almost transparent to the high-energy photons.

^{123}I-MIBG SPECT Acquisition

Thyroid blockage is usually administered to patients who undergo ^{123}I-MIBG imaging. It usually consists of potassium perchlorate (approximately 400 mg) or potassium iodate, potassium iodide, or Lugol's solution (equivalent of 100 mg of iodine) one hour before injection of ^{123}I-MIBG. The ^{123}I-MIBG dose is usually 10 mCi (370 MBq) per patient and is administered over 1-2 minutes.

^{123}I-MIBG SPECT images are usually acquired at 15-30 minutes (early scan) and 3-4 hours (late scan) post-tracer administration, respectively. The late scan is more commonly used, whereas the early scan is usually used to measure MIBG washout rate in comparison to the late scan. As noted in the previous section, collimator choice is an important issue in ^{123}I-MIBG SPECT [16, 17]. To reduce septal penetration, MEAP collimators are preferred; however, their sensitivity is lower than LEHR collimators requiring a longer scan, and they are less available than LEHR collimators in nuclear cardiology practice. Therefore, the largest clinical trial of ^{123}I-MIBG, AdreView Myocardial Imaging for Risk Evaluation in Heart Failure (ADMIRE-HF), used LEHR collimators for all image acquisition [19].

High-energy components of ^{123}I can also raise scatter contamination in the ^{123}I-MIBG SPECT images. Therefore, energy window configuration for ^{123}I imaging has been investigated for scatter compensation. In a phantom study[20], two energy window configurations with both MEAP and LEHR collimators were examined: 1) 20% photopeak window centered at 159 keV, 25% scatter window centered at 126 keV; and 2) 15% photopeak window centered at 159 keV, 28% scatter window centered at 128 keV. The optimal scatter compensation scaling factors were measured to be 0.55 and 0.3 for LEHR 20% and 15% photopeak window configurations, and 0.65 and 0.3 for MEAP 20% and 15% photopeak window configurations, respectively. The smaller optimal scaling factors for the 15% photopeak window configurations indicated that by reducing the width of the photopeak window, less scattered photons were acquired in the photopeak window. Nevertheless, with the optimal scaling factors there were no significant differences between the heart-to-mediastinum (H/M) ratios calculated from the two energy window configurations. Noteworthy, the MEAP SPECT H/M ratios were more accurate than the LEHR SPECT H/M ratios, confirming the findings of previous studies with ^{123}I planar imaging [16, 17].

Other than collimator choice and energy window configuration, ^{123}I-MIBG SPECT acquisition parameters are similar to conventional myocardial perfusion imaging using ^{99m}Tc tracers. ^{123}I-MIBG SPECT acquisition covers a 180° arc with 60 or more projections (~30 seconds/stop) from right-anterior orbit 45° to left-posterior orbit 45°. Images are stored in a 64 x 64 matrix with a nominal pixel size of 6-7 mm. Electrocardiogram (ECG) gating is not used for ^{123}I-MIBG SPECT.

^{123}I-MIBG SPECT Image Processing and Analysis

^{123}I-MIBG SPECT images can be reconstructed by the conventional techniques, such as filtered back-projection (FBP), maximum likelihood expectation maximization (MLEM), or ordered subsets expectation maximization (OSEM). Importantly, a deconvolution of the septal penetration (DSP) technique, based on the measured collimator-specific distance-dependent point-spread function (PSF), has been developed to improve quantification for ^{123}I-MIBG cardiac SPECT imaging [21]. Figure 10-2 shows ^{123}I point spread functions (PSFs) measured with LEHR and MEAP collimators, respectively. The ^{123}I PSFs included two effects: a) reduction of resolution with increased camera-source distance and b) septal penetration. As shown in these PSFs, the septal penetration component was a low but long, gradually decreasing plateau and was less distance-dependent. These ^{123}I PSFs allowed estimating the 3D collimator response to ^{123}I photons by convolution. Inclusion of this estimation in the projection used in iterative reconstruction, either MLEM or OSEM, septal penetration can be deconvoluted through a number of iterations and its impact can be reduced in the reconstructed images. The DSP technique was an additional process implemented in iterative reconstruction. It can be performed with or without other corrections for attenuation and scatter. In addition to reconstruction, Butterworth filtering is needed to reduce noise in the images. The optimal parameters of Butterworth filtering for ^{123}I-MIBG SPECT have been derived in a phantom experiment [20].

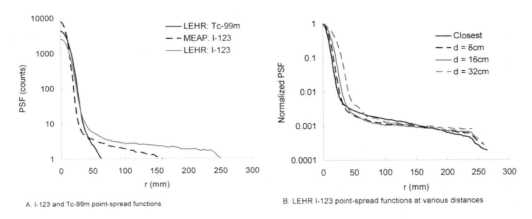

A. I-123 and Tc-99m point-spread functions   B. LEHR I-123 point-spread functions at various distances

Figure 10.2. ^{123}I point-spread functions (PSF). As compared to the ^{99m}Tc PSF, ^{123}I PSFs have a long plateau due to septal penetration of ^{123}I high-energy photons. The plateau is shorter and lower for a medium-energy all-purpose (MEAP) collimator than a low-energy high-resolution (LEHR) collimator, because the MEAP collimator has a thicker septa and is less transparent to ^{123}I high-energy photons. The height of the plateau does not vary much with the distance between the point source and camera.

The most widely used parameter in ^{123}I-MIBG imaging is the H/M ratio, which characterizes the global uptake of MIBG in the heart. The H/M ratio is conventionally measured by planar imaging as shown in Figure 10-3. A high H/M ratio denotes a greater tracer uptake and indicates normal heart conditions, while a lower value signifies reduced adrenergic density. H/M ratios can also be measured from the reconstructed ^{123}I-MIBG SPECT images. Figure 10-4 demonstrates a tool developed in the Emory Cardiac Toolbox for quantitation of ^{123}I-MIBG myocardial uptake from SPECT images [22].

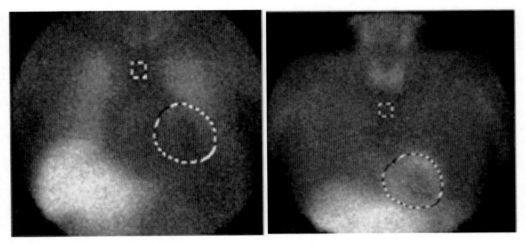

A. MIBG planar image of a HF patient.   B. MIBG planar image of a normal subject.

Figure 10.3. Measurement of H/M ratios from ^{123}I-MIBG planar imaging. Two regions-of-interest are drawn on the planar image, one including the entire heart and the other in the mediastinum between the two lungs.

In addition to global quantitation of cardiac ^{123}I-MIBG uptake, ^{123}I-MIBG SPECT can be used to assess regional uptake and provide insightful information about the condition of the sympathetic nervous system. A commonly measured parameter in ^{123}I-MIBG SPECT imaging is defect score. Defect score is calculated by the assessment of segmental ^{123}I-MIBG tracer uptake using the conventional 17-segment model. Each myocardial segment is visually scored according to the 5-point tracer uptake scale (0 representing normal tracer uptake and 4 representing no tracer uptake). Subsequently, MIBG defect score is obtained as the summation of all the segmental tracer uptake scores. Another important parameter is MIBG-perfusion mismatch score. Myocardial perfusion SPECT can be acquired in addition to ^{123}I-MIBG SPECT on a separate day. A similar method based on the 17-segment model is used to calculate a perfusion defect score. The MIBG-perfusion mismatch score can be calculated by subtracting the perfusion defect score from the MIBG defect score to represent the size of the mismatch. Noteworthy, these quantitative indices (MIBG defect score and MIBG-perfusion mismatch score) are measured by visual interpretation of ^{123}I-MIBG and perfusion SPECT images, and thus can be limited by significant intra- and inter-observer variability. Quantitative measurement of these parameters may improve their reproducibility and are currently under development.

Clinical Applications of ^{123}I-MIBG SPECT Imaging

The prognostic value of H/M ratios measured from ^{123}I-MIBG planar imaging has been extensively studied [23-29] and recently validated in the ADMIRE-HF trial [30]. A total of 961 subjects with NYHA functional class II or III HF and LVEF ≤35% were included in the ADMIRE-HF trial. Among them, a total of 237 subjects experienced cardiac events (NYHA class progression, potentially life-threatening arrhythmic event, or cardiac death) in a median follow-up period of 17 months. The hazard ratio for H/M ratio ≥1.60 was 0.40 ($p<0.001$), and the hazard ratio for continuous H/M ratio was 0.22 ($p<0.001$). Two-year event rate was 15% for H/M ratio ≥1.60 and 37% for H/M ratio <1.60. Importantly, a total of 86 subjects had either nonfatal arrhythmic events or sudden cardiac death. These combined "arrhythmic" events were significantly more common in subjects with H/M ratio <1.60 (79 of 760, 10.4%) than in subjects with H/M ratio ≥1.60 (7 of 201, 3.5%), indicating that there is a potential value of using ^{123}I-MIBG planar imaging to select HF patients for ICD therapy.

Table 10.2. Planar and SPECT H/M ratios

		Planar H/M	FBP H/M	OSEM H/M	DSP H/M
HF patients (N=926)	Mean	1.44	2.41	2.18	3.47
	SD	0.20	0.98	0.78	2.00
Controls (N=90)	Mean	1.77	3.87	3.67	6.49
	SD	0.23	1.48	1.20	2.93
P		<0.0001	<0.0001	<0.0001	<0.0001

FBP: filtered back-projection; OSEM: ordered subsets expectation maximization; DSP: deconvolution of septal penetration; HF: heart failure; SD: standard deviation; P: p value of the unpaired t test with unequal variance between the HF patients and controls.

The equivalency of H/M ratios measured by ^{123}I-MIBG SPECT to ^{123}I-MIBG planar imaging has been reported in a recent study with 1,016 subjects (926 HF patients and 90 controls) in the ADMIRE-HF trial [22]. Table 10-2 shows the planar and SPECT H/M ratios in the HF and control subjects.

For all SPECT reconstruction methods (FBP, OSEM, and DSP), the H/M ratios in the HF subjects were significantly smaller than those in the controls. Table 10-3 shows the optimal cutoff values, sensitivity, specificity, and area under the receiver operating characteristic (ROC) curves (AUC) of the planar and SPECT H/M ratios in differentiating the HF patients from the control subjects. There were no significant differences between the AUC values of the SPECT H/M ratios and planar H/M ratio.

Table 10.3. Optimal cutoff values, sensitivity, specificity, and AUC of planar and SPECT H/M ratios in differentiating the HF and control subjects

	Planar H/M	FBP H/M	OSEM H/M	DSP H/M
Optimal Cutoff	1.58	2.72	2.61	4.01
Sensitivity	0.78	0.72	0.76	0.72
Specificity	0.79	0.78	0.86	0.83
AUC	0.85	0.82	0.87	0.83
P (SPECT vs. Planar)		0.0892	0.7057	0.1310
P (FBP or DSP vs. OSEM)		<0.0001		0.0002

FBP: filtered back-projection; OSEM: ordered subsets expectation maximization; DSP: deconvolution of septal penetration; AUC: area under ROC curve; P: *p*-value.

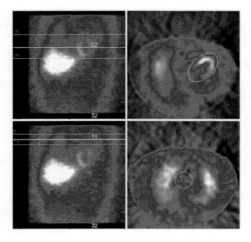 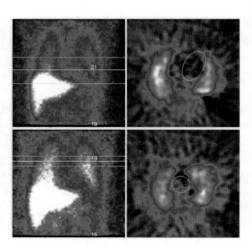

A. Patient with normal mIBG uptake   B. Patient with abnormal mIBG uptake

Figure 10.4. Examples of subjects with normal (panel A) and abnormal MIBG uptake (panel B) measured by ^{123}I-MIBG SPECT imaging. In each panel, the heart ROI was manually drawn and the mediastinum ROI was automatically determined on the heart and mediastinum transaxial images, which corresponded to the red lines on the planar images next to them, respectively. The H/M VOIs were then constructed to include the pixels within the H/M ROIs in between the corresponding green lines, respectively. SPECT H/M ratio was calculated by dividing the mean counts in the heart VOI by the mean counts in the mediastinum VOI.

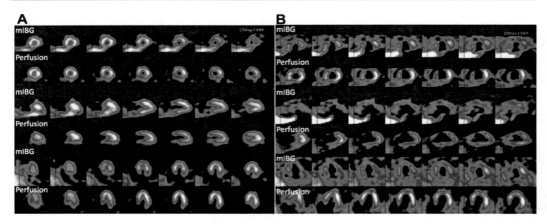

Figure 10.5. (A): Perfusion and ^{123}I-MIBG SPECT of a patient with ICD without experiencing ICD shock. (B): Perfusion and ^{123}I-MIBG SPECT of a patient with ICD and experiencing ICD shock. (Courtesy of Mark I. Travin, MD, Montefiore Medical Center, Bronx, NY, USA).

This study showed that the H/M ratios measured from ^{123}I-MIBG SPECT, regardless of the reconstruction method, have a similar capability for differentiating HF patients from normal controls. The prognostic value of H/M ratios measured from ^{123}I-MIBG SPECT remains to be established.

Sympathetic innervation is more sensitive to oxygen deprivation than myocytes, with the area of injury more widespread in the instance of transmural myocardial infarct or significant myocardial fibrosis, in part because the sympathetic nerve trunks traverse the area of injury. Neuronal dysfunction often persists longer than myocyte abnormalities [31]. An innervation-perfusion mismatch, i.e., denervated but viable myocardium, which creates innervation supersensitivity indicates dangerous ventricular arrhythmias [32]. ^{123}I-MIBG SPECT imaging in conjunction with myocardial perfusion imaging can be used to measure the size of MIBG defect and MIBG-perfusion mismatch. Figure 10-5 shows an example where a HF patient with ICD discharges had a more extensive MIBG defect as well as MIBG-perfusion mismatch. In a study with 116 HF patients referred for ICD therapy [33], appropriate ICD discharges (primary end point) were documented in 24 patients and appropriate ICD discharges or cardiac death (secondary end point) in 32 patients during a follow-up period of 23 ± 15 months. Late ^{123}I-MIBG defect score was an independent predictor for both end points. Patients with a large late ^{123}I-MIBG defect score (summed score >26) showed significantly more appropriate ICD discharges (52% vs. 5%, p<0.01) and more appropriate ICD discharges or cardiac death (57% vs. 10%, p<0.01) than patients with a small late ^{123}I-MIBG defect score (summed score $\leq$ 26) at 3-year follow-up. This study shows the potential value of using ^{123}I-MIBG SPECT to predict ventricular arrhythmia and cardiac death, and ultimately, to select HF patients for ICD therapy. A more complete review has recently been published in the Journal of Nuclear Cardiology [34].

Conclusion

The selection of HF patients for ICD therapy is a challenging clinical problem. The current methods are mainly based on LVEF, which has a number of limitations. ^{123}I-MIBG SPECT imaging provides a useful tool for assessment of the sympathetic nervous system. Several parameters given by ^{123}I-MIBG SPECT imaging, such as H/M ratio, MIBG defect score, and MIBG-perfusion mismatch score, have been shown to predict ventricular arrhythmia and are promising for the selection of HF patients for ICD therapy. Further studies are needed to establish these clinical applications of ^{123}I-MIBG SPECT imaging, which may require quantitative techniques to compensate for septal penetration of ^{123}I, to improve the image quality of ^{123}I-MIBG SPECT, and to explore new quantitative indices or comprehensive, multi-variant models to enhance the overall accuracy of using ^{123}I-MIBG SPECT parameters to predict ventricular arrhythmia and to select HF patients for ICD therapy.

Disclaimer

Dr. Chen is the principal investigator of an NIH/NHLBI grant (1R01HL094438, 5/1/2009-4/30/2013). Dr. Chen receives royalties from the sale of Emory Cardiac Toolbox with SyncTool. The terms of this arrangement have been reviewed and approved by Emory University in accordance with its conflict-of-interest practice.

References

[1]   McMurray JJ, Pfeffer MA. Heart failure. *Lancet* 2005; 365: 1877-89.
[2]   Roger VL, Go AS, Lloyd-Jones DM, Benjamin EJ, Berry JD et al. Heart disease and stroke statistics--2012 update: a report from the American Heart Association. *Circulation* 2012; 125: e2-e220.
[3]   Dickstein K, Cohen-Solal A, Filippatos G, McMurray JJ, Ponikowski P et al. ESC guidelines for the diagnosis and treatment of acute and chronic heart failure 2008: the Task Force for the diagnosis and treatment of acute and chronic heart failure 2008 of the European Society of Cardiology. Developed in collaboration with the Heart Failure Association of the ESC (HFA) and endorsed by the European Society of Intensive Care Medicine (ESICM). *European journal of heart failure* 2008; 10: 933-89.
[4]   Bardy GH, Lee KL, Mark DB, Poole JE, Packer DL et al. Amiodarone or an implantable cardioverter-defibrillator for congestive heart failure. *The New England journal of medicine* 2005; 352: 225-37.
[5]   Epstein AE, DiMarco JP, Ellenbogen KA, Estes NA, 3rd, Freedman RA et al. ACC/AHA/HRS 2008 Guidelines for Device-Based Therapy of Cardiac Rhythm Abnormalities: a report of the American College of Cardiology/American Heart Association Task Force on Practice Guidelines (Writing Committee to Revise the ACC/AHA/NASPE 2002 Guideline Update for Implantation of Cardiac Pacemakers

and Antiarrhythmia Devices): developed in collaboration with the American Association for Thoracic Surgery and Society of Thoracic Surgeons. *Circulation* 2008; 117: e350-408.

[6]   Stecker EC, Vickers C, Waltz J, Socoteanu C, John BT et al. Population-based analysis of sudden cardiac death with and without left ventricular systolic dysfunction: two-year findings from the Oregon Sudden Unexpected Death Study. *Journal of the American College of Cardiology* 2006; 47: 1161-6.

[7]   Podrid PJ, Fuchs T, Candinas R. Role of the sympathetic nervous system in the genesis of ventricular arrhythmia. *Circulation* 1990; 82: I103-13.

[8]   Zipes DP. Sympathetic stimulation and arrhythmias. *The New England journal of medicine* 1991; 325: 656-7.

[9]   Bax JJ, Kraft O, Buxton AE, Fjeld JG, Parizek P et al. 123 I-mIBG scintigraphy to predict inducibility of ventricular arrhythmias on cardiac electrophysiology testing: a prospective multicenter pilot study. *Circulation Cardiovascular imaging* 2008; 1: 131-40.

[10]   Bolmsjo MS, Persson BR, Strand SE. Imaging 123I with a scintillation camera. A study of detection performance and quality factor concepts. *Physics in medicine and biology* 1977; 22: 266-77.

[11]   Fleming JS, Alaamer AS. Influence of collimator characteristics on quantification in SPECT. *Journal of nuclear medicine : official publication, Society of Nuclear Medicine* 1996; 37: 1832-6.

[12]   Dobbeleir AA, Hambye AS, Franken PR. Influence of methodology on the presence and extent of mismatching between 99mTc-MIBI and 123I-BMIPP in myocardial viability studies. *Journal of nuclear medicine : official publication, Society of Nuclear Medicine* 1999; 40: 707-14.

[13]   Macey DJ, DeNardo GL, DeNardo SJ, Hines HH. Comparison of low- and medium-energy collimators for SPECT imaging with iodine-123-labeled antibodies. *Journal of nuclear medicine : official publication, Society of Nuclear Medicine* 1986; 27: 1467-74.

[14]   Geeter FD, Franken PR, Defrise M, Andries H, Saelens E et al. Optimal collimator choice for sequential iodine-123 and technetium-99m imaging. *Eur J Nucl Med* 1996; 23: 768-74.

[15]   Dobbeleir AA, Hambye AS, Franken PR. Influence of high-energy photons on the spectrum of iodine-123 with low- and medium-energy collimators: consequences for imaging with 123I-labelled compounds in clinical practice. *Eur J Nucl Med* 1999; 26: 655-8.

[16]   Inoue Y, Suzuki A, Shirouzu I, Machida T, Yoshizawa Y et al. Effect of collimator choice on quantitative assessment of cardiac iodine 123 MIBG uptake. *Journal of nuclear cardiology : official publication of the American Society of Nuclear Cardiology* 2003; 10: 623-32.

[17]   Inoue Y, Shirouzu I, Machida T, Yoshizawa Y, Akita F et al. Collimator choice in cardiac SPECT with I-123-labeled tracers. *Journal of nuclear cardiology : official publication of the American Society of Nuclear Cardiology* 2004; 11: 433-9.

[18]   Snay ER, Treves ST, Fahey FH. Improved quality of pediatric 123I-MIBG images with medium-energy collimators. *Journal of nuclear medicine technology* 2011; 39: 100-4.

[19]   Jacobson AF, Lombard J, Banerjee G, Camici PG. 123I-mIBG scintigraphy to predict risk for adverse cardiac outcomes in heart failure patients: design of two prospective

multicenter international trials. *Journal of nuclear cardiology : official publication of the American Society of Nuclear Cardiology* 2009; 16: 113-21.

[20] Chen J, Garcia EV, Galt JR, Folks RD, Carrio I. Optimized acquisition and processing protocols for I-123 cardiac SPECT imaging. *Journal of nuclear cardiology : official publication of the American Society of Nuclear Cardiology* 2006; 13: 251-60.

[21] Chen J, Garcia EV, Galt JR, Folks RD, Carrio I. Improved quantification in 123I cardiac SPECT imaging with deconvolution of septal penetration. *Nuclear medicine communications* 2006; 27: 551-8.

[22] Chen J, Folks RD, Verdes L, Manatunga DN, Jacobson AF et al. Quantitative I-123 mIBG SPECT in differentiating abnormal and normal mIBG myocardial uptake. *Journal of nuclear cardiology : official publication of the American Society of Nuclear Cardiology* 2012; 19: 92-9.

[23] Merlet P, Benvenuti C, Moyse D, Pouillart F, Dubois-Rande JL et al. Prognostic value of MIBG imaging in idiopathic dilated cardiomyopathy. *Journal of nuclear medicine : official publication, Society of Nuclear Medicine* 1999; 40: 917-23.

[24] Wakabayashi T, Nakata T, Hashimoto A, Yuda S, Tsuchihashi K et al. Assessment of underlying etiology and cardiac sympathetic innervation to identify patients at high risk of cardiac death. *Journal of nuclear medicine : official publication, Society of Nuclear Medicine* 2001; 42: 1757-67.

[25] Merlet P, Valette H, Dubois-Rande JL, Moyse D, Duboc D et al. Prognostic value of cardiac metaiodobenzylguanidine imaging in patients with heart failure. *Journal of nuclear medicine : official publication, Society of Nuclear Medicine* 1992; 33: 471-7.

[26] Cohen-Solal A, Esanu Y, Logeart D, Pessione F, Dubois C et al. Cardiac metaiodobenzylguanidine uptake in patients with moderate chronic heart failure: relationship with peak oxygen uptake and prognosis. *Journal of the American College of Cardiology* 1999; 33: 759-66.

[27] Nakata T, Miyamoto K, Doi A, Sasao H, Wakabayashi T et al. Cardiac death prediction and impaired cardiac sympathetic innervation assessed by MIBG in patients with failing and nonfailing hearts. *Journal of nuclear cardiology : official publication of the American Society of Nuclear Cardiology* 1998; 5: 579-90.

[28] Kasama S, Toyama T, Kumakura H, Takayama Y, Ichikawa S et al. Spironolactone improves cardiac sympathetic nerve activity and symptoms in patients with congestive heart failure. *Journal of nuclear medicine : official publication, Society of Nuclear Medicine* 2002; 43: 1279-85.

[29] Agostini D, Belin A, Amar MH, Darlas Y, Hamon M et al. Improvement of cardiac neuronal function after carvedilol treatment in dilated cardiomyopathy: a 123I-MIBG scintigraphic study. *Journal of nuclear medicine : official publication, Society of Nuclear Medicine* 2000; 41: 845-51.

[30] Jacobson AF, Senior R, Cerqueira MD, Wong ND, Thomas GS et al. Myocardial iodine-123 meta-iodobenzylguanidine imaging and cardiac events in heart failure. Results of the prospective ADMIRE-HF (AdreView Myocardial Imaging for Risk Evaluation in Heart Failure) study. *Journal of the American College of Cardiology* 2010; 55: 2212-21.

[31] Henneman MM, Bengel FM, Bax JJ. Will innervation imaging predict ventricular arrhythmias in ischaemic cardiomyopathy? *European journal of nuclear medicine and molecular imaging* 2006; 33: 862-5.

[32]   Minardo JD, Tuli MM, Mock BH, Weiner RE, Pride HP et al. Scintigraphic and electrophysiological evidence of canine myocardial sympathetic denervation and reinnervation produced by myocardial infarction or phenol application. *Circulation* 1988; 78: 1008-19.

[33]   Boogers MJ, Borleffs CJ, Henneman MM, van Bommel RJ, van Ramshorst J et al. Cardiac sympathetic denervation assessed with 123-iodine metaiodobenzylguanidine imaging predicts ventricular arrhythmias in implantable cardioverter-defibrillator patients. *Journal of the American College of Cardiology* 2010; 55: 2769-77.

[34]   Kelesidis I, Travin MI. Use of cardiac radionuclide imaging to identify patients at risk for arrhythmic sudden cardiac death. *Journal of nuclear cardiology : official publication of the American Society of Nuclear Cardiology* 2012; 19: 142-52; quiz 53-7.

In: SPECT
Editors: Hojjat Ahmadzadehfar and Elham Habibi

ISBN: 978-1-62808-344-6
© 2013 Nova Science Publishers, Inc.

Chapter XI

SPECT in Parkinson's Disease

Hong Zhang[*], *Mei Tian and Ling Wang*

Department of Nuclear Medicine, The Second Affiliated Hospital of Zhejiang University
School of Medicine, Hangzhou, China

Introduction

Parkinson's disease (PD) is a common neurodegenerative disorder characterized by the motor features of rigidity, tremors, akinesia, and changes in speech and gait which are associated with the loss of dopaminergic neurons in the substantia nigra pars compacta and the subsequent deficiency in striatal dopaminergic system. It has prevalence of 1-2 per 1,000 among the general population and of up to 2% among people aged over 65 years. The pathophysiological hallmark of PD is a slow, progressive degeneration of the nigrostriatal dopaminergic system. The widely accepted subcellular factor which underlies PD neuropathology is the presence of Lewy bodies [1] with characteristic inclusions of aggregated alpha-synuclein [2-4]. A recent study revealed that PD specific brain pathology extends far beyond the nigrostriatal dopaminergic system and affects widespread brain areas, including the olfactory system, autonomic and gain setting brainstem nuclei, and the cerebral cortex [5]. Physiological imaging techniques such as positron emission tomography (PET) or SPECT provide the means for detecting *in vivo* metabolic and neurochemical changes of PD. Motor symptoms such as tremor at rest, akinesia, rigidity, and postural instability are the cardinal signs in PD [6]. The type and severity of symptoms experienced by a person with PD vary with each individual and the stage of the disease. PD is the most common cause of parkinsonism. There are also many nonmotor features of PD including behavioral and psychiatric problems such as dementia [7], fatigue [8], anxiety [9], depression [10], autonomic dysfunction [11], addiction and compulsion [12], psychosis [13], olfactory

[*] Corresponding Author: Hong Zhang, MD, Professor of Nuclear Medicine, Chairman, Department of Nuclear Medicine, Second Affiliated Hospital of Zhejiang University School of Medicine; Chairman, Zhejiang University Medical PET Center; Chairman, Institute of Nuclear Medicine and Molecular Imaging, Zhejiang University; Chairman, Key Laboratory of Medical Molecular Imaging of Zhejiang Province; 88 Jiefang Road, Hangzhou, Zhejiang 310009, China. Tel/Fax: 0086-571-87767188.

dysfunction [14], and cognitive impairment [10]. These clinical features also occur in other neurodegenerative diseases and by dopamine receptor antagonist drugs, which means that with this main clinical application it is hard to diagnose patients with mild, incomplete, or uncertain parkinsonism [15]. In clinical practice, PD is diagnosed according to the criteria of the UK Parkinson 's Disease Society Brain Bank [16, 17]. The diagnosis is based on clinical criteria, but clinicopathological studies suggest that the accuracy of the clinical diagnosis in PD is only about 70%-80% in comparison with the "Gold-Standard", post-mortem neuropathologic examination [1, 18], therefore the diagnosis and treatment may be delayed for years until functional disability occurs. SPECT is an aid that can help diagnosing the disease earlier.

Imaging Agents of SPECT for PD

The ligands used for SPECT belong to a group of compounds derived from cocaine that bind to the dopamine transporter and include IPT, TRODAT-1, and FP-CIT tagged with either Iodine-123 (^{123}I; T1/2 = 13.2 h) or Technetium-99m (^{99m}Tc; T1/2 = 6 h) radioisotopes. Tracers used for SPECT imaging of PD patients are presented in Table 11.1.

Table 11.1. The tracer used for SPECT in Parkinson's disease

Dopamine reuptake (dopamine transport)	D2 dopamine receptor
[123]I-β-CIT	^{123}I-Iodospiperone,
^{123}I-FP-β-CIT	^{123}I-Iodobenzamide (^{123}I-IBZM),
^{123}I-IPT (presynaptic dopamine transporter)	(postsynaptic dopamine D2 receptor)
[123]I-Altropane	^{123}I-Iodolisuride, ^{123}I-IBF,
[123]I-β-PE2I	^{123}I-Epidepride (extrastriatal DA receptors)
^{99m}Tc-TRODAT-1	

Specific SPECT ligands for DAT (FP-CIT, beta-CIT, IPT, TRODAT-1) imaging provide a marker for presynaptic neuronal degeneration [19]. Postsynaptic receptor density is explored with dopamine receptor ligands, notably of the D2 type [20].

Dopamine Transporter Imaging

Prior to the scan patients should avoid taking any medications or drugs of abuse which could significantly influence the visual and quantitative analysis of DAT bindings ligands. Cocaine, amphetamine, CNS stimulants like phentermine, modafinil, antidepressants, anticholinergic drugs, opioids and anesthetics like ketamine may decrease striatal ^{123}I-FP-CIT binding, and adrenergic agonists like phenylephrine may increase striatal ^{123}I-FP-CITbinding [21], except, if the specific aim of the study is to assess the effect of such medications on DAT binding [22].

Antiparkinsonian medications (e.g. L-DOPA, dopamine agonists, NMDA receptor blockers, MAO-B inhibitors and COMT inhibitors) taken in standard dosages do not markedly affect DAT binding and therefore do not need to be withdrawn prior to DAT SPECT [22, 23]. In the case of using ^{123}I-labelled dopamine transporter ligands, the thyroid gland should be blocked by an adequate regimen (e.g. at least 200 mg of sodium perchlorate given at least 5 min prior to injection) to prevent free radioactive iodine accumulating in the thyroid [22].

[123]I-β-CIT

[123]I-2beta-carbomethoxy-3β -(4-iodophenyl) tropane (^{123}I-β-CIT) is a radiotracer which binds with nanomolar affinity to the serotonin transporter. It has a protracted period of striatal uptake enabling imaging 14–24 hours after injection of 150-250 MBq for stable quantitative measures of dopamine transporters [24].

^{123}I-FP-CIT

[123]I-N-ω-fluoropropyl-2β-carbomethoxy-3β-(4-iodophenyl) nortropane (^{123}I-FP-CIT) is an analogue of ^{123}I-β-CIT. It has been shown to achieve peak tracer uptake in the brain within hours after injection and to provide greater selectivity for the dopamine transporter. ^{123}I-FP-CIT washed out from striatal tissue 15–20 times faster than that of ^{123}I-β-CIT [24]. A clear decline in ^{123}I-FP-CIT binding was found with aging, amounting to 9.6%/ decade in the control group [25]. The recommended activity is 150-250 MBq. Data acquisition should be performed 3 to 6 hours after injection; however, it is recommended that a fixed time delay is used between injection and the beginning of data acquisition to ensure that data are comparable between subjects and intraindividual follow-up studies [22].

^{123}I-IPT

[123]I -N-(3-iodopropen-2-yl)-2 -carbomethoxy-3beta-(4-chlorophenyl) tropane (^{123}I-IPT) is a new cocaine analogue which allows the presynaptic dopamine transporters to be imaged with SPECT as early as 1-2 h after injection of 160-185 MBq of ^{123}I-IPT [26].

^{123}I-PE2I

[123]I -N-(3-iodoprop-2E-enyl)-2-β-carbomethoxy-3β-(4-methylphenyl) nortropane (^{123}I PE2I), a cocaine derivative, has good affinity for the DAT. ^{123}I-PE2I has revealed very intense and selective binding in the basal ganglia [27]. PE2I is a relatively new radioligand that has about 10-fold higher *in vitro* selectivity for the DAT than for the serotonin transporter (SERT) compared to ^{123}I-FP-CIT [28]. Further, ^{123}I-PE2I has faster kinetics than ^{123}I-FP-CIT. It is currently to be considered the best radioligand for imaging the DAT in the human brain with SPECT.

^{99m}Tc-TRODAT-1

^{99m}Tc-TRODAT-1 is a recently developed radiotracer that selectively binds to the dopamine transporters, which are significant because loss of these transporters corresponds with a loss of dopaminergic neurons. It is a potential agent for DAT SPECT. SPECT should be done 3 hours after injection of 740 MBq of ^{99m}Tc-TRODAT-1 [29].

Dopamine D2 Receptor Imaging

Many antiparkinsonian drugs (in particular dopamine agonists), neuroleptics and other medications (e.g. metoclopramide, cinnarizine, flunarizine, amphetamine and methylphenidate) compromise binding of the radioligand to the D2 receptors. The period of withdrawal of such drugs prior to the investigation depends on wash-out time and biological half-life of the respective drugs and may range from several hours to months [30]. L-DOPA therapy may be continued since interaction with D2 receptor ligands is relatively modest. Nevertheless when possible, patients should preferably be scanned during OFF conditions [30]. In the case of using ^{123}I-labelled dopamine transporter ligands the thyroid gland should be blocked by an adequate regimen (e.g. at least 200 mg of sodium perchlorate given at least 5 min prior to injection) to prevent free radioactive iodine accumulating in the thyroid [22].

^{123}I-IBZM

^{123}I-(S)-2-hydroxy-3-iodo-6-methoxy-(1-ethyl-2-pyrrolidinylmethyl)-benzamide   (^{123}I-IBZM) is a central nervous system (CNS) D-2 dopamine receptor imaging agent, and it has a high concentration in basal ganglia of brain [31]. The recommended activity is 150-250 MBq. Data acquisition should be performed 1.5 to 3 hours after injection [30].

^{123}I-IBF

^{123}I-5-iodo-7-N-((1-ethyl-2pyrrolidinyl)methyl)carbox-amido   2,3-dihydrobenzofuran (^{123}I-IBF) is an IBZM analogue. This agent concentrated in the striatum region and displayed a remarkably high target-to-nontarget ratio [32] and early time of peak uptake [33]. A study using P450 gene expression systems indicates that ^{123}I-IBF is enzymatically metabolized in the liver and rapidly excreted in the urine [34]. It is a potential agent for imaging D-2 dopamine receptors [35].

SPECT Imaging

For brain SPECT multiple detector cameras should be used for data acquisition with low energy high resolution (LEHR) or low energy ultra high resolution (LEUHR) parallel-hole collimators. The matrix size should be 128x128 or higher. The acquisition can be done in step and shoot mode with 120 projections. The scan time is for ^{123}I-labelled ligands about 40-50 s/projection and for ^{99m}Tc-TRODAT-1 30 s/projection [22, 29, 30]. The acquired data should be corrected for attenuation, scatter and partial volume effect.

Region of interest (ROI) techniques should be used to assess specific DAT or dopamine D2 receptor binding in the striatum and striatal subregions (caudate nucleus, putamen). Reference regions with absent (or low) DAT or D2 density (e.g. occipital cortex, cerebellum) are used to assess nonspecific binding [30].

Specific binding values [(mean counts of striatal ROI − mean counts of background ROI)/mean counts of background ROI] obtained from the patients are compared with those from normal subjects (preferably age matched) obtained with the same technique. The striatum may be subdivided into head of the caudate nucleus and anterior/posterior putamen to calculate anteroposterior gradients within the striatum. For intraindividual comparison (i.e. baseline vs. follow-up for therapy control or assessment of disease progression), standardized evaluation using approaches based on, for example, stereotactic normalization is most useful. It allows even subtle changes to be detected more reliably [30].

The Use of SPECT in PD

The Course and the Pathogenesis of PD

Brain SPECT imaging of DAT with specific radioligands provides a useful tool of *in vivo* investigation of the pathogenesis of PD, and it is a sensitive method for examining the integrity of the presynaptic dopaminergic system [15]. Cerebral and extracranial Lewy-body-type degeneration in PD does not develop independently from each other but develop in a strongly coupled manner. The cerebral and extracranial changes are driven by at least similar pathomechanisms [36]. Patients with PD have markedly reduced DAT levels in striatum, which correlated with disease severity and disease progression [24], whereas postsynaptic striatal D2 receptors are upregulated [37]. Similarly, another study reported that the mean ^{123}I-IBZM striatal-occipital ratio of binding was significantly higher in PD patients than in controls. In PD patients, higher values were found contralateral to the clinically most affected side, suggesting D2 receptor upregulation and the reverse was seen using ^{123}I-FP-CIT SPECT [38]. Dual isotope imaging using ^{99m}Tc-TRODAT-1 and ^{123}I-IBZM is also a useful means in evaluating the changes of both pre- and postsynaptic dopamine system in a primate model of parkinsonism [39]. There was a significant association of visually analyzed shapes of the striatum in FP-CIT SPECT and clinical PD subtype. It suggested that factors other than nigrostriatal degeneration may contribute to disease severity [40]. One study including 122 patients confirmed neuropathological models for reduced dopaminergic projection to the dorsal putamen in akinetic-rigid patients as well as the lateral putamen and caudate nucleus in tremor-dominant patients *in vivo* [41], and the serotonergic system is suggested to be implicated in PD [42]. Furthermore, another study showed that SERT-dependent ^{123}I-FP-CIT uptake may allow a more comprehensive assessment of neurochemical disturbances in degenerative parkinsonisms [43]; this study suggested that the neurodegenerative process extends beyond nigrostriatal system and affects serotoninergic neurons in parkinsonisms.

Early Diagnosis of PD

Since the *in vivo* molecular imaging techniques using SPECT have been introduced, the diagnosis of PD became more reliable by assessing dopaminergic and even nondopaminergic systems. SPECT is a very sensitive technique to detect nigrostriatal degeneration in PD. Various radiotracers have been used in the diagnosis of PD. DAT imaging is abnormal even in the earliest clinical presentation of PD [15]. A study using ^{123}I-β-CIT found that the relative uptake reduction in the hemi-PD patients was greater in the putamen than in the caudate in patients with early PD and suggested that it may be useful in identifying individuals with developing dopaminergic pathology before onset of motor symptoms [44]. It was reported that ^{123}I-β-CIT SPECT was 100% sensitive and specific for the diagnosis in younger patients (age <55 years). In older patients (age >55 years), specificity was substantially lower (68.5%) [45]. More recently, a prospective, longitudinal study using ^{123}I-FP-CIT had investigated 99 patients with tremor and/or parkinsonism over 3 years, and the results showed a mean sensitivity of 78% and a specificity of 97% [46]. A 2-year followed-up SPECT study using [99m]Tc- TRODAT-1 was performed in patients with clinically unclear Parkinsonian syndromes (CUPSs) and found that the rate of disagreement of SPECT in the patients was of 20%. The sensitivity of this technique was 100%, and specificity was 70%. It indicated that TRODAT-1 helps the diagnosis of patients with CUPS [47]. DAT SPECT is sensitive enough to detect a loss of nigrostriatal neurons *in vivo* even in preclinical phases of sporadic PD.

^{123}I-FP-CIT SPECT has been successfully used to detect the loss of dopaminergic nigrostriatal neurons in Parkinson's disease at an early stage. But the results reported were controversial. Tissingh et al. reported that striatal ^{123}I-FP-CIT uptake is markedly decreased in PD, more in the putamen than in the caudate nucleus, and the mean reduction in the putamen and caudate nucleus was 57% and 29% of the control mean, respectively. However, no significant correlations were found between striatal ^{123}I-FP-CIT binding ratios and disease severity [25]. Spiegel et al. found that the striatal ^{123}I-FP-CIT binding correlated significantly with the motor part of the unified Parkinson's disease rating scale (UPDRS) but not with age, disease duration, or gender [48]. Another study indicated that in patients with PD, the striatum, caudate, and putamen uptake was correlated with disease severity assessed by UPDRS and duration of disease [40]. More studies are needed to confirm these findings.

Patients with unilateral PD showed a bilateral loss of striatal DAT [25]. A study using semiquantitative ^{123}I-FP-CIT SPECT detected a bilateral dopaminergic deficit in early PD with unilateral symptoms and preclinical DAT loss in the ipsilateral striatal binding, corresponding to the side not yet affected by motor signs. It suggested that semi-quantitative analysis may be used to diagnose PD at early stage as well as to identify individuals developing bilateral dopaminergic damage [49]. The decrease of striatal uptake contralateral to the more affected side of the body was more prominent compared to the ip–silateral side (Fig. 11.1) [50]. Moreover, another study showed a significant loss of putaminal uptake ipsilateral to the symptoms was found in the stage I group compared with the healthy volunteers [51]. The mean reduction of binding was found in the order of putamen and caudate nucleus. DAT imaging is a sensitive method to detect presynaptic dopamine neuronal dysfunction. Normal DAT-SPECT can be used to exclude underlying true nigrostriatal dysfunction [52]. SPECT also contributes to the assessment of the nonmotor symptoms of PD. ^{123}I-MIBG was used in the diagnosis of damaged tissue of the heart. However, Sawada et al. [47] found that a reduction in MIBG cardiac accumulation reflects the systemic pathological process of the disease. Both early and delayed images showed that the heart to mediastinum ratios were significantly lower in the PD group than in the non-PD group (Figure 11.2) [53].

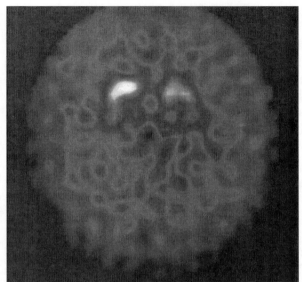

Courtesy of Elham Habibi, Department of Nuclear Medicine, University Hospital Bonn, Germany.

Figure 11.1. Patient with idiopathic PD. ^{123}I-FP-CIT SPECT of a 77 y/o patient with resting tremor, accentuated on the right side, and postural instability, shows reduced DAT uptake in the basal ganglia (especially on the left side).

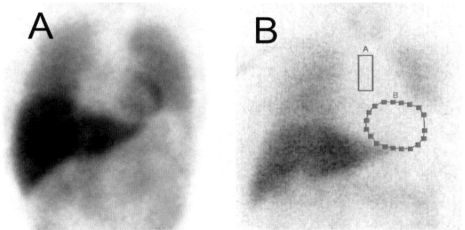

Courtesy of Elham Habibi, Department of Nuclear Medicine, University Hospital Bonn, Germany.

Figure 11.2. ^{123}I-MIBG scintigraphy of two patients. A: shows a late scan of a patient with multiple system atrophy with a normal heart uptake of ^{123}I-MIBG. B: shows a late scan of a patient with idiopathic Parkinson's disease without any heart uptake.

Sakakibara et al. [54] first reported the correlation of urinary dysfunction with nigrostriatal dopaminergic deficit in PD, which was studied by ^{123}I-β-CIT SPECT. The tracer uptake in patients with urinary dysfunction was significantly reduced than in those without urinary dysfunction.

Differential Diagnosis of PD

Clinical features of PD may be shared with other disorders; thus, the differential diagnosis of PD is extensive. Idiopathic Parkinson's disease is associated with Lewy body degeneration of nigrostriatal dopaminergic neurons [55]. Atypical parkinsonian syndromes (APSs) such as multiple system atrophy (MSA), progressive supranuclear palsy (PSP), and corticobasal degeneration are characterized by poor response to antiparkinsonian medication and rapid clinical deterioration, which one often confused with PD. Other diseases, for example, drug-induced parkinsonism (DIP), essential tremor (ET), vascular parkinsonism (VP), or dementia with Lewy bodies (DLBs) may also share common features with PD. ET is a slowly progressive neurological disorder. DIP is developed when patients are treated with neuroleptic or dopamine receptor blocking agents. In most patients, Parkinsonism is reversible upon stopping the offending drug, though it may take several months to resolve fully but in some patients it may even persist. The differentiation between PD and DIP is difficult to assess on clinical grounds alone. Functional imaging of the DAT defines integrity of the dopaminergic system, and a normal scan suggests an alternative diagnosis such as ET, VP (unless there is focal basal ganglia infarction), DIP, or psychogenic parkinsonism [19, 56]. Furthermore, a semiquantitative analysis with a cut-off of striatal asymmetry index greater than 14.08 could differentiate PD from VP with a 100% specificity [57]. ^{123}I-FP-CIT SPECT images demonstrate that SPECT imaging with DAT ligands is useful to determine whether parkinsonism is entirely drug induced [58] and showed high levels of accuracy [59]. Cuberas-Borros et al. performed FP-CIT images in 3 different groups of ET, DIP, and PD patients. Lower uptake was found in the PD group in comparison with the ET and DIP groups both in the putamen and in the caudate nucleus, but the differences between DIP and ET populations were only found in the putamen. There was an optimal discrimination threshold value between the reference population and the pathologic population for the putamen ratio by using volumes of interests, (VOIs) analysis [60].

SERT-dependent ^{123}I-FP-CIT imaging showed a mild decrease in SERT levels in PD compared to ET and healthy control, and reduced to undetectable levels of SERT in PSP and DLB patients were displayed markedly [43]. To improve diagnostic accuracy, non-DAT tracers (i.e., D2 dopamine receptors) are necessary together with long-term clinical follow-up and rescans [61]. MSA is a neurodegenerative disorder characterized by neuropathologic demonstration of CNS alpha-synucleinpositive glial cytoplasmic inclusions with neurodegenerative changes in striatonigral or olivopontocerebellar structures [62]. Clinically, MSA is characterized by autonomic dysfunction and/or urinary dysfunction which may be associated with parkinsonian symptoms in 80% of patients (MSA-P) or with cerebellar ataxia in 20% of patients (MSA-C). It is difficult to differentiate it from other movement disorders, particularly in the early course of disease. Voxel wise analysis of ^{123}I-β-CIT SPECT revealed more widespread decline of monoaminergic transporter availability in MSA-P compared with idiopathic Parkinson's disease (IPD) [63], matching the underlying pathological features.

They suggest that a quantification of midbrain DAT signal should be included in the routine clinical analysis of ^{123}I-β-CIT SPECT in patients with uncertain parkinsonism. A combined ^{99m}Tc-ECD/^{123}I-FP-CIT brain SPECT protocols have been proven to improve the differential diagnosis of IPD and MSA as well as corticobasal degeneration and PSP [64]. SPECT with the tracer ^{123}I-Ioflupane can also give an accurate and highly sensitive measure of dopamine degeneration [65].

A study showed that the degree of loss was higher in putamen than caudate in both PD and MSA patients. However, MSA patients showed a more symmetric loss (ipsilateral versus contralateral side) of striatal DAT in both caudate and putamen than PD patients (Figure 11.3) [66]. It was also reported that patients with a side-to-side difference of reduced striatal ^{123}I-β-CIT binding greater than 15% are likely to suffer from IPD, while the patients with the difference between 5% and 15% are more likely to have MSA [67]. Another study showed that mean distribution volume ratios (DVRs) in the basal ganglia of MSA patients were significantly less than in controls, but generally higher than in PD patients. Furthermore, the MSA patients had significantly increased DVRs in the posterior putamen (mean 0.49 ± 0.30) compared with PD patients (0.74 ± 0.25) [68]. Another study which used both ^{123}I-β-CIT (for DAT) and ^{123}I-IBF (for D2) reported that DAT binding in the posterior putamen was markedly reduced in all patients. However, D2 binding in posterior putamen was significantly increased in dopa-untreated PD, and it was significantly reduced in MSA. These findings suggested that DAT SPECT may be useful in differentiating parkinsonism from controls and D2 SPECT in further differentiating MSA from PD [69]. IBZM SPECT using recently introduced three dimensional automated quantification method calculating the Striatal/frontal cortex binding ratios [70] and voxel-by-voxel binding potential parametric imaging also can discriminate among extrapyramidal diseases such as PD and PSP [71]. ^{123}I-IBZM SPECT is an effective diagnostic tool in the establishment of the differential diagnosis in patients with PD and Parkinson-plus syndromes. Quantification of these studies had limited utility since the overlapping of index values between normal and pathological restricts their use in individual cases [72]. Vlaar et al. reported that FP-CIT SPECT is accurate to differentiate patients with IPD from those with ET, and IPD from VP and DIP, but the accuracy of both FP-CIT and IBZM SPECT scans to differentiate between IPD and APS is low [56]. However, a study suggested that using multidimensional combination of FP-CIT, IBZM, and MIBG scintigraphy was likely to significantly increase test accuracy (94%) in differentiating PD from APS [73]. More recently, a study using ^{123}I-PE2I indicated that dopamine transporter scan has a high sensitivity and specificity in distinguishing between patients with and without striatal neurodegeneration. Calculation of the striatal anterior-posterior ratio can assist in differentiating between idiopathic PD and APS [74]. Moreover, study with ^{123}I-FP-CIT in 165 patients with a clinical diagnosis of PD ($n = 120$) or APS ($n = 45$) suggested that a global and severe degeneration pattern had a high positive predictive value of APS within the first 5 years of the disease [75]. A ^{123}I-FP-CIT and ^{123}I-IBZM SPECT study, in which seven subjects were all from a Spanish family with G309D mutation in the PINK1 gene, showed that striatal DAT binding was reduced in all three PARK6 patients. But in two of the siblings, DAT binding was markedly increased. It suggested that the increased DAT binding may be an early preclinical finding [76]. SPECT is also useful for distinguishing PD from Dopa responsive dystonia (DRD), or for assessing the integrity of the nigrostriatal dopaminergic pathway in atypical cases of postural tremor or iatrogenic parkinsonian syndromes. The imaging with ^{99m}Tc-TRODAT-1/^{123}I-IBZM in a 39-year-old woman with a 24-year history of DRD indicated that ^{99m}Tc-TRODAT-1 is helpful in differentiating DRD from early-onset idiopathic parkinsonism and the ^{123}I-IBZM SPECT is also helpful in differentiating these two conditions in the later clinical course [77]. In IPD, two different clinical phenotypes are usually distinguished: a tremor-dominant variant (TD) and an akinetic-rigid type (ART). TD patients compared to ART patients are characterized by a slower disease progression and a minor cognitive impairment. For different phenotypes of PD, ^{123}I-FP-CIT SPECT has indicated that the dopaminergic system in ART patients is more involved compared to that in the TD patients and that this kind of difference is present from the initial stage of the disease [78-80]. There was a significantly higher FP-CIT uptake in contralateral putamen and a higher but not statistically significant uptake in all the other striatal regions in TD patients when compared to ART patients [79]. Similarly, Spiegel et al. reported a greater impairment in ART patients in all striatal regions analyzed [80].

These results suggest that further systems besides the nigrostriatal dopaminergic system may contribute to generation of parkinsonian tremor.

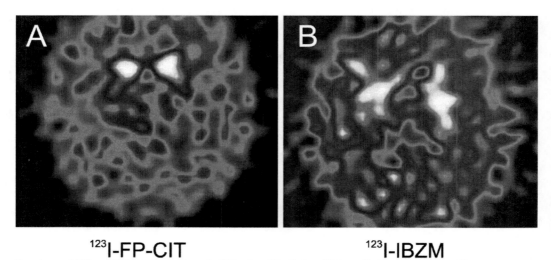

^{123}I-FP-CIT   ^{123}I-IBZM

Courtesy of Elham Habibi, Department of Nuclear Medicine, University Hospital Bonn, Germany.

Figure 11.3. 69 y/o patient with multiple system atrophy. Both DAT SPECT and D2-SPECT show pathological reduced uptake. A: ^{123}I-FP-CIT SPECT shows a symmetrical reduced uptake in the basal ganglia, especially in the putamen. B: ^{123}I-IBZM SPECT shows also reduced D2 receptors.

Monitoring the Progression of the PD

Pathologic studies investigating the rate of PD progression have been limited to patients with severe illness of long duration and rely entirely on cross-sectional data. The UPDRS or other functional clinical endpoints are used to monitor disease progression. It makes it difficult to isolate clinical changes solely due to disease progression [81]. The rate of progression of dopaminergic degeneration is much faster in PD than in normal aging [82]. Patients with PD present first with unilateral symptoms that gradually progress to involve both sides [6]. Clinical progression has been investigated with SPECT, which could prove to be an objective tool for monitoring the disease progression. ^{123}I-β-CIT SPECT imaging of the dopamine transporter is a sensitive biomarker of PD onset and severity. A group of 50 early-stage PD patients was examined [83]. Two SPECT imaging series were obtained 12 months apart. The average decrease in ^{123}I-β-CIT binding ratios was about 8% in the whole striatum, 8% in the putaminal region, and 4% in the caudate region. This finding supported the feasibility of using ^{123}I-β-CIT in the evaluation of disease progression in PD [84]. Moreover, sequential SPECT scans using ^{123}I-β-CIT in PD subjects demonstrated a decline in striatal uptake of approximately 11.2%/year from the baseline scan, compared with 0.8%/year in the healthy controls [81]. Another SPECT study with ^{123}I-β-CIT demonstrated a rapid decline of striatal binding in patients with APS, exceeding the reduction in PD, and the dopaminergic degeneration in PD slows down during the course of the disease [85]. Combined ^{123}I-β-CIT and ^{123}I-IBZM SPECT studies have demonstrated that postsynaptic dopamine receptor up-regulation contralateral to the presenting side occurs in untreated unilateral PD and disappears in untreated bilateral (asymmetric) PD despite a greater loss of dopamine transporter function [86]. This may be helpful in monitoring the progression of nigrostriatal dysfunction in early PD. Tatsch et al. [26] found that specific ^{123}I-IPT uptake in the caudate and putamen, and putamen to caudate ratios, decreased with increasing Hoehn and Yahr stage (H-Y). These findings indicated that ^{123}I-IPT SPECT also may be a useful imaging to estimate the extent of nigrostriatal degeneration in PD patients. Tissingh et al. reported that disease severity correlated negatively and highly significantly with the ^{123}I-β-CIT binding in patients with early PD. Tremor ratings did not correlate with the ^{123}I-β-CIT uptake, whereas rigidity and bradykinesia did [87]. The striatal ^{123}I-β-CIT uptake in a large cohort of PD subjects significantly correlated with severity of PD as measured by UPDRS [81]. The mean reduction of ^{99m}Tc-TRODAT-1 uptake was found in the order of putamen (contralateral side, -81%; ipsilateral side, -67%) and caudate nucleus (contralateral side, -46%; ipsilateral side, -40%), and it correlated negatively with the UPDRS and H-Y staging [88]. Winogrodzka et al. [82] used ^{123}I-FP-CIT SPECT for the assessment of the rate of dopaminergic degeneration in PD. The mean annual decrease in striatal binding ratios in PD patients was found to be about 8% of the baseline mean, indicating that ^{123}I-FP-CIT SPECT was applicable to investigate the progression of dopaminergic degeneration. The specific to nonspecific ^{123}I-FP-CIT uptake ratios were calculated for striatum, caudate, and putamen, all of which were correlated with disease severity assessed by UPDRS and the duration of disease, suggesting that tremor may origins from other systems instead of the dopamine transporter system. Meanwhile, these ratios correlated with the bradykinesia subscore but not with rigidity or tremor subscore. It suggested that factors other than nigrostriatal degeneration may contribute to disease severity [40].

Evaluation of the Treatment Effect of PD

Current therapies include drug therapy, surgical procedures, and stem cell transplantation. Drug therapy such as DA replacement therapy with levodopa fails to prevent the progression of the disease process and only alleviates the clinical symptoms. Once the diagnosis is made, the neurologist with the patient must decide whether to institute treatment at the time of diagnosis or when functional disability occurs [89]. To evaluate the effectiveness of treatment, it is critical to develop methods that can reliably measure the progression of dopaminergic degeneration. Postsynaptic imaging has been helpful in predicting therapeutic response to dopaminergic medication early in the course of Parkinson's disease. Studies have demonstrated that PD patients receiving treatment do better than those who do not, and those receiving treatment earlier do better in long term [90]. Schwarz et al. performed a follow-up study of 2–4 years including 55 patients with parkinsonism and prior dopaminomimetic therapy and found that IBZM-SPECT accurately predicted the response to apomorphine and levodopa, The sensitivity and specificity was 96.3%/64.7%, and 100%/75%, respectively [91]. Thus, ^{123}I-IBZM can be used routinely to identify which PD patients will benefit from dopaminergic medication [92]. Another study including 20 PD patients who undergone short-term levodopa test and SPECT imaging found there was a relationship between responsiveness to levodopa and asymmetry detected with ^{123}I-FP-CIT. This technique can predict dopaminergic responsiveness in patients with PD [93]. Recently, a ^{99m}Tc-TRODAT-1 SPECT indicated that levodopa did not interfere with DAT binding, suggesting that differences between clinical assessment and radiotracer imaging in clinical trials may not be specifically related to levodopa treatment [94]. Similarly, the effect of subchronic treatment on striatal DAT was examined in patients who were not currently being treated with these medications. These results suggested that typical clinical doses of levodopa/carbidopa and L-selegiline did not induce significant occupancy of the ^{123}I-β-CIT binding site and that 4–6 weeks of treatment caused no significant modulation of DAT levels. These results supported the validity of measuring DAT levels with ^{123}I-β-CIT without the need to withdraw patients from medication treatment [95]. ^{123}I-β-CIT SPECT imaging provides a quantitative biomarker for the progressive nigrostriatal dopaminergic degeneration in PD. As new protective and restorative therapies for PD are developed, dopamine transporter imaging offers the potential to provide an objective endpoint for these therapeutic trials [81, 82]. Hwang et al. found that the PD patients with fluctuating levodopa response showed a significant decrease in [123]IIBZM uptake (D2 receptor densities) than early levodopa-naïve PD and chronic PD with stable levodopa response which contributed to the development of motor fluctuation [96].

Conclusion

SPECT imaging has proven to be a useful tool to investigate the many facets of PD *in vivo*. This technique helps understand the pathogenesis, the differential diagnosis, and the progression of the PD. The disadvantage of SPECT compared to PET is that it is difficult to obtain a reliable quantification. Furthermore, the resolution of images is a limitation for the visualization of basal ganglia in PD. However, SPECT is more practical as a

routine procedure than PET. Imaging agents like dopamine transporter or D2 receptor ligands assess only part of aspects of the dopamine neurons. New tracers need to be synthesized to detect other aspects of dopamine neurons. The SPECT imaging of the nigrostriatal dopaminergic pathway can be used to monitor therapeutic effects in Parkinson's disease. As new protective and restorative therapies for PD are developed, dopamine transporter imaging offers the potential to provide an objective endpoint for these therapeutic trials. Further studies are needed to evaluate the possible effects of the therapy, especially for the delayed-onset bilateral symptoms. Moreover, there is a pressing need to improve our understanding of the pathogenesis to enable development of disease modifying treatments.

References

[1] Hughes AJ, Daniel SE, Kilford L, Lees AJ. Accuracy of clinical diagnosis of idiopathic Parkinson's disease: a clinico-pathological study of 100 cases. *J Neurol Neurosurg Psychiatry* 1992; 55: 181-4.

[2] Ruiperez V, Darios F, Davletov B. Alpha-synuclein, lipids and Parkinson's disease. *Progress in lipid research* 2010; 49: 420-8.

[3] Leong SL, Cappai R, Barnham KJ, Pham CL. Modulation of alpha-synuclein aggregation by dopamine: a review. *Neurochemical research* 2009; 34: 1838-46.

[4] Bellucci A, Collo G, Sarnico I, Battistin L, Missale C et al. Alpha-synuclein aggregation and cell death triggered by energy deprivation and dopamine overload are counteracted by D2/D3 receptor activation. *Journal of neurochemistry* 2008; 106: 560-77.

[5] Braak H, Del Tredici K, Rub U, de Vos RA, Jansen Steur EN et al. Staging of brain pathology related to sporadic Parkinson's disease. *Neurobiology of aging* 2003; 24: 197-211.

[6] Larsen JP, Beiske AG, Bekkelund SI, Dietrichs E, Tysnes OB et al. [Motor symptoms in Parkinson disease]. *Tidsskr Nor Laegeforen* 2008; 128: 2068-71.

[7] Peppard RF, Martin WR, Carr GD, Grochowski E, Schulzer M et al. Cerebral glucose metabolism in Parkinson's disease with and without dementia. *Archives of neurology* 1992; 49: 1262-8.

[8] Kummer A, Scalzo P, Cardoso F, Teixeira AL. Evaluation of fatigue in Parkinson's disease using the Brazilian version of Parkinson's Fatigue Scale. *Acta Neurol Scand* 2011; 123: 130-6.

[9] Prediger RD, Matheus FC, Schwarzbold ML, Lima MM, Vital MA. Anxiety in Parkinson's disease: a critical review of experimental and clinical studies. *Neuropharmacology* 2012; 62: 115-24.

[10] Aarsland D, Bronnick K, Larsen JP, Tysnes OB, Alves G. Cognitive impairment in incident, untreated Parkinson disease: the Norwegian ParkWest study. *Neurology* 2009; 72: 1121-6.

[11] Magerkurth C, Schnitzer R, Braune S. Symptoms of autonomic failure in Parkinson's disease: prevalence and impact on daily life. *Clin Auton Res* 2005; 15: 76-82.

[12] O'Sullivan SS, Wu K, Politis M, Lawrence AD, Evans AH et al. Cue-induced striatal dopamine release in Parkinson's disease-associated impulsive-compulsive behaviours. *Brain : a journal of neurology* 2011; 134: 969-78.

[13] Morgante L, Colosimo C, Antonini A, Marconi R, Meco G et al. Psychosis associated to Parkinson's disease in the early stages: relevance of cognitive decline and depression. *J Neurol Neurosurg Psychiatry* 2012; 83: 76-82.

[14] Berendse HW, Roos DS, Raijmakers P, Doty RL. Motor and non-motor correlates of olfactory dysfunction in Parkinson's disease. *Journal of the neurological sciences* 2011; 310: 21-4.

[15] Cohenpour M, Golan H. [Nuclear neuroimaging of dopamine transporter in Parkinsonism--role in routine clinical practice]. *Harefuah* 2007; 146: 698-702, 33.

[16] Meara J, Bhowmick BK, Hobson P. Accuracy of diagnosis in patients with presumed Parkinson's disease. *Age and ageing* 1999; 28: 99-102.

[17] Gelb DJ, Oliver E, Gilman S. Diagnostic criteria for Parkinson disease. *Archives of neurology* 1999; 56: 33-9.

[18] Rajput AH, Rozdilsky B, Rajput A. Accuracy of clinical diagnosis in parkinsonism--a prospective study. *The Canadian journal of neurological sciences Le journal canadien des sciences neurologiques* 1991; 18: 275-8.

[19] Marshall V, Grosset D. Role of dopamine transporter imaging in routine clinical practice. *Movement disorders : official journal of the Movement Disorder Society* 2003; 18: 1415-23.

[20] Thobois S, Guillouet S, Broussolle E. Contributions of PET and SPECT to the understanding of the pathophysiology of Parkinson's disease. *Neurophysiologie clinique = Clinical neurophysiology* 2001; 31: 321-40.

[21] Booij J, Kemp P. Dopamine transporter imaging with [(123)I]FP-CIT SPECT: potential effects of drugs. *Eur J Nucl Med Mol Imaging* 2008; 35: 424-38.

[22] Darcourt J, Booij J, Tatsch K, Varrone A, Vander Borght T et al. EANM procedure guidelines for brain neurotransmission SPECT using (123)I-labelled dopamine transporter ligands, version 2. *Eur J Nucl Med Mol Imaging* 2010; 37: 443-50.

[23] Schillaci O, Pierantozzi M, Filippi L, Manni C, Brusa L et al. The effect of levodopa therapy on dopamine transporter SPECT imaging with(123)I-FP-CIT in patients with Parkinson's disease. *Eur J Nucl Med Mol Imaging* 2005; 32: 1452-6.

[24] Seibyl JP, Marek K, Sheff K, Zoghbi S, Baldwin RM et al. Iodine-123-beta-CIT and iodine-123-FPCIT SPECT measurement of dopamine transporters in healthy subjects and Parkinson's patients. *J Nucl Med* 1998; 39: 1500-8.

[25] Tissingh G, Booij J, Bergmans P, Winogrodzka A, Janssen AG et al. Iodine-123-N-omega-fluoropropyl-2beta-carbomethoxy-3beta-(4-iod ophenyl)tropane SPECT in healthy controls and early-stage, drug-naive Parkinson's disease. *J Nucl Med* 1998; 39: 1143-8.

[26] Tatsch K, Schwarz J, Mozley PD, Linke R, Pogarell O et al. Relationship between clinical features of Parkinson's disease and presynaptic dopamine transporter binding assessed with [123I]IPT and single-photon emission tomography. *Eur J Nucl Med* 1997; 24: 415-21.

[27] Emond P, Guilloteau D, Chalon S. PE2I: a radiopharmaceutical for in vivo exploration of the dopamine transporter. *CNS neuroscience & therapeutics* 2008; 14: 47-64.

[28] Page G, Chalon S, Emond P, Maloteaux JM, Hermans E. Pharmacological characterisation of (E)-N-(3-iodoprop-2-enyl)-2beta-carbomethoxy-3beta-(4'-methylphenyl)nortropane (PE2I) binding to the rat neuronal dopamine transporter expressed in COS cells. *Neurochemistry international* 2002; 40: 105-13.

[29] Huang WS, Chiang YH, Lin JC, Chou YH, Cheng CY et al. Crossover study of (99m)Tc-TRODAT-1 SPECT and (18)F-FDOPA PET in Parkinson's disease patients. *J Nucl Med* 2003; 44: 999-1005.

[30] Van Laere K, Varrone A, Booij J, Vander Borght T, Nobili F et al. EANM procedure guidelines for brain neurotransmission SPECT/PET using dopamine D2 receptor ligands, version 2. *Eur J Nucl Med Mol Imaging* 2010; 37: 434-42.

[31] Kung HF, Pan S, Kung MP, Billings J, Kasliwal R et al. In vitro and in vivo evaluation of [123I]IBZM: a potential CNS D-2 dopamine receptor imaging agent. *J Nucl Med* 1989; 30: 88-92.

[32] Kung MP, Kung HF, Billings J, Yang Y, Murphy RA et al. The characterization of IBF as a new selective dopamine D-2 receptor imaging agent. *J Nucl Med* 1990; 31: 648-54.

[33] al-Tikriti MS, Baldwin RM, Zea-Ponce Y, Sybirska E, Zoghbi SS et al. Comparison of three high affinity SPECT radiotracers for the dopamine D2 receptor. *Nucl Med Biol* 1994; 21: 179-88.

[34] Matsumoto H, Tanaka A, Suzuki N, Kondo S, KatoAzuma M et al. [Metabolism of 123I-IBF in humans]. *Kaku Igaku* 1999; 36: 169-77.

[35] Murphy RA, Kung HF, Kung MP, Billings J. Synthesis and characterization of iodobenzamide analogues: potential D-2 dopamine receptor imaging agents. *J Med Chem* 1990; 33: 171-8.

[36] Spiegel J, Hellwig D, Jost WH, Farmakis G, Samnick S et al. Cerebral and Extracranial Neurodegeneration are Strongly Coupled in Parkinson's Disease. *The open neurology journal* 2007; 1: 1-4.

[37] Ichise M, Kim YJ, Ballinger JR, Vines D, Erami SS et al. SPECT imaging of pre- and postsynaptic dopaminergic alterations in L-dopa-untreated PD. *Neurology* 1999; 52: 1206-14.

[38] Verstappen CC, Bloem BR, Haaxma CA, Oyen WJ, Horstink MW. Diagnostic value of asymmetric striatal D2 receptor upregulation in Parkinson's disease: an [123I]IBZM and [123I]FP-CIT SPECT study. *Eur J Nucl Med Mol Imaging* 2007; 34: 502-7.

[39] Ma KH, Huang WS, Chen CH, Lin SZ, Wey SP et al. Dual SPECT of dopamine system using [99mTc]TRODAT-1 and [123I]IBZM in normal and 6-OHDA-lesioned formosan rock monkeys. *Nucl Med Biol* 2002; 29: 561-7.

[40] Benamer HT, Patterson J, Wyper DJ, Hadley DM, Macphee GJ et al. Correlation of Parkinson's disease severity and duration with 123I-FP-CIT SPECT striatal uptake. *Movement disorders : official journal of the Movement Disorder Society* 2000; 15: 692-8.

[41] Eggers C, Kahraman D, Fink GR, Schmidt M, Timmermann L. Akinetic-rigid and tremor-dominant Parkinson's disease patients show different patterns of FP-CIT single photon emission computed tomography. *Movement disorders : official journal of the Movement Disorder Society* 2011; 26: 416-23.

[42] Kish SJ, Tong J, Hornykiewicz O, Rajput A, Chang LJ et al. Preferential loss of serotonin markers in caudate versus putamen in Parkinson's disease. *Brain : a journal of neurology* 2008; 131: 120-31.

[43] Roselli F, Pisciotta NM, Pennelli M, Aniello MS, Gigante A et al. Midbrain SERT in degenerative parkinsonisms: a 123I-FP-CIT SPECT study. *Movement disorders : official journal of the Movement Disorder Society* 2010; 25: 1853-9.

[44] Marek KL, Seibyl JP, Zoghbi SS, Zea-Ponce Y, Baldwin RM et al. [123I] beta-CIT/SPECT imaging demonstrates bilateral loss of dopamine transporters in hemi-Parkinson's disease. *Neurology* 1996; 46: 231-7.

[45] Eerola J, Tienari PJ, Kaakkola S, Nikkinen P, Launes J. How useful is [123I]beta-CIT SPECT in clinical practice? *J Neurol Neurosurg Psychiatry* 2005; 76: 1211-6.

[46] Marshall VL, Reininger CB, Marquardt M, Patterson J, Hadley DM et al. Parkinson's disease is overdiagnosed clinically at baseline in diagnostically uncertain cases: a 3-year European multicenter study with repeat [123I]FP-CIT SPECT. *Movement disorders : official journal of the Movement Disorder Society* 2009; 24: 500-8.

[47] Sawada H, Oeda T, Yamamoto K, Kitagawa N, Mizuta E et al. Diagnostic accuracy of cardiac metaiodobenzylguanidine scintigraphy in Parkinson disease. *European journal of neurology : the official journal of the European Federation of Neurological Societies* 2009; 16: 174-82.

[48] Spiegel J, Mollers MO, Jost WH, Fuss G, Samnick S et al. FP-CIT and MIBG scintigraphy in early Parkinson's disease. *Movement disorders : official journal of the Movement Disorder Society* 2005; 20: 552-61.

[49] Filippi L, Manni C, Pierantozzi M, Brusa L, Danieli R et al. 123I-FP-CIT semi-quantitative SPECT detects preclinical bilateral dopaminergic deficit in early Parkinson's disease with unilateral symptoms. *Nucl Med Commun* 2005; 26: 421-6.

[50] Huang WS, Ma KH, Chou YH, Chen CY, Liu RS et al. 99mTc-TRODAT-1 SPECT in healthy and 6-OHDA lesioned parkinsonian monkeys: comparison with 18F-FDOPA PET. *Nucl Med Commun* 2003; 24: 77-83.

[51] Huang WS, Lin SZ, Lin JC, Wey SP, Ting G et al. Evaluation of early-stage Parkinson's disease with 99mTc-TRODAT-1 imaging. *J Nucl Med* 2001; 42: 1303-8.

[52] Kagi G, Bhatia KP, Tolosa E. The role of DAT-SPECT in movement disorders. *J Neurol Neurosurg Psychiatry* 2010; 81: 5-12.

[53] Ishibashi K, Saito Y, Murayama S, Kanemaru K, Oda K et al. Validation of cardiac (123)I-MIBG scintigraphy in patients with Parkinson's disease who were diagnosed with dopamine PET. *Eur J Nucl Med Mol Imaging* 2010; 37: 3-11.

[54] Sakakibara R, Shinotoh H, Uchiyama T, Yoshiyama M, Hattori T et al. SPECT imaging of the dopamine transporter with [(123)I]-beta-CIT reveals marked decline of nigrostriatal dopaminergic function in Parkinson's disease with urinary dysfunction. *Journal of the neurological sciences* 2001; 187: 55-9.

[55] Agid Y. Parkinson's disease: pathophysiology. *Lancet* 1991; 337: 1321-4.

[56] Vlaar AM, de Nijs T, Kessels AG, Vreeling FW, Winogrodzka A et al. Diagnostic value of 123I-ioflupane and 123I-iodobenzamide SPECT scans in 248 patients with parkinsonian syndromes. *Eur Neurol* 2008; 59: 258-66.

[57] Contrafatto D, Mostile G, Nicoletti A, Dibilio V, Raciti L et al. [(123) I]FP-CIT-SPECT asymmetry index to differentiate Parkinson's disease from vascular parkinsonism. *Acta Neurol Scand* 2012; 126: 12-6.

[58] Lorberboym M, Treves TA, Melamed E, Lampl Y, Hellmann M et al. [123I]-FP/CIT SPECT imaging for distinguishing drug-induced parkinsonism from Parkinson's disease. *Movement disorders : official journal of the Movement Disorder Society* 2006; 21: 510-4.

[59] Diaz-Corrales FJ, Sanz-Viedma S, Garcia-Solis D, Escobar-Delgado T, Mir P. Clinical features and 123I-FP-CIT SPECT imaging in drug-induced parkinsonism and Parkinson's disease. *Eur J Nucl Med Mol Imaging* 2010; 37: 556-64.

[60] Cuberas-Borros G, Lorenzo-Bosquet C, Aguade-Bruix S, Hernandez-Vara J, Pifarre-Montaner P et al. Quantitative evaluation of striatal I-123-FP-CIT uptake in essential tremor and parkinsonism. *Clin Nucl Med* 2011; 36: 991-6.

[61] Felicio AC, Shih MC, Godeiro-Junior C, Andrade LA, Bressan RA et al. Molecular imaging studies in Parkinson disease: reducing diagnostic uncertainty. *The neurologist* 2009; 15: 6-16.

[62] Gilman S, Wenning GK, Low PA, Brooks DJ, Mathias CJ et al. Second consensus statement on the diagnosis of multiple system atrophy. *Neurology* 2008; 71: 670-6.

[63] Scherfler C, Seppi K, Donnemiller E, Goebel G, Brenneis C et al. Voxel-wise analysis of [123I]beta-CIT SPECT differentiates the Parkinson variant of multiple system atrophy from idiopathic Parkinson's disease. *Brain : a journal of neurology* 2005; 128: 1605-12.

[64] El Fakhri G, Ouyang J. Dual-radionuclide brain SPECT for the differential diagnosis of parkinsonism. *Methods Mol Biol* 2011; 680: 237-46.

[65] Antonini A, Benti R, De Notaris R, Tesei S, Zecchinelli A et al. 123I-Ioflupane/SPECT binding to striatal dopamine transporter (DAT) uptake in patients with Parkinson's disease, multiple system atrophy, and progressive supranuclear palsy. *Neurological sciences : official journal of the Italian Neurological Society and of the Italian Society of Clinical Neurophysiology* 2003; 24: 149-50.

[66] Varrone A, Marek KL, Jennings D, Innis RB, Seibyl JP. [(123)I]beta-CIT SPECT imaging demonstrates reduced density of striatal dopamine transporters in Parkinson's disease and multiple system atrophy. *Movement disorders : official journal of the Movement Disorder Society* 2001; 16: 1023-32.

[67] Knudsen GM, Karlsborg M, Thomsen G, Krabbe K, Regeur L et al. Imaging of dopamine transporters and D2 receptors in patients with Parkinson's disease and multiple system atrophy. *Eur J Nucl Med Mol Imaging* 2004; 31: 1631-8.

[68] Swanson RL, Newberg AB, Acton PD, Siderowf A, Wintering N et al. Differences in [99mTc]TRODAT-1 SPECT binding to dopamine transporters in patients with multiple system atrophy and Parkinson's disease. *Eur J Nucl Med Mol Imaging* 2005; 32: 302-7.

[69] Kim YJ, Ichise M, Ballinger JR, Vines D, Erami SS et al. Combination of dopamine transporter and D2 receptor SPECT in the diagnostic evaluation of PD, MSA, and PSP. *Movement disorders : official journal of the Movement Disorder Society* 2002; 17: 303-12.

[70] Popperl G, Radau P, Linke R, Hahn K, Tatsch K. Diagnostic performance of a 3-D automated quantification method of dopamine D2 receptor SPECT studies in the differential diagnosis of parkinsonism. *Nucl Med Commun* 2005; 26: 39-43.

[71] Oyanagi C, Katsumi Y, Hanakawa T, Hayashi T, Thuy D et al. Comparison of striatal dopamine D2 receptors in Parkinson's disease and progressive supranuclear palsy patients using [123I] iodobenzofuran single-photon emission computed tomography. *Journal of neuroimaging : official journal of the American Society of Neuroimaging* 2002; 12: 316-24.

[72] Poblete Garcia V, Garcia Vicente A, Ruiz Solis S, Martinez Delgado C, Vaamonde J et al. [SPECT with 123I-IBZM: utility in differential diagnosis of degenerative Parkinsonisms and establishment of quantification method]. *Revista espanola de medicina nuclear* 2005; 24: 234-43.

[73] Sudmeyer M, Antke C, Zizek T, Beu M, Nikolaus S et al. Diagnostic accuracy of combined FP-CIT, IBZM, and MIBG scintigraphy in the differential diagnosis of degenerative parkinsonism: a multidimensional statistical approach. *J Nucl Med* 2011; 52: 733-40.

[74] Ziebell M, Andersen BB, Thomsen G, Pinborg LH, Karlsborg M et al. Predictive value of dopamine transporter SPECT imaging with [(1)(2)(3)I]PE2I in patients with subtle parkinsonian symptoms. *Eur J Nucl Med Mol Imaging* 2012; 39: 242-50.

[75] Kahraman D, Eggers C, Schicha H, Timmermann L, Schmidt M. Visual assessment of dopaminergic degeneration pattern in 123I-FP-CIT SPECT differentiates patients with

atypical parkinsonian syndromes and idiopathic Parkinson's disease. *J Neurol* 2012; 259: 251-60.

[76] Kessler KR, Hamscho N, Morales B, Menzel C, Barrero F et al. Dopaminergic function in a family with the PARK6 form of autosomal recessive Parkinson's syndrome. *J Neural Transm* 2005; 112: 1345-53.

[77] Hwang WJ, Yao WJ, Wey SP, Ting G. Clinical and [99mTc]TRODAT-1/[123I]IBZM SPECT imaging findings in dopa-responsive dystonia. *Eur Neurol* 2004; 51: 26-9.

[78] Schillaci O, Chiaravalloti A, Pierantozzi M, Di Pietro B, Koch G et al. Different patterns of nigrostriatal degeneration in tremor type versus the akinetic-rigid and mixed types of Parkinson's disease at the early stages: molecular imaging with 123I-FP-CIT SPECT. *Int J Mol Med* 2011; 28: 881-6.

[79] Rossi C, Frosini D, Volterrani D, De Feo P, Unti E et al. Differences in nigro-striatal impairment in clinical variants of early Parkinson's disease: evidence from a FP-CIT SPECT study. *European journal of neurology : the official journal of the European Federation of Neurological Societies* 2010; 17: 626-30.

[80] Spiegel J, Hellwig D, Samnick S, Jost W, Mollers MO et al. Striatal FP-CIT uptake differs in the subtypes of early Parkinson's disease. *J Neural Transm* 2007; 114: 331-5.

[81] Marek K, Innis R, van Dyck C, Fussell B, Early M et al. [123I]beta-CIT SPECT imaging assessment of the rate of Parkinson's disease progression. *Neurology* 2001; 57: 2089-94.

[82] Winogrodzka A, Bergmans P, Booij J, van Royen EA, Janssen AG et al. [123I]FP-CIT SPECT is a useful method to monitor the rate of dopaminergic degeneration in early-stage Parkinson's disease. *J Neural Transm* 2001; 108: 1011-9.

[83] Winogrodzka A, Bergmans P, Booij J, van Royen EA, Stoof JC et al. [(123)I]beta-CIT SPECT is a useful method for monitoring dopaminergic degeneration in early stage Parkinson's disease. *J Neurol Neurosurg Psychiatry* 2003; 74: 294-8.

[84] Seibyl JP, Marek K, Sheff K, Baldwin RM, Zoghbi S et al. Test/retest reproducibility of iodine-123-betaCIT SPECT brain measurement of dopamine transporters in Parkinson's patients. *J Nucl Med* 1997; 38: 1453-9.

[85] Pirker W, Djamshidian S, Asenbaum S, Gerschlager W, Tribl G et al. Progression of dopaminergic degeneration in Parkinson's disease and atypical parkinsonism: a longitudinal beta-CIT SPECT study. *Movement disorders : official journal of the Movement Disorder Society* 2002; 17: 45-53.

[86] Wenning GK, Donnemiller E, Granata R, Riccabona G, Poewe W. 123I-beta-CIT and 123I-IBZM-SPECT scanning in levodopa-naive Parkinson's disease. *Movement disorders : official journal of the Movement Disorder Society* 1998; 13: 438-45.

[87] Tissingh G, Bergmans P, Booij J, Winogrodzka A, van Royen EA et al. Drug-naive patients with Parkinson's disease in Hoehn and Yahr stages I and II show a bilateral decrease in striatal dopamine transporters as revealed by [123I]beta-CIT SPECT. *J Neurol* 1998; 245: 14-20.

[88] Weng YH, Yen TC, Chen MC, Kao PF, Tzen KY et al. Sensitivity and specificity of 99mTc-TRODAT-1 SPECT imaging in differentiating patients with idiopathic Parkinson's disease from healthy subjects. *J Nucl Med* 2004; 45: 393-401.

[89] Weiner WJ. Early diagnosis of Parkinson's disease and initiation of treatment. *Reviews in neurological diseases* 2008; 5: 46-53; quiz 4-5.

[90] Lyons KE, Pahwa R. Diagnosis and initiation of treatment in Parkinson's disease. *Int J Neurosci* 2011; 121 Suppl 2: 27-36.

[91] Schwarz J, Tatsch K, Gasser T, Arnold G, Oertel WH. [123]IBZM binding predicts dopaminergic responsiveness in patients with parkinsonism and previous dopaminomimetic therapy. *Movement disorders : official journal of the Movement Disorder Society* 1997; 12: 898-902.

[92] Hertel A, Weppner M, Baas H, Schreiner M, Maul FD et al. Quantification of IBZM dopamine receptor SPET in de novo Parkinson patients before and during therapy. *Nucl Med Commun* 1997; 18: 811-22.

[93] Contrafatto D, Mostile G, Nicoletti A, Raciti L, Luca A et al. Single photon emission computed tomography striatal asymmetry index may predict dopaminergic responsiveness in Parkinson disease. *Clinical neuropharmacology* 2011; 34: 71-3.

[94] Fernagut PO, Li Q, Dovero S, Chan P, Wu T et al. Dopamine transporter binding is unaffected by L-DOPA administration in normal and MPTP-treated monkeys. *PLoS One* 2010; 5: e14053.

[95] Innis RB, Marek KL, Sheff K, Zoghbi S, Castronuovo J et al. Effect of treatment with L-dopa/carbidopa or L-selegiline on striatal dopamine transporter SPECT imaging with [123I]beta-CIT. *Movement disorders : official journal of the Movement Disorder Society* 1999; 14: 436-42.

[96] Hwang WJ, Yao WJ, Wey SP, Shen LH, Ting G. Downregulation of striatal dopamine D2 receptors in advanced Parkinson's disease contributes to the development of motor fluctuation. *Eur Neurol* 2002; 47: 113-7.

In: SPECT
Editors: Hojjat Ahmadzadehfar and Elham Habibi

ISBN: 978-1-62808-344-6
© 2013 Nova Science Publishers, Inc.

Chapter XII

SPECT in Epilepsy

Hojjat Ahmadzadehfar[1] and *Michael P. Malter[2]*

[1]Department of Nuclear Medicine, UniversityHospital Bonn, Germany
[2]Department of Neurology, Marien Hospital
BergischGladbach, Germany

Introduction

An epileptic seizure is defined as an excessive burst of abnormally synchronized neuronal activity affecting small or large neuronal networks that results in clinical manifestations that are sudden, transient and usually brief. Epilepsy is defined as a disorder of the brain characterized by an ongoing predisposition toward recurrent epileptic seizures [1, 2].

About 1–2% of the general population has epilepsy. About 50 million people worldwide are affected by epileptic seizures. The point prevalence of epilepsy in developed populations is approximately 4–10 cases per 1000 persons [3, 4].

The incidence rate is age dependent, with the highest rates in childhood, especially in the first year of life (100 cases per 100,000 per year). The rate declines until adolescence (30–40/100,000 per year) and rises again in the elderly (100/100,000 per year). Males have a slightly higher incidence of epilepsy than females. Epilepsy is more likely to occur in socially disadvantaged populations. Causes of epilepsy are multifaceted. Partial seizures seem to occur more often than generalized seizures and individuals with underlying risk factors such as cerebral palsy or mental retardation have a higher risk of developing epilepsy [5].

Classification of Seizures and Epilepsies

Seizures are classified according to the International League against Epilepsy (ILAE). In 2010 the ILAE Task Force proposed a new classification for seizures and epileptic syndromes

* Email: Hojjat.ahmadzadehfar@ukb.uni-bonn.de.

[6]. The aim of the new classification was to incorporate new insights into epileptic pathomechanisms into the terminology. These changes remain under debate in the epileptological society and are not commonly accepted. To avoid misunderstandings, we use the terms from the established classification from 1981 [7] and 1989 [8] herein.

Seizures can principally be divided into partial and generalized seizures. Partial seizures arise in specific loci of the cortex in one hemisphere. They are further divided according to the extent to which awareness is affected. If it is unaffected, then it is a simple partial seizure; otherwise it is a complex partial seizure. Clinical manifestations can be motor, sensory, autonomic, or psychic. A partial seizure may spread within the brain – a process known as secondary generalization.

Generalized seizures are those that arise from large areas of the cortex in both hemispheres and are classified according to their effect on the body, but all involve loss of consciousness. These include absence, myoclonic, clonic, tonic, tonic-clonic, and atonic seizures [7].

The definition of epileptic syndromes is based on two axes. The first axis reflects the type of seizure: epilepsies with generalized seizures vs. those with partial seizures. The second axis comprises etiological aspects: symptomatic or "secondary" epilepsies, idiopathic or "primary" epilepsies and those of cryptogenic origin [8].

In idiopathic epilepsy with generalized seizures, the seizure is the only clinical manifestation of the cerebral malfunction and no underlying morphological cause of the epileptic seizures is apparent. Most other seizures, including most epileptic syndromes with partial seizures, are acquired secondary to some form of acquired or inherited cerebral lesion [9].

Therapy

Antiepileptic drugs are a symptomatic not a causative treatment option. Medical treatment can be started after first seizure if diagnostic work-up reveals a high prevalence of subsequent seizures, i.e. typical EEG features, epileptogenic morphological lesions. It should be started after the second seizure if provocative factors can be excluded. Around 70% of medically treated epilepsy patients reach seizure freedom but almost 30% do not become consistently seizure free under antiepileptic drug treatment [10]. The term pharmacoresistant epilepsy is used for these patients. Definitions of pharmacoresistance were given by the ILAE [10]. In clinical practice, the likelihood of achieving seizure freedom under drug treatment is low if two adequate drug trials have failed. In cases of partial epilepsy, alternative treatment options such as epilepsy surgery may be a promising option.

The aim of resective epilepsy surgery is to identify and resect seizure onset zone to obtain sustained seizure freedom, to identify the peri-operative risks, and to estimate the postsurgical functional neurological outcome [11, 12]. The epileptogenic zone is conceptualized as the area of brain responsible for the generation of focal seizures, the complete removal of which is necessary to achieve seizure freedom [1]. The epileptogenic zone can overlap with the morphological lesion. Precise localization of the epileptogenic zone often requires a combination of surface and invasive simultaneous video electroencephalography (EEG) recordings, morphological (MRI) and functional imaging (magneto encephalography (MEG), Wada-Test, SPECT and PET) [13].

Eligibility for epilepsy surgery can be graded according to the chance of post-surgical seizure freedom.

Candidates with the highest chance of seizure freedom are those with a clear-cut epileptogenic lesion, such as hippocampal atrophy or dysplasia, and evidence of seizure onset therein from surface EEG recordings.

At the next level are those with suspected lesions that have to be proven by additional diagnostics, such as functional imaging and invasive EEG recordings. At the most challenging level are patients with multiple or without detectable lesions.

Those patients that benefit the most from epilepsy surgery are individuals with partial seizures arising from the temporal lobe; however, on occasion extratemporal seizures are amenable to surgical treatment [13].

Experienced epilepsy surgery centers can achieve a 70% or greater seizure-free outcome with anterior temporal lobectomy with low associated morbidity [14, 15]. Wiebe et al. showed that in temporal lobe epilepsy due to any cause, surgery is superior to prolonged medical therapy [16]. Resection of extra temporal foci is less effective and more hazardous than temporal lobectomy, with only 40–50 % of operated patients rendered seizure free. Success is much higher with resection of a structural lesion that has been confirmed as the seizure onset zone. In a single center study only 38% of all non-lesional patients obtained seizure-freedom after epilepsy surgery [17]. In cases of unspecific non-localizing ictal signs and symptoms and lack of ictal surface EEG findings, in which the epileptogenic lesion can only be suspected on morphological MRI, or in cases of non-lesional functional epilepsy, extended diagnostic work-up is required to create a sufficient surgical hypothesis. Nuclear medicine imaging techniques such as ictal and interictal SPECT and interictal PET have demonstrated their usefulness in these cases [15, 18, 19]. In a minority of cases epilepsy surgery will proceed directly according to these functional imaging findings. But they can be a corner stone for implantation hypothesis for invasive EEG recordings.

In a study performed at a tertiary referral center, an underlying structural cause of chronic epilepsy was found in only 254 out of 341 (74%) of the patients [20]. These results suggest that the number of patients with no structural abnormality on the MRI is significant and that, in such patients, functional imaging can contribute to identifying a possible epileptogenic focus [11].

A broad single center analysis revealed that the proportion of difficult patients for epilepsy surgery as outlined above has increased over the last 25 years as has the need for differentiated and advanced diagnostic techniques [21].

Brain SPECT for the Evaluation of Epileptic Foci

In general, cerebral metabolism and blood flow are increased by up to 300% during an epileptic seizure [22], and may be normal or reduced between seizures (interictal period). The most common histologic abnormality in patients with temporal lobe epilepsy is mesial temporal sclerosis, with loss of neurons and gliosis in the hippocampus and amygdale [23]. In contrast to this localized abnormality, interictalhypoperfusion and hypometabolism may extend well into the lateral temporal, frontal and parietal cortex [15, 24].

The optimum brain SPECT approach for localizing a seizure focus involves performing ictal and interictal imaging studies, on separate days, followed by subtraction of the co-registered images. This method is reported to have an accuracy rate in the range of 89–94% (25) with incorrect lateralization in less than 5% [26, 27].

Radiopharmaceuticals Used for Brain Perfusion SPECT Imaging

1. Stabilized ^{99m}Tc-HMPAO (hexamethyl propylene amine oxime) (Ceretec):

HMPAO is not only lipid soluble and able to penetrate the intact blood–brain barrier, it also displays very high in vivo instability. It reacts in seconds after intravenous injection, probably with intracellular glutathione, and is trapped inside the brain. Uptake in the brain reaches a maximum of 3.5–7.0% of the injected dose within one minute of injection. It is rapidly cleared from the blood after intravenous injection. Up to 15% of its activity is eliminated from the brain within 2 minutes post injection, after which little activity is lost for the following 24 hours except by physical decay of ^{99m}Tc(28). Regional uptake and retention are generally related to regional perfusion [28]. ^{99m}Tc-HMPAO should be injected no sooner than 10 min after radioligand reconstitution and no more than 4 hours after reconstitution [29]. A 90-min delay from injection to imaging gives the best image quality. However images obtained after a 40-min delay will be interpretable [29].

2. ^{99m}Tc-ECD (ethylcysteinate dimer) (Neurolite):

^{99m}Tc-ECD is also a lipophilic complex with a high first-pass extraction fraction and deposition and retention in the brain in proportion to cerebral blood flow. It shows high initial cerebral uptake with rapid blood clearance after intravenous injection (less than 10% of the administered activity remains in the blood after 5 minutes) [30]. Approximately 5 to 8% of administered activity localizes in the brain within 5 minutes after injection and exhibits little change for one hour after injection. Brain washout is approximately 20% between 5 and 60 minutes after injection and approximately 10% per hour thereafter [30]. ^{99m}Tc-ECD should not be injected earlier than 10 min before and no more than 6 h after reconstitution [29]. Approximately a 45-min delay from injection to imaging gives the best image quality. Images obtained after a 20-min delay will be interpretable [29]. The rapid urinary excretion of ^{99m}Tc-ECD favors its dosimetry, so high doses can be administered. The dosimetry is similar to lower doses of ^{99m}Tc-HMPAO if patients are instructed to force diuresis and void after the scan procedure. The use of higherdoses, together with the higher gray-matter–to–white-matter ratio, contributes to the better image quality obtained with ^{99m}Tc-ECD in comparison with ^{99m}Tc-HMPAO [31]. Imaging with both these radiopharmaceuticals should be completed within 4 h after injection. Excessive delay should be avoided because of radioactive decay.

Other suitable radiopharmaceuticals for brain perfusion SPECT, such as ^{123}I-IMP and ^{123}I-HIPDM, are more costly and less readily available.

Dosage

Adults, 555–1,110 MBq for ^{99m}Tc-HMPAO or ^{99m}Tc-ECD (typically 740 MBqfor^{99m}Tc-HMPAO or 1,110 MBq for ^{99m}Tc-ECD); in children, 7.4–11.1 MBq/kg. Minimum recommended dose is 110 MBq [32].

Contraindications

   1. Pregnancy.

   2. Breast feeding: mothers should interrupt breast feeding for 24 h if SPECT is indicated.

   3. Lack of cooperation, or inability to cooperate, with procedure.

Ictal and Interictal SPECT

Ictal SPECT is a time-consuming investigation. Patients have to undergo video-EEG monitoring for several days until a seizure occurs within the time frame during which the radioactive labeled SPECT tracer is available. In most centers, this is restricted to normal daytime working hours. A considerable number of patients fail to have a seizure within this dedicated time period, particularly those who have nocturnal seizures. For a patient to be injected during the ictal phase, the radio labeled product should be prepared in advance and stored in a shielded syringe next to the patient's bedside. The injection should be performed by a trained technologist or other personnel immediately available at the time of seizure onset. The ictal injection should be performed in a rapid bolus fashion such that the entire tracer is injected before the seizure abates [1].

The injection can also be performed by an automatic injector, incorporating a lead cover for the tracer syringe to protect patients and staff from radioactivity. The injector is operated remotely from the monitoring workstation where EEG and/or video are used to determine the beginning of the seizure [19].

The patient is then stabilized and transferred to the SPECT camera to receive a brain SPECT scan, which will indicate the regional cerebral perfusion at the time of ictus.

Knowledge of the timing of tracer injection before an ictal SPECT scan is essential for proper interpretation of the images. With an injection at the very onset of a seizure, there is an increased probability of visualizing an epileptogenic focus seen as a focal area of increased uptake. In the event of a delayed injection, the probability of capturing the epileptogenic focus is decreased as the seizure will have already propagated; the ictal scan may then show several areas of slightly increased tracer uptake corresponding to areas of electrical discharge during seizure propagation.

The duration of the seizure is also important: it is difficult to capture short-lived seizures using SPECT, as it is likely that the electrical discharge will have already propagated to the remainder of the brain when the tracer reaches the brain cells. In this case, the SPECT findings may be those of widespread hyperperfusion or of different focal areas of increased uptake in the regions into which the seizure has spread.

Each epilepsy subtype shows a different pattern of spread, which translates into different patterns of ictal hyperperfusion on the SPECT scan [11]. There should be a gap of 48 hours between ictal and interictal SPECT.

For interictal SPECT, because of the sensitivity of brain perfusion SPECT in detecting regional cerebral blood flow (rCBF) changes coupled with neuronal activity, sensorial and cognitive stimuli must be kept to a minimum during tracer injection and uptake. Injection in a quiet room and no interaction with the patient is desirable at this time. An intravenous cannula should be placed 10 to 15 min prior to injection. If the patient's eyes are open in a bright room during injection, high tracer uptake in the calcarine cortex is an expected SPECT pattern. On the other hand, if the patient's eyes are closed in a dimly lit room during injection, low tracer uptake is found in the calcarine cortex. Thus injecting conditions should be recorded and considered in the evaluation of the SPECT images. Patient cooperation is of particular importance. To avoid head movement during scanning (20–30 min), the patient should be comfortable [31].

Patients should void prior to acquisition for maximum comfort during the study and they should be advised to void again after the acquisition to help reduce radiation exposure. They should be instructed not to speak, read, or move for at least 5 min before to 5 min after injection. Patients should also have no interaction with staff for at least 5 min before to 5 min after injection. If a patient needs sedation, tracer injection must precede sedation to avoid sedation-induced metabolism/blood flow changes in the SPECT images. In uncooperative children, sedation is not recommended until other strategies to facilitate sleep during the scan procedure have been exhausted [31]. Patient positioning greatly contributes to the final quality of SPECT images.

Image Acquisition

Images should be acquired using multiple detectors or other dedicated small to medium field-of-view SPECT. Low energy high resolution (LEHR) or low energy ultra-high resolution (LEUHR) parallel-hole collimators are the most readily available collimator sets for brain imaging. All-purpose collimators are not suitable [32]. A 128x128 matrix should be chosen. A low counting rate would require smoother filtering during reconstruction, which would result in loss of spatial resolution. The matrix and pixel size should be assessed on each specific SPECT device [31].

Total Scan Time

Depending on the imaging device, the typical scan time for triple head cameras is around 20–25 min; for dual head cameras it is closer to 30 min. Segmentation of data acquisition into multiple sequential acquisitions (e.g. 6×5 min) may permit the exclusion of bad data, e.g. removing segments of projection data with patient motion [32]. Excluding shoulders from the field of view keeps the radius of rotation to a minimum, thus maintaining the collimators as close as possible to the patient's head. Belts at the forearm level help to hold the patient's arms if the imaging bed is narrow. Keeping the head at flexion helps to reduce the radius of rotation. Lowering the chin to the chest helps to include the entire cerebellum within the field of view and allows a better reorientation plane for oblique slices during reconstruction [31]. For reconstruction, we refer to the current guidelines from the EANM [32] and SNMMI [29].

Patterns of Ictal Cerebral Blood Flow

Ictal SPECT typically demonstrates focal hyperperfusion in brain regions involved in seizure activity. A successful injection early in a seizure usually gives the best results with clear localization of the ictal onset zone seen as the most prominent area of hyperperfusion. Injections given late into a seizure may fail to localize the epileptogenic focus and/or may show areas with uptake of variable grade, related to the spread of electrical discharge from seizure propagation [11].

Propagation often occurs from the posterior (parieto-occipital lobes) to anterior cerebral regions (mainly to the temporal and frontal lobe) [32]. Another propagation pattern is from the temporal to the frontal lobe [11].

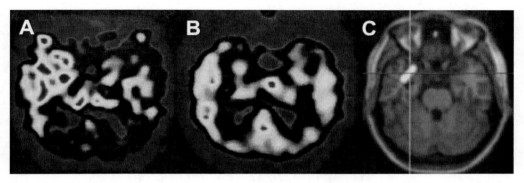

Figure 12.1.[99m]Tc-HMPAO Ictal SPECT (A) of a patient with temporal lobe epilepsy shows hyperperfusion in the right temporal lobe, especially in the temporal pole and medial temporal lobe. In this region shows the interictal SPECT (B) relatively less perfusion compared to icatl SPECT. Image C shows the SISCOM analysis after co-registration with MRI of the patient prior to surgery (SISCOM-image by courtesy of Dr. Carlos M Quesada, Department of Epileptology, University Hospital Bonn, Germany).

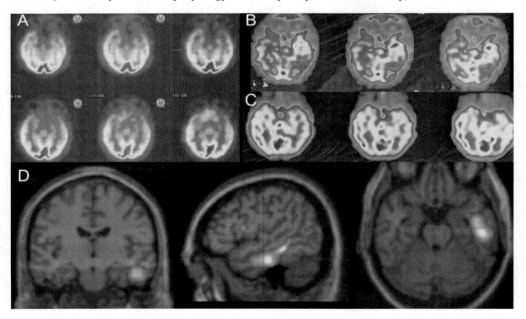

Figure 12.2. Interictal[18]F-FDG PET of a patient with temporal lobe epilepsy shows hypometabolism in left temporal pole (A), hyperperfusion on ictal ^{99m}Tc-HMPAO SPECT. Image C shows the SISCOM analysis after co-registration with MRI of this patient prior to surgery (SISCOM-image by courtesy of Dr. Carlos M Quesada, Department of Epileptology, University Hospital Bonn, Germany).

In temporal lobe epilepsy (TLE) the area of hyperperfusion typically involves the anterior pole and medial temporal lobe with a variable degree of lateral temporal cortex(15) (Figure

12.1and Figure 12.2). Ictal studies can be used to clearly distinguish between temporal and extra temporal epilepsy [33, 34]. Ictal dystonia is associated with relative hyperperfusion of the basal ganglia opposite the dystonic limb [32]. Increased perfusion of lesser extent may also be seen in the ipsilateral thalamus [15]. Propagation of the seizure frequently leads to a variable degree of hyperperfusion from the ipsilateral temporal lobe to the contra-lateral temporal lobe, insula, basal ganglia, and frontal lobe. Thus to determine the hyperperfusion pattern of ictal SPECT both the radiotracer injection time and semiologic progression after the injection are important issues [32]. Cerebellar hyperperfusion (CH) contra-lateral to the supratentorial epileptogenicarea is frequently revealed on ictal SPECT of epilepsy patients [35, 36]; however, Shin et al. Reported that during TLE seizures, hemispheric CH occurred not only in contra-lateral but also in ipsilateral or bilateral cerebellar hemispheres to the side of seizure origin [37].

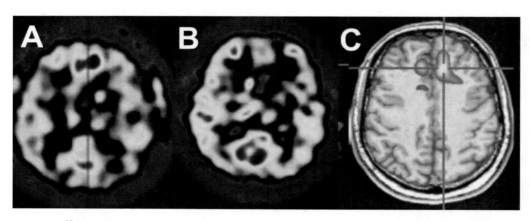

Figure 12.3. ^{99m}Tc-HMPAO Ictal SPECT (A) of a patient with frontal lobe epilepsy shows hyperperfusion in the frontal lobes (L>R). In this region shows the interictal SPECT (B) relatively less perfusion compared to icatl SPECT. Image C shows the SISCOM analysis after co-registration with MRI of the patient. In this patient no pathologic changes could be detected on the MRI (SISCOM-image by courtesy of Dr. Carlos M Quesada, Department of Epileptology, University Hospital Bonn, Germany).

The diagnostic yield of ictal SPECT studies in extra temporal epilepsies amounted to 92% [36, 38-40]. However, propagation of epileptic seizure activity is more variable in patients with extra temporal epilepsies and often develops rapidly. It therefore seems conceivable that in some patients the ictal increase in CBF as demonstrated by ictal SPECT scans reflects propagation of epileptic seizure activity rather than the seizure onset zone [40].

Of all partial seizures, those of frontal lobe origin (FLPS) are the most bizarre and are often mistaken for psychogenic seizures [41]. Ictal SPECT has the potential to localize seizures in patients with intractable frontal lobe epilepsy, and advance understanding of the in vivo anatomico-clinical relationships of frontal lobe seizures [36]. Unlike the diffuse hyperperfusion changes reported during temporal lobe seizures, ictal hyperperfusion in frontal lobe epilepsy is well circumscribed and is often accompanied by contralateral cerebellar and ipsilateral basal ganglia hyperperfusion (Figure 12-3) [36, 42].

Ictal SPECT is also helpful for the localization of parietal seizures. Ictal SPECT localization correlated with two main clinical seizure patterns: an anterior syndrome characterized by sensorimotor manifestations and a posterior syndrome characterized by complex partial seizures of the psychoparetic type. Parietal hyperperfusion is discrete and short-lived, demanding true ictal injections for diagnostic studies [39].

Gupta et al. [43] showed that ictal SPECT is a useful adjunctive test in presurgical evaluation of children with refractory partial epilepsy due to focal cortical dysplasia, especially when MRI is normal.

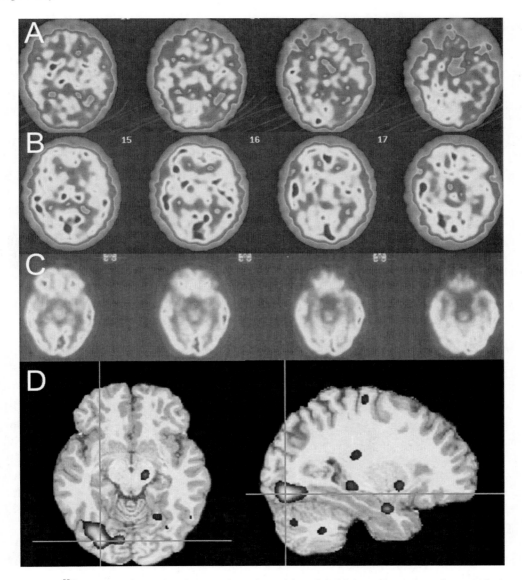

Figure 12.4. ^{99m}Tc-HMPAO Ictal SPECT (A) of a patient with occipital lobe epilepsy shows hyperperfusion in the occipital lobe (right). In this region show the interictal SPECT (B) and ^{18}F-FDG PET (C) relatively less perfusion and hypometabolism, respectively. Image D shows the SISCOM analysis after co-registration with MRI of the patient. In this patient no pathologic changes could be detected on the MRI (SISCOM-image by courtesy of Dr. Carlos M Quesada, Department of Epileptology, University Hospital Bonn, Germany).

Ictal SPECT can provide novel localizing data in MRI-negative occipital lobe epilepsy patients [44]. In occipital lobe epilepsy a very early ictal injection is required to find a focus and to avoid incorrect localization to the temporal lobe, because propagation of the seizure to one or both temporal lobes usually occurs in occipital lobe epilepsy (Figure 12.4) [15].

Patterns of Interictal Cerebral Blood Flow

The tracer for the interictal scan is injected in the nuclear medicine unit when the patient has not had a seizure for at least 30 minutes [11]. During the interictal phase, the epileptogenic zone normally shows reduced cerebral blood flow and is seen as an area of hypoperfusion on the interictal SPECT scan. However, the epileptogenic focus may occasionally show normal tracer uptake. Individual variability is possible, with different degrees of hypoperfusion [11]. Hypoperfusion most commonly involves the anterior pole of the temporal lobe and medial temporal region (Figure 12.1), but involvement of the lateral temporal cortex and ipsilateral frontal and parietal cortex is not uncommon. Hypoperfusion is occasionally observed [15].

Ictal SPECT studies are more sensitive than interictal studies [38, 45]. The superiority of ictal SPECT compared with interictal SPECT for identification of the location or the lateralization of epileptic seizures has been demonstrated by several studies of patients with temporal lobe epilepsy, indicating sensitivities of between 73and 97% for ictal SPECT and 50% for interictal SPECT [33, 46-48].

The principal role of the interictal SPECT is to aid localization of the seizure focus by comparison to the ictal scan, either visually or by subtraction of the interictal from the ictal images.

SISCOM Analysis

Subtraction of the interictal from ictal SPECT and coregistration of the result with MRI (SISCOM) is the best way to study propagation patterns; this technique enhances the sensitivity and spatial accuracy of the ictal SPECT [49] (Figure 12.1 and 12.2). With SISCOM, the first step involves the coregistration of the ictal and interictal SPECT images by matching surface points of each scan. The scans are then normalized. The transformed interictal scan is subtracted from the ictal scan. The subtraction image shows only those pixels whose intensity is above a set threshold. The image is then co-registered with the MRI after matching the cerebral surface to give an anatomical correlate [11].

Co-registration with the MRI allows accurate anatomic localization. This allows comparison with intracranial electrocorticography recordings and has shown high concordance [46]. This multimodality imaging, which combines the structural and functional imaging information, improves the ability to detect and define the extent of epileptogenic lesions and to regionalize potentially epileptogenic regions in patients who have normal MRI scans. In addition, a remarkable predictive value of SISCOM with respect to surgical outcome has been described, and could assist in the decision making for epilepsy surgery: among patients whose SISCOM findings fell within the margins of the resected tissue or in the disconnected hemisphere, 75% were rendered seizure free; among those whose SISCOM findings fell outside the margins of surgery, 100% continued to have seizures [50].

In a recent prospective study, von Oertzen et al. showed that SISCOM is a highly valuable diagnostic tool for localizing the seizure-onset zone in non-lesional and extra temporal epilepsies. Outcome in this patient group was unexpectedly good, even in patients with non-lesional MRI. The high correlation with intracranial electrocorticography and site of successful surgery is a strong indicator that outcome prediction in this patient group should be adapted accordingly, which may encourage more patients to undergo electrode implantation and subsequent successful surgery. Statistical analysis showed that SISCOM with a shorter duration of seizures, focal seizures, and lesional MRI was more likely to generate an implantation hypothesis [19].

Statistical Parametric Mapping

Statistical parametric mapping (SPM) compares an ictal SPECT scan to a series of normal regional cerebral blood flow SPECT studies with the aim of identifying regions of significantly increased cerebral blood flow, indicative of seizure activity [11]. The usefulness of SPM over visual analysis has been demonstrated by several studies [51-53]. One important advantage of SPM is that it can obviate the need for an interictal scan, with the resulting reduction in radiation exposure. Inherent disadvantages include false localization caused by regional alterations in cerebral blood flow unrelated to seizure activity, technical factors in image processing that may induce artifacts, and the developmental stage/maturation of the brain with poor localization of the epileptogenic focus in children under 6 years of age [11, 54].

References

[1]   Tamber MS, Mountz JM. Advances in the diagnosis and treatment of epilepsy. *Semin. Nucl. Med.* 2012;42(6):371-386.

[2]   Fisher RS, van Emde Boas W, Blume W, et al. Epileptic seizures and epilepsy: definitions proposed by the International League Against Epilepsy (ILAE) and the International Bureau for Epilepsy (IBE). *Epilepsia.* 2005;46(4):470-472.

[3]   Cockerell OC, Eckle I, Goodridge DM, Sander JW, Shorvon SD. Epilepsy in a population of 6000 re-examined: secular trends in first attendance rates, prevalence, and prognosis. *J. Neurol. Neurosurg. Psychiatry.* 1995;58(5):570-576.

[4]   Hauser WA, Annegers JF, Elveback LR. Mortality in patients with epilepsy. Epilepsia. 1980;21(4):399-412.

[5]   Kotsopoulos IA, van Merode T, Kessels FG, de Krom MC, Knottnerus JA. Systematic review and meta-analysis of incidence studies of epilepsy and unprovoked seizures. *Epilepsia.* 2002;43(11):1402-1409.

[6]   Berg AT, Berkovic SF, Brodie MJ, et al. Revised terminology and concepts for organization of seizures and epilepsies: report of the ILAE Commission on Classification and Terminology, 2005-2009. *Epilepsia.* 2010;51(4):676-685.

[7]   Proposal for revised clinical and electroencephalographic classification of epileptic seizures. From the Commission on Classification and Terminology of the International League Against Epilepsy. *Epilepsia.* 1981;22(4):489-501.

[8]   Proposal for revised classification of epilepsies and epileptic syndromes. Commission on Classification and Terminology of the International League Against Epilepsy. *Epilepsia.* 1989;30(4):389-399.

[9]   Tikofsky RS, Van Heertum RL. Seizure disorders. In: Van Heertum RL, Tikofsky RS, eds. Functional cerebral SPECT and PET imaging. 3rd ed: Lippincott Williams and Wilkins, Philadelphia; 2000. 189-228.

[10] Kwan P, Brodie MJ. Early identification of refractory epilepsy. *N. Engl. J. Med.* 2000;342(5):314-319.

[11] Patil S, Biassoni L, Borgwardt L. Nuclear medicine in pediatric neurology and neurosurgery: epilepsy and brain tumors. *Semin. Nucl. Med.* 2007;37(5):357-381.

[12] Clusmann H, Kral T, Schramm J. Present practice and perspective of evaluation and surgery for temporal lobe epilepsy. *Zentralblatt fur Neurochirurgie.* 2006;67(4):165-182.

[13] Duncan JS. Imaging and epilepsy. *Brain : a journal of neurology.* 1997;120 (Pt 2):339-377.

[14] Rapport RL, 2nd, Ojemann GA, Wyler AR, Ward AA, Jr. Surgical management of epilepsy. *West J. Med.* 1977;127(3):185-189.

[15] Rowe CC. Nuclear Medicine in the managment of a patient with epilepsy. In: Ell PJ, Gambhir S, eds. Nuclear Medicine in clinical diagnosis and treatment. 3rd ed: Churchill Livingstone; 2004. 1371-1385.

[16] Wiebe S, Blume WT, Girvin JP, Eliasziw M. A randomized, controlled trial of surgery for temporal-lobe epilepsy. *N. Engl. J. Med.* 2001;345(5):311-318.

[17] Bien CG, Szinay M, Wagner J, Clusmann H, Becker AJ, Urbach H. Characteristics and surgical outcomes of patients with refractory magnetic resonance imaging-negative epilepsies. *Archives of neurology.* 2009;66(12):1491-1499.

[18] Lee KK, Salamon N. [18F] fluorodeoxyglucose-positron-emission tomography and MR imaging coregistration for presurgical evaluation of medically refractory epilepsy. *AJNR Am. J. Neuroradiol.* 2009;30(10):1811-1816.

[19] von Oertzen TJ, Mormann F, Urbach H, et al. Prospective use of subtraction ictal SPECT coregistered to MRI (SISCOM) in presurgical evaluation of epilepsy. *Epilepsia.* 2011;52(12):2239-2248.

[20] Li LM, Fish DR, Sisodiya SM, Shorvon SD, Alsanjari N, Stevens JM. High resolution magnetic resonance imaging in adults with partial or secondary generalised epilepsy attending a tertiary referral unit. J Neurol Neurosurg Psychiatry. 1995;59(4):384-387.

[21] Bien CG, Raabe AL, Schramm J, Becker A, Urbach H, Elger CE. Trends in presurgical evaluation and surgical treatment of epilepsy at one centre from 1988-2009. *J. Neurol. Neurosurg Psychiatry.* 2013;84(1):54-61.

[22] Hougaard K, Oikawa T, Sveinsdottir E, Skinoj E, Ingvar DH, Lassen NA. Regional cerebral blood flow in focal cortical epilepsy. *Archives of neurology.* 1976;33(8):527-535.

[23] Hudson LP, Munoz DG, Miller L, McLachlan RS, Girvin JP, Blume WT. Amygdaloid sclerosis in temporal lobe epilepsy. *Annals of neurology.* 1993;33(6):622-631.

[24] Engel J, Jr., Brown WJ, Kuhl DE, Phelps ME, Mazziotta JC, Crandall PH. Pathological findings underlying focal temporal lobe hypometabolism in partial epilepsy. *Annals of neurology.* 1982;12(6):518-528.

[25] Henry TR, Van Heertum RL. Positron emission tomography and single photon emission computed tomography in epilepsy care. *Semin Nucl Med.* 2003;33(2):88-104.

[26] Duncan R, Patterson J, Roberts R, Hadley DM, Bone I. Ictal/postictal SPECT in the pre-surgical localisation of complex partial seizures. *J. Neurol. Neurosurg. Psychiatry.* 1993;56(2):141-148.

[27] Shen W, Lee BI, Park HM, et al. HIPDM-SPECT brain imaging in the presurgical evaluation of patients with intractable seizures. *J. Nucl. Med.* 1990;31(8):1280-1284.

[28] Kung HF. New technetium 99m-labeled brain perfusion imaging agents. Semin Nucl Med. 1990;20(2):150-158.

[29] Juni JE, Waxman AD, Devous MD, Sr., et al. Procedure guideline for brain perfusion SPECT using (99m)Tc radiopharmaceuticals 3.0. *J. Nucl. Med. Technol.* 2009;37(3):191-195.

[30] Holman BL, Hellman RS, Goldsmith SJ, et al. Biodistribution, dosimetry, and clinical evaluation of technetium-99m ethyl cysteinate dimer in normal subjects and in patients with chronic cerebral infarction. J. Nucl. Med. 1989;30(6):1018-1024.

[31] Catafau AM. Brain SPECT in clinical practice. *Part I: perfusion. J. Nucl. Med.* 2001;42(2):259-271.

[32] Kapucu OL, Nobili F, Varrone A, et al. EANM procedure guideline for brain perfusion SPECT using (99m)Tc-labelled radiopharmaceuticals, version 2. *Eur. J. Nucl. Med. Mol. Imaging.* 2009;36(12):2093-2102.

[33] Weil S, Noachtar S, Arnold S, Yousry TA, Winkler PA, Tatsch K. Ictal ECD-SPECT differentiates between temporal and extratemporal epilepsy: confirmation by excellent postoperative seizure control. *Nucl. Med. Commun.* 2001;22(2):233-237.

[34] Stefan H, Bauer J, Feistel H, et al. Regional cerebral blood flow during focal seizures of temporal and frontocentral onset. *Annals of neurology.* 1990;27(2):162-166.

[35] Won JH, Lee JD, Chung TS, Park CY, Lee BI. Increased contralateral cerebellar uptake of technetium-99m-HMPAO on ictal brain SPECT. *J. Nucl. Med.* 1996;37(3):426-429.

[36] Harvey AS, Hopkins IJ, Bowe JM, Cook DJ, Shield LK, Berkovic SF. Frontal lobe epilepsy: clinical seizure characteristics and localization with ictal 99mTc-HMPAO SPECT. *Neurology.* 1993;43(10):1966-1980.

[37] Shin WC, Hong SB, Tae WS, Seo DW, Kim SE. Ictal hyperperfusion of cerebellum and basal ganglia in temporal lobe epilepsy: SPECT subtraction with MRI coregistration. *J. Nucl Med.* 2001;42(6):853-858.

[38] Newton MR, Berkovic SF, Austin MC, Rowe CC, McKay WJ, Bladin PF. SPECT in the localisation of extratemporal and temporal seizure foci. *J. Neurol. Neurosurg. Psychiatry.* 1995;59(1):26-30.

[39] Ho SS, Berkovic SF, Newton MR, Austin MC, McKay WJ, Bladin PF. Parietal lobe epilepsy: clinical features and seizure localization by ictal SPECT. *Neurology.* 1994;44(12):2277-2284.

[40] Noachtar S, Arnold S, Yousry TA, Bartenstein P, Werhahn KJ, Tatsch K. Ictal technetium-99m ethyl cysteinate dimer single-photon emission tomographic findings and propagation of epileptic seizure activity in patients with extratemporal epilepsies. *Eur. J. Nucl. Med.* 1998;25(2):166-172.

[41] Saygi S, Katz A, Marks DA, Spencer SS. Frontal lobe partial seizures and psychogenic seizures: comparison of clinical and ictal characteristics. *Neurology.* 1992;42(7):1274-1277.

[42] Marks DA, Katz A, Hoffer P, Spencer SS. Localization of extratemporal epileptic foci during ictal single photon emission computed tomography. *Annals of neurology.* 1992;31(3):250-255.

[43] Gupta A, Raja S, Kotagal P, Lachhwani D, Wyllie E, Bingaman WB. Ictal SPECT in children with partial epilepsy due to focal cortical dysplasia. *Pediatr. Neurol.* 2004;31(2):89-95.

[44] Sturm JW, Newton MR, Chinvarun Y, Berlangieri SU, Berkovic SF. Ictal SPECT and interictal PET in the localization of occipital lobe epilepsy. *Epilepsia.* 2000;41(4):463-466.

[45] Berkovic SF, Andermann F, Olivier A, et al. Hippocampal sclerosis in temporal lobe epilepsy demonstrated by magnetic resonance imaging. *Annals of neurology.* 1991;29(2):175-182.

[46] Spanaki MV, Spencer SS, Corsi M, MacMullan J, Seibyl J, Zubal IG. Sensitivity and specificity of quantitative difference SPECT analysis in seizure localization. *J. Nucl. Med.* 1999;40(5):730-736.

[47] Devous MD, Sr., Thisted RA, Morgan GF, Leroy RF, Rowe CC. SPECT brain imaging in epilepsy: a meta-analysis. *J. Nucl. Med.* 1998;39(2):285-293.

[48] Zaknun JJ, Bal C, Maes A, et al. Comparative analysis of MR imaging, ictal SPECT and EEG in temporal lobe epilepsy: a prospective IAEA multi-center study. *Eur. J. Nucl. Med. Mol. Imaging.* 2008;35(1):107-115.

[49] O'Brien TJ, So EL, Mullan BP, et al. Subtraction ictal SPECT co-registered to MRI improves clinical usefulness of SPECT in localizing the surgical seizure focus. *Neurology.* 1998;50(2):445-454.

[50] Wichert-Ana L, de Azevedo-Marques PM, Oliveira LF, et al. Interictal hyperemia correlates with epileptogenicity in polymicrogyric cortex. *Epilepsy research.* 2008;79(1):39-48.

[51] Tae WS, Joo EY, Kim JH, et al. Cerebral perfusion changes in mesial temporal lobe epilepsy: SPM analysis of ictal and interictal SPECT. *Neuroimage.* 2005;24(1):101-110.

[52] Lee JD, Kim HJ, Lee BI, Kim OJ, Jeon TJ, Kim MJ. Evaluation of ictal brain SPET using statistical parametric mapping in temporal lobe epilepsy. *Eur. J. Nucl. Med.* 2000;27(11):1658-1665.

[53] Bruggemann JM, Som SS, Lawson JA, Haindl W, Cunningham AM, Bye AM. Application of statistical parametric mapping to SPET in the assessment of intractable childhood epilepsy. Eur. *J. Nucl. Med. Mol. Imaging.* 2004;31(3):369-377.

[54] Muzik O, Chugani DC, Juhasz C, Shen C, Chugani HT. Statistical parametric mapping: assessment of application in children. *Neuroimage.* 2000;12(5):538-549.

In: SPECT
Editors: Hojjat Ahmadzadehfar and Elham Habibi

ISBN: 978-1-62808-344-6
© 2013 Nova Science Publishers, Inc.

Chapter XIII

SPECT in the Evaluation of Brain Tumors

Yasushi Shibata[*]

Department of Neurosurgery, Mito Medical Center,
University of Tsukuba, Japan

Introduction

A brain tumor is an intracranial neoplasm that has various pathologies [1]. Using diagnostic information, a tumor can be classified as least aggressive (benign) to most aggressive (malignant). In most cases, a brain tumor is named for the cell type of origin or its location. Identifying the type of brain tumor helps to determine the most appropriate course of treatment.

There are three main types of brain tumors: intra-medullary, extra-medullary, and metastatic. Most intra-medullary tumors originate from glial cells and are called gliomas. A glioma is generally infiltrative into the brain parenchyma; therefore, a complete surgical excision is usually difficult. The prognosis of patients with a glioma depends on the malignancy grade of the tumor although it is generally poor. On the other hand, most extra-medullary brain tumors are benign and complete surgical removal results in a good prognosis. Metastatic brain tumors are always malignant and although the prognosis depends on a patient's systemic condition, it is generally poor.

Diagnosis of Brain Tumors

The main symptoms of brain tumors are headache, paresis, and epileptic seizures. A progressive clinical course suggests a brain tumor. An accurate preoperative diagnosis of the tumor pathology and malignancy grade is often challenging. Most intra-medullary tumors are

---
[*] Corresponding author: Yasushi Shibata. E-mail: yshibata@md.tsukuba.ac.jp.

malignant; however, they may be benign; while, the majority of extra-medullary tumors are benign, but malignant tumors also exist.

Selecting an appropriate treatment depends on the malignancy grade and prognosis of the tumor; thus, a correct preoperative diagnosis is important. The final diagnosis depends on the pathological analysis of the surgical specimen.

Radiological Diagnosis of Brain Tumors

Brain magnetic resonance imaging (MRI) is the modality of choice for evaluating patients who have symptoms and signs suggesting a brain tumor and for assessing the tumor location and extent. Even if most clinical questions can be answered by MRI and computed tomography (CT), these techniques have limitations in the characterization of brain lesions, defining the tumor extent, therapy monitoring, and in detecting the recurrence or progression of tumors.

High contrast enhancement in a tumor means high blood flow but not necessarily malignancy. Meningioma and pituitary adenomas are typical benign extra-medullary tumors with high contrast enhancement. In addition, complete visualization of infiltrating malignant glioma cells is difficult, even with high resolution MRI.

The brain neoplasms are treated with various combinations of surgery, radiation, and chemotherapy. Changes that follow treatment may include edema and radiation necrosis, and it is often challenging to differentiate between tumor recurrence and such benign physical changes with CT or MRI [2-5]. Nuclear medicine imaging allows *in vivo* investigation of tumor metabolism, given the wide availability of radiotracers, and plays a major role in the diagnosis and follow-up of patients with brain tumors.

SPECT for the Diagnosis and Evaluation of Brain Tumors

Single photon emission computed tomography (SPECT) is a valuable diagnostic modality for the evaluation of the brain tumor malignancy grade and activity. ^{201}Thallium-chloride (^{201}Tl) and two ^{99m}Technetium labeled radiopharmaceuticals (methoxyisobutylisonitrile (^{99m}Tc-MIBI) and tetrofosmin (^{99m}Tc-Tetrofosmin)) have been clinically used with SPECT to evaluate brain tumors. SPECT has also been used with the radioactive labeled amino acid 3-[123I] iodo-a-methyl-L-tyrosine for the diagnosis of brain tumors and evaluation of tumor response to radiation therapy.

^{201}Thallium SPECT

^{201}Tl, a potassium analog, is taken up by viable tumor cells but not by necrotic tissue or non-proliferating glial cells [6]. It is cyclotron produced with a physical half-life of 73 hours. ^{201}Tl has been used in myocardial scintigraphy and in evaluating lung carcinomas and brain tumors. ^{201}Tl SPECT is useful for identifying the presence of a tumor [7], grading of the tumor malignancy [3, 4, 6], and distinguishing tumor recurrence from radiation necrosis [2-4] (Figure 13-1). The SPECT procedure involves imaging approximately 20-30 minutes following injection of 74-148 MBq of ^{201}Tl.

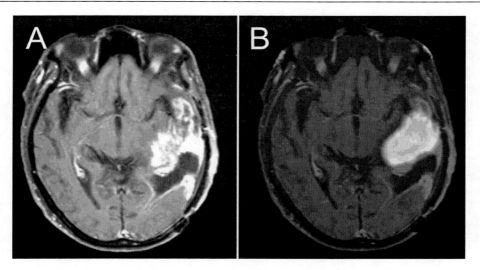

Figure 13-1. 72 year-old-women with glioblastma. Gd enhanced MRI (A) and fusion image of ^{201}Tl SPECT and Gd enhanced MRI (B).

Occasionally, a 2-hour delayed ^{201}Tl acquisition may be helpful as the abnormal tumor tissue would be expected to washout more slowly than normal brain tissue [8, 9]. The SPECT imaging should be done using a low energy general purpose collimator. The photopeak should be centered at 80 and 167 keV.

The ^{201}Tl index, the ratio of counts in the lesion region of interest (ROI) to counts in the contralateral ROI, is used to differentiate between low and high grade gliomas [6] as well as between recurrence and radiation necrosis [11, 12]. The value of these ratios varies according to the identification of the ROI, the location and size of the lesion, and whether or not there is a central necrosis.

Some investigators recommend drawing the ROI over the highest pixel counts of ^{201}Tl uptake; while, others recommend drawing it over the inner and outer border of the tumor and averaging the pixel counts. Ratios above 1.6-2.4 may indicate malignant lesions; while, lower ratios indicate either benign lesions or early recurrence [13]. In a population of 90 patients with supratentorial brain tumors, the overall sensitivity and specificity of ^{201}Tl in detecting the lesions were 71.7% and 80.9% respectively [14]. Dynamic ^{201}Tl SPECT is useful to evaluate tumor vascularity, histopathology, and malignancy [15, 16]. The utility of ^{201}Tl SPECT in differentiating toxoplasmosis from lymphoma in AIDS patients was demonstrated by Kessler et al. with a sensitivity of 100% and specificity of 93% [17].

The utility of ^{201}Tl SPECT as an early predictor of outcome in patients with recurrent gliomas has been shown by Vos et al. They reported that at baseline and follow-up, maximal tumor intensity by ^{201}Tl SPECT was the strongest predictive variable and was inversely related to overall survival as well as progression-free survival.

They also showed a progression of maximal tumor intensity after two courses of chemotherapy was a powerful predictor of poor outcome. For a [201]Tl -avid lesion that has been treated and shown to be ^{201}Tl negative on follow-up, any ^{201}Tl uptake is an indicator of tumor recurrence [13]. Glioma surgery may improve the prognosis, but this is controversial, possibly due to the method of evaluating glioma surgical extent.

In a study from our group, we evaluated the glioma surgical extent using fusion images of preoperative ^{201}Tl SPECT with postoperative MRI to predict the prognosis of the patients regarding the removal rate and postsurgical residual tumor. All patients received standard adjuvant radiation and chemotherapy after surgery. We found the fusion image of preoperative ^{201}Tl SPECT and postoperative MRI was more useful for evaluating glioma removal extent than just MRI. Patients with partial removal had a poor prognosis; thus, the aim should be for maximum surgical removal using multimodal images including MRI and ^{201}Tl SPECT. The total removal of ^{201}Tl SPECT positive lesions improves the prognosis and prevents early recurrence [18].

Inflammation after surgery or radiation is a major cause of false positives [3, 4, 19-21]. Other inflammatory lesions, like brain abscesses, can be also a source of a false positive scan [22] (Figure 13-2). Using combined ^{201}Tl and ^{99m}Tc–hexamethylpropyleneamine oxime (^{99m}Tc-HMPAO) for brain tumors has been recommended to increase the specificity of ^{201}Tl SPECT [2, 23]. Carvalho et al. assessed the ability of sequential ^{201}Tl and ^{99m}Tc-HMPAO SPECT to distinguish tumor recurrence from radiation changes after high-dose radiation therapy for malignant gliomas. The authors found ^{99m}Tc-HMPAO SPECT is useful for identifying the absence of solid tumor recurrence in patients with low to moderate ^{201}Tl uptake (ratio 1.1 to 3.4) and low perfusion to that site (less than 0.5.) [23]. Some causes of false negative findings may include small tumor size; located centrally or adjacent to areas of physiological tracer uptake, such as choroid plexus; histological heterogeneity; and cystic or necrotic components [24, 25]. Young et al. [25] reported that when using a [201]Tl -index > 2 in lesions bigger than 2 cm, ^{201}Tl SPECT has a 100% sensitivity and 89% specificity for the differentiation between brain lymphoma and toxoplasmosis in patients with AIDS; while, the sensitivity and specificity were 50% and 82%, respectively, in lesions smaller than 2 cm.

Both central neurocytomas and gangliogliomas are benign gliomas with a high ^{201}Tl uptake [26, 27]. High cell density and high metabolic rate are thought to explain the high ^{201}Tl uptake in these low proliferative tumors. In our series, one patient with a central neurocytoma showed high ^{201}Tl uptake and no ^{99m}Tc-MIBI uptake (Figure 13-3).

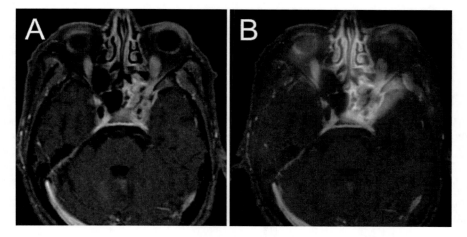

Figure 13-2. 70 year-old man with cavernous sinusitis. Gd enhanced MRI (A) and fusion image of ^{201}Tl SPECT and Gd enhanced MRI (B).

In this case, ^{99m}Tc-MIBI SPECT was more accurate than ^{201}Tl SPECT to evaluate tumor malignancy. Pilocytic astrocytoma is one of the most benign gliomas and the ^{201}Tl SPECT findings show variable uptake [28]. Lower ^{201}Tl uptake is also observed in early follow-up studies after surgical excisions and/or aggressive chemotherapy. This is due to granulation tissue and new vascularity associated with treatment [13]

^{99m}Tc-MIBI SPECT

^{99m}Tc-MIBI is a lipophilic cationic complex with a physical half-life of 6 hours, initially designed for myocardial perfusion SPECT. ^{99m}Tc-MIBI SPECT is also useful to diagnose brain tumor recurrence [29, 30]; evaluate the biological characteristics of brain tumors [31], tumor volume, and survival [32, 33]; and in the differential diagnosis of radiation necrosis [5]. As with ^{201}Tl imaging, the ^{99m}Tc-MIBI index can be used to differentiate between low and high grade gliomas [34] as well as recurrence and radiation necrosis [29], and to estimate the prognosis [32, 33]. ^{99m}Tc-MIBI index is concentrated in the mitochondria as the result of active diffusion due to increased metabolic needs [29]. Its uptake is affected by tumor malignancy, viability, density, oxygenation, vascular supply, and blood brain barrier (BBB) disruption [35]. These factors are not linearly correlated because glioblastoma, the most malignant form of glioma, is pathologically heterogeneous and includes internal necrosis.

In ^{99m}Tc-MIBI SPECT, tumor imaging occurs approximately 20-30 minutes following injection of about 740 MBq ^{99m}Tc-MIBI. Delayed images (2-4 h p.i.) have been also recommended. The SPECT imaging should be done using a low energy general purpose collimator and the photopeak should be centered at 140 keV. In the brain, ^{99m}Tc-MIBI is taken up by normal choroid plexus, scalp, the pituitary gland, and nasopharyngeal tissues [36].

With respect to the histological type, a higher ^{99m}Tc-MIBI retention index has been noted in glioblastoma multiforme compared with metastatic tumors. In addition, while ^{99m}Tc-MIBI SPECT shows high uptake and retention in malignant gliomas, washout from metastatic brain tumors is faster than from glioblastomas [37]. ^{99m}Tc-MIBI has also been successfully used in high-grade gliomas to distinguish recurrent tumor from radionecrosis [30] and when the results of both CT and MRI are difficult to interpret, because of inflammation resulting from surgery or radiation, and offer only an imperfect indication of tumor viability [38]. A false negative finding by ^{99m}Tc-MIBI SPECT may occur due to an intact BBB. [30]. In a study on patients in the pre-surgical phase for interparenchymal brain tumors, ^{99m}Tc-MIBI SPECT identified tumors in the fronto-temporal regions more easily than in the temporal regions or in the posterior fossa [36]. P-glycoprotein is a drug efflux pump in the cell membrane and it acts to remove ^{99m}Tc-MIBI from tumor cells [40, 41]. Other studies have suggested that p-glycoprotein expression in malignant gliomas may cause false negative results in ^{99m}Tc-MIBI SPECT [42-44]. However, the effect of p-glycoprotein expression on clinical ^{99m}Tc-MIBI SPECT images has been investigated, and the effect was negligible in the diagnosis of brain tumor malignancy [45]. Henze also reported that p-glycoprotein efflux does not contribute to falsely negative ^{99m}Tc-MIBI SPECT, since ^{99m}Tc-MIBI washout did not occur between the early and late SPECT scans [46].

Some of the false positive results were due to recent radiation induced local disruption of the BBB [30].

^{99m}Tc-MIBI shows early accumulation into the normal choroid plexus and good wash out from it. Choroid plexus papillomas show slower tracer wash out than the normal choroid plexus; hence, the delayed ^{99m}Tc-MIBI index is higher than the early ^{99m}Tc-MIBI index [47].

Comparison of 201Tl and 99mTc-MIBIBrain SPECT in Patients with Gliomas

The diagnostic values of brain ^{201}Tl and ^{99m}Tc-MIBI SPECT have been evaluated by other group using sensitivities and specificities with arbitrary cut off values. The diagnostic ability of ^{201}Tl SPECT and ^{99m}Tc-MIBI SPECT were directly compared for patients with an initial glioma using ROC analysis. The study population included 59 patients with gliomas. The benign group included patients with low grade astrocytomas and central neurocytomas; while, the malignant group included patients with anaplastic astrocytomas and glioblastomas. All patients underwent ^{201}Tl and ^{99m}Tc-MIBI SPECT and tumor/not-tumor (T/N) ratios were calculated. The area z-score (A_z) values were calculated from the areas under the ROC curves (Figure 13-4). The delayed ^{99m}Tc-MIBI had the highest A_z while the early ^{99m}Tc-MIBI had the lowest A_z. Both ^{201}Tl and ^{99m}Tc-MIBI SPECT are considered useful imaging modalities for the evaluation of glioma malignancies. Delayed ^{99m}Tc-MIBI SPECT demonstrated better diagnostic value in patients with gliomas based on ROC analysis although the difference was not statistically significant [48].

Some studies have reported that ^{99m}Tc-MIBI SPECT has higher sensitivity and specificity than ^{201}Tl SPECT for adult and childhood brain tumors and for the differential diagnosis of recurrence and radiation necrosis [5, 33, 28]; however, other studies disagree [37]. This discrepancy may be caused by small and heterogeneous patient populations and arbitrarily selected cut off values. In ^{201}Tl SPECT, there is some normal brain uptake, which makes the T/N ratio low. ^{99m}Tc-MIBI has a high photon energy level and higher T/N ratio in comparison with ^{201}Tl SPECT and yields clear SPECT images with high sensitivity for malignant brain tumors [5, 29, 38].

^{99m}Tc-Tetrofosmin SPECT

^{99m}Tc-Tetrofosmin is a lipophilic cationic tracer with a physical half-life of 6 hours that was initially used for myocardial perfusion SPECT. The utility of ^{99m}Tc-Tetrofosmin in evaluation of brain tumors has been demonstrated [49-52]. Soricelli et al. [49] showed significant agreement among ^{201}Tl and ^{99m}Tc-Tetrofosmin SPECT for the diagnosis of brain tumors; however, the image quality, contrast, and the definition of tumor margins obtained by ^{99m}Tc-Tetrofosmin were superior to those with ^{201}Tl. ^{99m}Tc-Tetrofosmin is also useful for non-invasive grading. There was a striking difference between the ^{99m}Tc-Tetrofosmin index in low grade and high grade gliomas, which was not the case for ^{201}Tl, ^{99m}Tc-MIBI, and ^{18}F-FDG PET [53]. ^{99m}Tc-Tetrofosmin can also distinguish tumor recurrence from radiation necrosis [50-52].We compared the radiological image findings from ^{99m}Tc-Tetrofosmin and ^{201}Tl SPECT for 11 patients with brain tumors. The tracer uptakes of ^{99m}Tc-Tetrofosmin and

^{201}Tl were almost matched. In the patients with meningioma, both ^{99m}Tc-Tetrofosmin and ^{201}Tl early images showed high uptake and these tracers were washed out in delayed images, except of atypical meningioma. Both ^{99m}Tc-Tetrofosmin and ^{201}Tl delayed SPECT images showed high uptake in tumors from patients with glioblastomas (Figure 13-5).

There is physiological ^{99m}Tc-Tetrofosmin uptake in the normal choroid plexus, which contributes to the spatial correlation between tumors and ventricles. ^{99m}Tc-Tetrofosmin SPECT is better and more useful than ^{201}Tl SPECT to diagnose tumor location, extent, malignancy, viability, and effects from therapies [54].

3-[^{123}I]Iodo-A-Methyl-L-Tyrosine SPECT

3-[^{123}I]iodo-a-methyl-L-tyrosine (^{123}I-IMT) is an amino acid SPECT tracer for brain imaging. Tumors are imaged with SPECT approximately 10 minutes after the injection of 370-740 MBq ^{123}I-IMT. To prevent the uptake of free iodine, the thyroid should be blocked with 400-600 mg sodium perchlorate 30 minutes before tracer application. The SPECT imaging should be done using a low energy high resolution collimator using a 20% energy window centered on the 159-keV photopeak. ^{123}I-IMT SPECT was directly compared with [methyl-^{11}C]-L-methionine (^{11}C-MET) PET in 14 patients with cerebral gliomas [55]. Visual comparison of the scans yielded no differences in tumor size and shape with both methods. The tumor to brain ratios of ^{123}I-IMT SPECT and ^{11}C-MET PET showed a significant correlation especially in the early, transport dominated phase at 15 min after injection.

Kuwert et al. [56] showed that ^{123}I-IMT SPECT may aid in differentiating high-grade gliomas from histologically benign brain tumors and non-neoplastic brain lesions; however, this modality was inappropriate for distinguishing non-neoplastic from benign lesions. In this study, the sensitivity and specificity of ^{123}I-IMT SPECT were 71% and 83%, respectively, for differentiating high grade from low grade gliomas, 82% and 100%, respectively, for distinguishing high-grade gliomas from non-neoplastic lesions, and 50% and 100%, respectively, for discriminating low-grade gliomas from non-neoplastic lesions [56].

The utility of ^{123}I-IMT SPECT for determining tumor grade and prognosis of the disease is controversial [56-60]. A strong correlation between tracer uptake and tumor proliferative activity was reported by Kuwert et al. [59].

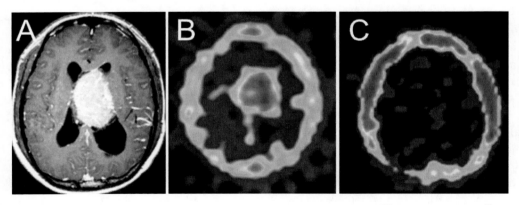

Figure 13-3. 18 year-old man with central neurocytoma. Gd enhanced MRI (A), ^{201}Tl SPECT (B) and ^{99m}Tc-MIBI SPECT (C).

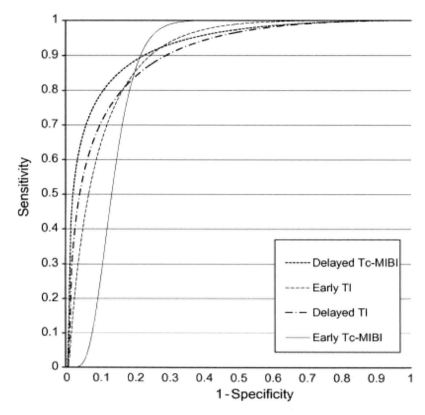

Figure 13-4. ROC curves.

In contrast, Weber et al. [61] reported that ^{123}I-IMT uptake appeared not to correlate with the biological aggressiveness of tumor cells in patients with unresectable high-grade gliomas. Nevertheless, the clear association between focal ^{123}I-IMT uptake after tumor resection and poor survival suggests that ^{123}I-IMT is a specific marker for residual tumor tissue [61].

It is very important to precisely determine the tumor extent for planning surgery or radiation. ^{123}I-IMT is taken up in brain areas with an intact blood-brain barrier and ^{123}I-IMT SPECT appears to be able to image the infiltrating tissue of cerebral gliomas like ^{11}C-MET [62]. In a study using ^{123}I-IMT SPECT in addition to MRI for planning radiation therapy, a larger tumor volume was detected by ^{123}I-IMT SPECT than by conventional MRI. The authors highlighted that ^{123}I-IMT SPECT investigations improved tumor detection and delineation in the treatment planning process [63].

Several studies yielded good sensitivity and specificity of ^{123}I-IMT SPECT for the detection of viable tumor tissue in previously treated patients [57, 58, 64]. Bader et al. showed that ^{123}I-IMT SPECT was equivalent to a stereotactic biopsy in its ability to identify high-grade tumors at recurrence [57]. The fusion of ^{123}I-IMT SPECT images with MRI improves the interpretation of the findings and may increase the specificity of the investigation [65]. In addition, ^{123}I-IMT SPECT was a promising complementary imaging tool for the detection of recurrences of non-astrocytic intracranial tumors and for distinguishing them from treatment induced changes [66]. Several studies indicate the utility of ^{123}I-IMT in the follow-up of patients with brain tumors [57, 64, 67].

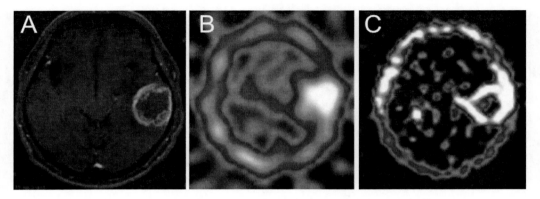

Figure 13-5. 58 year-old man with glioblastoma. Gd enhanced MRI (A), ^{201}Tl SPECT (B) and ^{99m}Tc-Tetrofosmin SPECT (C).

Patients with recurrence had significantly higher ratios of ^{123}I-IMT uptake in the tumor area to that in the background region than patients without recurrence. The majority of brain metastases exhibit high ^{123}I-IMT uptake, which does not allow differentiation from gliomas. A combination of ^{123}I-IMT and ^{201}Tl SPECT, however, may be able to distinguish high-grade gliomas from other malignant brain lesions, like metastases, with high accuracy [68].

References

[1]   Louis, D. N., Ohgaki, H., Wiestler, O. D., Cavenee, W. K., Burger, P. C., et al. The 2007 WHO classification of tumours of the central nervous system. *Acta Neuropathol.* 2007; 114: 97-109.

[2]   Schwartz, R. B., Carvalho, P. A., Alexander, E., 3rd, Loeffler, J. S., Folkerth, R., et al. Radiation necrosis vs high-grade recurrent glioma: differentiation by using dual-isotope SPECT with 201TI and 99mTc-HMPAO. *AJNR Am. J. Neuroradiol.* 1991; 12: 1187-92.

[3]   Yoshii, Y., Satou, M., Yamamoto, T., Yamada, Y., Hyodo, A., et al. The role of thallium-201 single photon emission tomography in the investigation and characterisation of brain tumours in man and their response to treatment. *Eur. J. Nucl. Med.* 1993; 20: 39-45.

[4]   Staffen, W., Hondl, N., Trinka, E., Iglseder, B., Unterrainer, J., et al. Clinical relevance of 201Tl-chloride SPET in the differential diagnosis of brain tumours. *Nucl. Med. Commun.* 1998; 19: 335-40.

[5]   Yamamoto, Y., Nishiyama, Y., Toyama, Y., Kunishio, K., Satoh, K., et al. 99mTc-MIBI and 201Tl SPET in the detection of recurrent brain tumours after radiation therapy. *Nucl. Med. Commun.* 2002; 23: 1183-90.

[6]   Black, K. L., Hawkins, R. A., Kim, K. T., Becker, D. P., Lerner, C., et al. Use of thallium-201 SPECT to quantitate malignancy grade of gliomas. *J. Neurosurg.* 1989; 71: 342-6.

[7]   O'Tuama, L. A., Janicek, M. J., Barnes, P. D., Scott, R. M., Black, P. M., et al. 201Tl/99mTc-HMPAO SPECT imaging of treated childhood brain tumors. *Pediatr. Neurol.* 1991; 7: 249-57.

[8]   Sehweil, A., McKillop, J. H., Ziada, G., Al-Sayed, M., Abdel-Dayem, H., et al. The optimum time for tumour imaging with thallium-201. *Eur. J. Nucl. Med.* 1988; 13: 527-9.

[9]   Sehweil, A. M., McKillop, J. H., Milroy, R., Wilson, R., Abdel-Dayem, H. M., et al. Mechanism of 201Tl uptake in tumours. *Eur. J. Nucl. Med.* 1989; 15: 376-9.

[10]   Fukumoto M. Single-photon agents for tumor imaging: 201Tl, 99mTc-MIBI, and 99mTc-tetrofosmin. *Ann Nucl Med.* Apr 2004;18(2):79-95

[11]   Kosuda, S., Shioyama, Y., Kamata, N., Suzuki, K., Tanaka, Y., et al. [Differential diagnosis between recurrence of brain tumor and radiation necrosis by 201Tl SPECT]. *Nippon Igaku Hoshasen Gakkai Zasshi* 1991; 51: 415-21.

[12]   Kosuda, S., Fujii, H., Aoki, S., Suzuki, K., Tanaka, Y., et al. Reassessment of quantitative thallium-201 brain SPECT for miscellaneous brain tumors. *Ann. Nucl. Med.* 1993; 7: 257-63.

[13]   Abdel Dayem, H., Scott, A., Macapinlac, H. Thallium-201 chloride: a tumor imaging agent. In: Ell, P. J., Gambhir, S., eds. *Nuclear Medicine in clinical diagnosis and treatment.* 3 ed: Churchill Livinstone 2004:71-81.

[14]   Stathaki, M. I., Koukouraki, S. I., Karkavitsas, N. S. The role of scintigraphy in the evaluation of brain malignancies. *Hell J. Nucl. Med.* 2010; 13: 264-72.

[15]   Ueda, T., Kaji, Y., Wakisaka, S., Watanabe, K., Hoshi, H., et al. Time sequential single photon emission computed tomography studies in brain tumour using thallium-201. *Eur. J. Nucl. Med.* 1993; 20: 138-45.

[16]   Sugo, N., Yokota, K., Kondo, K., Harada, N., Aoki, Y., et al. Early dynamic 201Tl SPECT in the evaluation of brain tumours. *Nucl. Med. Commun.* 2006; 27: 143-9.

[17]. Kessler LS, Ruiz A, Donovan Post MJ, Ganz WI, Brandon AH, Foss JN. Thallium-201 brain SPECT of lymphoma in AIDS patients: pitfalls and technique optimization. *AJNR Am J Neuroradiol.* Jun-Jul 1998;19(6):1105-1109.

[18]   Shibata, Y., Matsushita, A., Akimoto, M., Yamamoto, T., Takano, S., et al. [Evaluation of surgical removal with fusion image of Tl SPECT and MRI]In Japanese. *CIresearch* 2010; 32: 19-24.

[19]   Buchpiguel, C. A., Alavi, J. B., Alavi, A., Kenyon, L. C. PET versus SPECT in distinguishing radiation necrosis from tumor recurrence in the brain. *J. Nucl. Med.* 1995; 36: 159-64.

[20]   Rollins, N. K., Lowry, P. A., Shapiro, K. N. Comparison of gadolinium-enhanced MR and thallium-201 single photon emission computed tomography in pediatric brain tumors. *Pediatr. Neurosurg.* 1995; 22: 8-14.

[21]   Serizawa, T., Saeki, N., Higuchi, Y., Ono, J., Matsuda, S., et al. Diagnostic value of thallium-201 chloride single-photon emission computerized tomography in differentiating tumor recurrence from radiation injury after gamma knife surgery for metastatic brain tumors. *J. Neurosurg.* 2005; 102 Suppl.: 266-71.

[22]   Martinez del Valle, M. D., Gomez-Rio, M., Horcajadas, A., Rodriguez-Fernandez, A., Muros de Fuentes, M. A., et al. False positive thallium-201 SPECT imaging in brain abscess. *Br. J. Radiol.* 2000; 73: 160-4.

[23] Carvalho, P. A., Schwartz, R. B., Alexander, E., 3rd, Garada, B. M., Zimmerman, R. E., et al. Detection of recurrent gliomas with quantitative thallium-201/technetium-99m HMPAO single-photon emission computerized tomography. *J. Neurosurg.* 1992; 77: 565-70.

[24] Kallen K, Burtscher IM, Holtas S, Ryding E, Rosen I. 201Thallium SPECT and 1H-MRS compared with MRI in chemotherapy monitoring of high-grade malignant astrocytomas. *J Neurooncol.* 2000;46(2):173-185.

[25] Young RJ, Ghesani MV, Kagetsu NJ, Derogatis AJ. Lesion size determines accuracy of thallium-201 brain single-photon emission tomography in differentiating between intracranial malignancy and infection in AIDS patients. *AJNR Am J Neuroradiol.* Sep 2005;26(8):1973-1979. [26]Kumabe, T., Shimizu, H., Sonoda, Y., Shirane, R. Thallium-201 single-photon emission computed tomographic and proton magnetic resonance spectroscopic characteristics of intracranial ganglioglioma: three technical case reports. *Neurosurgery* 1999; 45: 183-7.

[27] Kanamori, M., Kumabe, T., Shimizu, H., Yoshimoto, T. (201)Tl-SPECT, (1)H-MRS, and MIB-1 labeling index of central neurocytomas: three case reports. *Acta Neurochir. (Wien)* 2002; 144: 157-63.

[28] Comte, F., Bauchet, L., Rigau, V., Hauet, J. R., Fabbro, M., et al. Correlation of preoperative thallium SPECT with histological grading and overall survival in adult gliomas. *Nucl. Med. Commun.* 2006; 27: 137-42.

[29] Soler, C., Beauchesne, P., Maatougui, K., Schmitt, T., Barral, F. G., et al. Technetium-99m sestamibi brain single-photon emission tomography for detection of recurrent gliomas after radiation therapy. *Eur. J. Nucl. Med.* 1998; 25: 1649-57.

[30] Le Jeune FP, Dubois F, Blond S, Steinling M. Sestamibi technetium-99m brain single-photon emission computed tomography to identify recurrent glioma in adults: 201 studies. *J Neurooncol.* Apr 2006;77(2):177-183.

[31] Ak I, Gulbas Z, Altinel F, Vardareli E. Tc-99m MIBI uptake and its relation to the proliferative potential of brain tumors. *Clin Nucl Med.* Jan 2003;28(1):29-33.

[32] Beauchesne P, Soler C. Correlation of 99mTc-MIBI brain spect (functional index ratios) and survival after treatment failure in malignant glioma patients. *Anticancer Res.* Sep-Oct 2002;22(5):3081-3085.

[33] Beauchesne P, Pedeux R, Boniol M, Soler C. 99mTc-sestamibi brain SPECT after chemoradiotherapy is prognostic of survival in patients with high-grade glioma. *J Nucl Med.* 2004;45(3):409-413.

[34] Baillet, G., Albuquerque, L., Chen, Q., Poisson, M., Delattre, J. Y. Evaluation of single-photon emission tomography imaging of supratentorial brain gliomas with technetium-99m sestamibi. *Eur. J. Nucl. Med.* 1994; 21: 1061-6.

[35] Henze, M., Mohammed, A., Schlemmer, H. P., Herfarth, K. K., Hoffner, S., et al. PET and SPECT for Detection of Tumor Progression in Irradiated Low-Grade Astrocytoma: A Receiver-Operating-Characteristic Analysis. *J. Nucl. Med.* 2004; 45: 579-86.

[36] Bagni, B., Pinna, L., Tamarozzi, R., Cattaruzzi, E., Marzola, M. C., et al. SPET imaging of intracranial tumours with 99Tcm-sestamibi. *Nucl. Med. Commun.* 1995; 16: 258-64.

[37] Nishiyama, Y., Yamamoto, Y., Fukunaga, K., Satoh, K., Kunishio, K., et al. Comparison of 99Tcm-MIBI with 201Tl chloride SPET in patients with malignant brain tumours. *Nucl. Med. Commun.* 2001; 22: 631-9.

[38]   O'Tuama, L. A., Treves, S. T., Larar, J. N., Packard, A. B., Kwan, A. J., et al. Thallium-201 versus technetium-99m-MIBI SPECT in evaluation of childhood brain tumors: a within-subject comparison. *J. Nucl. Med.* 1993; 34: 1045-51.

[39]   Kirton A, Kloiber R, Rigel J, Wolff J. Evaluation of pediatric CNS malignancies with (99m)Tc-methoxyisobutylisonitrile SPECT. *J Nucl Med.* 2002;43(11):1438-1443.

[40]   Feun, L. G., Savaraj, N., Landy, H. J. Drug resistance in brain tumors. *J. Neurooncol.* 1994; 20(2): 165-76.

[41]   Lehnert, M. Multidrug resistance in human cancer. *J. Neurooncol.* 1994; 22(3): 239-43.

[42]   Andrews, D. W., Das, R., Kim, S., Zhang, J., Curtis, M. Technetium-MIBI as a glioma imaging agent for the assessment of multi-drug resistance. *Neurosurgery* 1997; 40(6): 1323-32.

[43]   Ballinger, J. R., Sheldon, K. M., Boxen, I., Erlichman, C., Ling, V. Differences between accumulation of 99mTc-MIBI and 201Tl-thallous chloride in tumour cells: role of P-glycoprotein. *Q. J. Nucl. Med.* 1995; 39(2): 122-8.

[44]   Piwnica-Worms, D., Chiu, M. L., Budding, M., Kronauge, J. F., Kramer, R. A., et al. Functional imaging of multidrug-resistant P-glycoprotein with an organotechnetium complex. *Cancer Res.* 1993; 53(5): 977-84.

[45]   Shibata, Y., Matsumura, A., Nose, T. Effect of expression of P-glycoprotein on technetium-99m methoxyisobutylisonitrile single photon emission computed tomography of brain tumors. *Neurol. Med. Chir. (Tokyo)* 2002; 42: 325-30.

[46]   Henze, M., Mohammed, A., Schlemmer, H., Herfarth, K. K., Mier, W., et al. Detection of tumour progression in the follow-up of irradiated low-grade astrocytomas: comparison of 3-[123I]iodo-alpha-methyl- L-tyrosine and 99mTc-MIBI SPET. *Eur. J. Nucl. Med. Mol. Imaging* 2002; 29: 1455-61.

[47]   Shibata, Y., Katayama, W., Kawamura, H., Anno, I., Matsumura, A. Proton Magnetic Resonance Spectroscopy and 201Thallium-, 99m Technetium methoxyisobutylisonitrile Single Photon Emission Computed Tomography findings of a patient with choroids plexus papilloma. *Neuroradiology* 2008; 50: 741-2.

[48]   Shibata, Y., Yamamoto, T., Takano, S., Katayama, W., Takeda, T., et al. Direct comparison of thallium-201 and technetium-99m MIBI SPECT of a glioma by receiver operating characteristic analysis. *J. Clin. Neurosci.* 2009; 16: 264-9.

[49]   Soricelli, A., Cuocolo, A., Varrone, A., Discepolo, A., Tedeschi, E., et al. Technetium-99m-tetrofosmin uptake in brain tumors by SPECT: comparison with thallium-201 imaging. *J. Nucl. Med.* 1998; 39: 802-6.

[50]   Alexiou, G. A., Tsiouris, S., Goussia, A., Papadopoulos, A., Kyritsis, A. P., et al. Evaluation of glioma proliferation by 99mTc-Tetrofosmin. *Neuro-oncology* 2008; 10: 104-5.

[51]   Alexiou, G. A., Tsiouris, S., Kyritsis, A. P., Polyzoidis, K. S., Fotopoulos, A. D. Classic tumour imaging agents for glioma evaluation: 99mTc-tetrofosmin. *Eur. J. Nucl. Med. Mol. Imaging* 2007; 34: 2143-4.

[52]   Alexiou, G. A., Fotopoulos, A. D., Papadopoulos, A., Kyritsis, A. P., Polyzoidis, K. S., et al. Evaluation of brain tumor recurrence by (99m)Tc-tetrofosmin SPECT: a prospective pilot study. *Ann. Nucl. Med.* 2007; 21: 293-8.

[53]   Choi, J. Y., Kim, S. E., Shin, H. J., Kim, B. T., Kim, J. H. Brain tumor imaging with 99mTc-tetrofosmin: comparison with 201Tl, 99mTc-MIBI, and 18F-fluorodeoxyglucose. *J. Neurooncol.* 2000; 46: 63-70.

[54] Shibata, Y., Endo, K. [Evaluation of brain tumors with Tc-Tetrofosmin SPECT] In Japanese. *CI research* 2011; 33: 175-80.

[55] Langen, K. J., Ziemons, K., Kiwit, J. C., Herzog, H., Kuwert, T., et al. 3-[123I]iodo-alpha-methyltyrosine and [methyl-11C]-L-methionine uptake in cerebral gliomas: a comparative study using SPECT and PET. *J. Nucl. Med.* 1997; 38: 517-22.

[56] Kuwert, T., Morgenroth, C., Woesler, B., Matheja, P., Palkovic, S., et al. Uptake of iodine-123-alpha-methyl tyrosine by gliomas and non-neoplastic brain lesions. *Eur. J. Nucl. Med.* 1996; 23: 1345-53.

[57] Bader, J. B., Samnick, S., Moringlane, J. R., Feiden, W., Schaefer, A., et al. Evaluation of l-3-[123I]iodo-alpha-methyltyrosine SPET and [18F]fluorodeoxyglucose PET in the detection and grading of recurrences in patients pretreated for gliomas at follow-up: a comparative study with stereotactic biopsy. *Eur. J. Nucl. Med.* 1999; 26: 144-51.

[58] Kuwert, T., Probst-Cousin, S., Woesler, B., Morgenroth, C., Lerch H et al. Iodine-123-alpha-methyl tyrosine in gliomas: correlation with cellular density and proliferative activity. *J. Nucl. Med.* 1997; 38: 1551-5.

[59] Woesler, B., Kuwert, T., Morgenroth, C., Matheja, P., Palkovic, S., et al. Non-invasive grading of primary brain tumours: results of a comparative study between SPET with 123I-alpha-methyl tyrosine and PET with 18F-deoxyglucose. *Eur. J. Nucl. Med.* 1997; 24: 428-34.

[60] Weber, W., Bartenstein, P., Gross, M. W., Kinzel, D., Daschner, H., et al. Fluorine-18-FDG PET and iodine-123-IMT SPECT in the evaluation of brain tumors. *J. Nucl. Med.* 1997; 38: 802-8.

[61] Weber, W. A., Dick, S., Reidl, G., Dzewas, B., Busch, R., et al. Correlation between postoperative 3-[(123)I]iodo-L-alpha-methyltyrosine uptake and survival in patients with gliomas. *J. Nucl. Med.* 2001; 42: 1144-50. [62] Langen, K. J., Pauleit, D., Coenen, H. H. 3-[(123)I]Iodo-alpha-methyl-L-tyrosine: uptake mechanisms and clinical applications. *Nucl. Med. Biol.* 2002; 29: 625-31.

[63] Grosu, A. L., Weber, W., Feldmann, H. J., Wuttke, B., Bartenstein, P., et al. First experience with I-123-alpha-methyl-tyrosine spect in the 3-D radiation treatment planning of brain gliomas. *Int. J. Radiat. Oncol. Biol. Phys.* 2000; 47: 517-26.

[64] Guth-Tougelidis, B., Muller, S., Mehdorn, M. M., Knust, E. J., Dutschka, K., et al. [Uptake of DL-3-123I-iodo-alpha-methyltyrosine in recurrent brain tumors]. *Nuklearmedizin* 1995; 34: 71-5.

[65] Amthauer, H., Wurm, R., Kuczer, D., Ruf, J., Michel, R., et al. Relevance of image fusion with MRI for the interpretation of I-123 iodo-methyl-tyrosine scans in patients with suspected recurrent or residual brain tumor. *Clin. Nucl. Med.* 2006; 31: 189-92.

[66] Plotkin, M., Eisenacher, J., Bruhn, H., Wurm, R., Michel, R., et al. 123I-IMT SPECT and 1H MR-spectroscopy at 3.0 T in the differential diagnosis of recurrent or residual gliomas: a comparative study. *J. Neurooncol.* 2004; 70: 49-58.

[67] Kuwert, T., Woesler, B., Morgenroth, C., Lerch, H., Schafers, M., et al. Diagnosis of recurrent glioma with SPECT and iodine-123-alpha-methyl tyrosine. *J. Nucl. Med.* 1998; 39: 23-7.

[68] Matheja, P., Rickert, C., Weckesser, M., Palkovic, S., Lottgen, J., et al. Sequential scintigraphic strategy for the differentiation of brain tumosur. *Eur. J. Nucl. Med.* 2000; 27: 550-8.

Index

A

activation pattern, 7
active transport, 164
adenoma, 45, 46, 48, 49, 50, 51, 52, 53, 54, 55, 56, 59, 61, 65, 67, 68, 69, 70, 72, 73, 127, 143
adenosine, 148, 163, 164, 173
adenosine triphosphate, 164, 173
adrenal gland, 114, 119, 123, 135, 136, 141, 143, 144
adrenal hyperplasia, 135
aerosols, 93, 97
alveoli, 93
American Heart Association, 154, 179, 187, 197
angina, 151, 156, 157, 158
angiogenesis, 161, 165, 168, 176, 184
angiography, 88, 100, 104, 105, 106, 149, 153
angiotensin II, 178
annihilation, 1, 2, 162
apoptosis, 112, 161, 165, 167, 168, 170, 174, 176, 180, 181, 184
arousal, 122
arthritis, 81
astrocytoma, 239
ataxia, 208
atherogenesis, 169
atherosclerosis, 160, 165, 169, 170, 172, 182, 183, 184
atherosclerotic plaque, 160, 161, 165, 166, 169, 170, 171, 172, 182, 183, 184
utonomic nervous system, 190

B

basal ganglia, 203, 204, 207, 208, 209, 210, 212, 228, 233
blood-brain barrier, 242

bone scan, 76, 78, 81, 82, 85, 86, 87, 88, 89
bone tumors, 76, 81, 84, 88
brain abscess, 238
brain tumor, ix, 232, 235, 236, 237, 238, 239, 240, 241, 242, 243
breast cancer, 78, 79, 81, 86, 87, 117
bronchial asthma, 148

C

calibration, 38, 39
carcinoembryonic antigen, 130
carcinoid tumor, 49, 129, 131, 134
cardiac output, 178
cardiac risk, 150, 152
cardiomyopathy, 133, 134, 148, 180, 186, 199
central nervous system, 111, 122, 151, 204
choroid, 238, 239, 240, 241
chromatography, 136
chronic heart failure, 155, 156, 158, 197, 199
chronic obstructive pulmonary disease, 105
cocaine, 202, 203
cognitive impairment, 202, 210
collimators, 8, 10, 11, 12, 13, 14, 41, 57, 65, 68, 71, 94, 124, 139, 153, 190, 191, 192, 198, 204, 226
Compton effect, 29
congestive heart failure, 155, 156, 197, 199
COPD, 92, 93, 96, 97, 102, 103, 105, 148
coronary angioplasty, 156, 157
coronary artery disease, 147, 148, 149, 150, 151, 152, 153, 155, 156, 157, 158
coronary heart disease, 179
corticobasal degeneration, 208, 209

D

degenerative joint disease, 78

dementia, 201, 208, 213
depression, 201, 213
dilated cardiomyopathy, 155, 156, 180, 181, 189, 199
dopamine agonist, 202, 204
dopaminergic, 201, 204, 205, 206, 208, 209, 210, 211, 212, 215, 216, 217, 218, 219
dystonia, 209, 218, 228

E

electrocardiogram, 148
electroencephalography, 222
emboli, 92, 104
embolism, 91, 96, 104
embolus, 106
emphysema, 105
epilepsy, ix, 221, 222, 223, 225, 228, 229, 230, 231, 232, 233, 234
essential tremor, 208, 216

F

false negative, 48, 50, 53, 55, 65, 113, 118, 124, 238, 239
filters, 28
fine tuning, 27
focal seizure, 222, 231, 233
free radicals, 173, 185
frontal cortex, 209
frontal lobe, 227, 228

G

gadolinium, 35, 161, 176
gamma camera, 1, 3, 4, 8, 14, 18, 19, 20, 21, 31, 50, 94, 101, 112, 113, 117, 118, 123, 124, 134, 137, 139, 140, 191
gamma radiation, 4
gamma rays, 17, 29
ganglioneuroblastoma, 134
ganglioneuroma, 134
gastrin, 122
gastrointestinal tract, 110, 136, 164
generalized seizures, 221, 222
glioblastoma, 239, 243
glioblastoma multiforme, 239
glioma, 235, 236, 238, 239, 240
goiter, 49, 53, 57, 69, 71

H

heart disease, 106, 154, 166, 175, 179, 185, 189
heart failure, 92, 98, 99, 103, 147, 148, 150, 155, 156, 160, 175, 176, 177, 178, 179, 180, 181, 186, 187, 194, 197, 198, 199
hemangioma, 85, 127, 143
hepatocellular carcinoma, 143
hippocampus, 223
hyperparathyroidism, 46, 49, 53, 59, 66, 68, 71
hyperthyroidism, 44
hypothalamus, 111

I

idiopathic, 133, 134, 136, 155, 156, 199, 207, 208, 209, 213, 217, 218, 222
IFN, 169
image interpretation, 110, 136
imaging modalities, 64, 78, 83, 147, 161, 240
imaging systems, 40, 79
immobilization, 50
infarction, 160, 164, 169, 173, 174, 181, 185, 186, 208, 233
insulinoma, 113, 118
iodinated contrast, 57
ischemia, 148, 149, 150, 151, 153, 157, 160, 163, 164, 167, 173, 176, 184, 186
isotope, 11, 42, 180, 205
iteration, 26

L

liver, 38, 39, 41, 87, 110, 111, 114, 117, 119, 120, 121, 123, 125, 126, 127, 131, 140, 141, 142, 143, 151, 204
liver metastases, 119
lumbar spine, 82
lung cancer, 115, 121
lung function, 96, 105

M

macrophages, 165, 166, 168, 169, 170, 171, 172, 175, 176, 177, 183
magnetic resonance imaging, 41, 45, 77, 111, 146, 160, 168, 176, 182, 184, 232, 234, 236
melanoma, 117
meningioma, 241
mental retardation, 221meta-analysis, 100, 155, 231, 234